Comparative Materia Medica

Eugenio F. Candegabe
MD

Translated from *Materia Medica Comparada*
by Rosalind Shapiro, RSHom

COMPARATIVE MATERIA MEDICA
Dr Eugenio F. Candegabe
UK £24.50, pub. date 4/97
Beaconsfield Publishers Ltd
20 Chiltern Hills Road
Beaconsfield HP9 1PL, UK
Tel/Fax: +44-(0)1494-672118

BEACONSFIELD PUBLISHERS LTD
Beaconsfield, Bucks, UK

Original edition © Editorial Albatros SACI, Buenos Aires,
    Argentina, 1989
New material © Eugenio Federico Candegabe 1997
This translation © Rosalind Shapiro 1997

British Library Cataloguing in Publication Data
Candegabe, E. F.
    Comparative materia medica. – (Beaconsfield homoeopathic
    library; no. 18)
    1. Homeopathy
    I. Title
    615.5'32

ISBN 0–906584–36–1

Phototypeset by Gem Graphics, Trenance, Mawgan Porth, Cornwall
in 10 on 12 point Times.
Printed and bound in Great Britain at The Bath Press, Bath

Contents

Contents

Contents

Contents

Contents

Contents

Contents

Contents

Miscellaneous Studies

Acknowledgements

Some time ago, Mr John Churchill of Beaconsfield Publishers Ltd told me that Rosalind Shapiro, who was both an exceptional translator and a practising homoeopath, was going to undertake the translation of this book. I was confident that any translator chosen by Mr Churchill would produce work of the highest standard, but I must confess that I have been both surprised and delighted at the singular dedication and thoroughness demonstrated by the translator in bringing to light the many errors in the original text.

I wish to express my gratitude to my translator and my publisher for their excellent collaboration and for all the hard work they have put into the publication of the English-language edition of my *Comparative Materia Medica*.

I should also like to take this opportunity to pay tribute to the standard of homoeopathy in Great Britain.

E. F. Candegabe

Foreword

by Dr Tomás Pablo Paschero

Dr Candegabe has made a most valuable contribution to the study of homoeopathy with his long-awaited *Comparative Materia Medica*.

As he demonstrates in this text, the study of homoeopathy must encompass an understanding of the nature of the action of the remedy – in other words, of the essential characteristics which determine what is curative in the medicine and correspondingly what is to be cured in the patient. Hence it follows that what is to be cured in the individual patient is the miasmatic predisposition, according to the principles of chronic disease. It is this which determines the structure and development of each case, over and above the presenting pathology.

The art of case-taking is a skill which the homoeopathic practitioner must master if he or she is to construct a faithful image of the symptomatology and medical history of the patient.

By 'medical history' I do not mean a factual account of the subjective and objective symptoms of the presenting pathology, which have brought about certain changes in the organism of a mental or physical nature. Rather, the recording of an individual's life – his disease, his state of mind and emotions, his relationships with his fellow creatures, his attitudes, priorities and values.

The homoeopath must bring a deep understanding of the problems of the human psyche to each and every case if he is to make a clear appraisal of the symptoms presented to him; he must be able to discern those symptoms which are unique to the patient and unusual to the disease, those strange, rare and peculiar symptoms which are the characteristics of the disease. It should then be possible to find the simillimum – that remedy which most closely covers the central core of the case, and without which the patient would be unable to overcome the negative factors in his life which inhibit his development as a person. Lack of love is one negative factor which underlies the whole human condition.

Foreword

It is our past conditioning which determines our experience of life and the sort of individual we are. From childhood we learn the emotional responses and patterns of behaviour which govern the way we develop, mature and adapt to circumstances and situations. When a person gets stuck at one of the developmental stages of childhood, this can give rise to mental disturbance, which is a fundamental cause of all disease. If the complex mechanism of conditioned reflexes originating in childhood is stimulated by mental or emotional stress, then pathology, according to our miasmatic inheritance or congenital predisposition, will be the result.

Mental symptoms are not only those of which the patient is conscious: they must also include those of a subconscious nature. We cannot expect the patient, who is doing his best to cope with his reality, to be clear about his mental symptoms when he would rather believe that his innermost conflicts did not exist.

His true self – a being of dynamism, depth and intuition – is masked by the personality, and it can be detected only through observation of his behaviour, the way he relates to those around him, his dreams, fantasies and ambitions, and his weaknesses. The homoeopath must take note of all of these, not for their dramatic interest but for the clues which will lead to an understanding of the patient's inner being. It is the subconscious workings of the psyche which determine the nature and functioning of the conscious mind.

The general symptoms and modalities of the case, such as food desires and aversions, the reactions to certain kinds of weather, to heat and to cold, all serve to maintain and defend the patient's status quo. Disease is a reaction of the defence mechanism, and mental disturbance – the foundation of all physical symptomatology – arises from the conflict created between the promptings of the syphilitic miasm to destruction and death, or of the sycotic miasm to selfishness and egotism, and the constraints imposed upon the individual by society.

Dr Candegabe uses his comparison of remedies and his repertory work to demonstrate that the essential mental symptoms of the patient must be contained in the Minimum Characteristic Syndrome of the remedy. The depth and definition of the individual personality will thus be revealed, and what is curative in the remedy will correlate to what is to be cured in the patient.

The question as to which of the mental symptoms of the patient can be taken to be the characteristic symptoms becomes clear when taken in conjunction with the rest of the symptoms elicited during the case-taking. Similarly, the individual traits brought out by the provings can

xiii

be understood by their relationship to the symptom picture as a whole; and by combining our knowledge of the particular and the general we can achieve a true understanding of the personality and action of the dynamic remedy.

In this comprehensive work, Dr Candegabe has made a comparative study of several similar remedies, identifying and translating their essential characteristics into repertory language, and exploring the dynamic interplay of symptoms which go to make up our remedy pictures.

Dr Candegabe, a true master of the art of homoeopathy, confirms that we must find the simillimum for each patient. It is only this that will bring about the lasting cure which will cause the patient to change his attitude to life, so that the meaning of his existence alters, and his capacity for intelligent thought, energetic action and love grows and develops, and he becomes of service to his fellow human beings.

T. P. Paschero

Preface

As a result of the homoeopathic treatment of both my wife and my son Marcelo, I came to realise that I had found a system of medicine that could live up to my highest aspirations as a physician; it provided me with the tools to understand my patients in all their aspects – physical, mental, emotional and spiritual – and it enabled me to help them to grow and develop into self-fulfilled individuals.

However, the first obstacle which the practitioner of homoeopathy will encounter is his inability to apply his knowledge of materia medica to clinical practice. If we want to understand the essential nature of the remedy it will be of little benefit to study a mere catalogue of its symptoms, no matter how complete.

I came up against this problem time and time again in the early days of my practice; the remedy pictures I had learnt bore no resemblance to the patient sitting in front of me. I knew nothing of arranging symptoms in hierarchy and so had to resort to using several symptoms in the case. I had studied the teachings of such masters as Hahnemann, Clarke, Kent, Nash, Hering, Allen and Voisin, and my head was full of symptom pictures ranging from the basic lesion-based approach of Vannier to the purified mental/emotional/symptom-based images taught by Gallavardin, Clarke and Kent.

But it was not until I came across the lectures on materia medica by Dr Tomás Pablo Paschero, which were published in the journal *Homeopatía* between 1955 and 1960, that I became aware of the essential living being which pervades each individual remedy. Even now, while my understanding of humanity and medicine may have grown with the years, I still gain a great deal from re-reading these articles, and I learn more from them with every reading. I remember with affection a professor of medicine at the Faculty who once commented on my inaccurate observation of a preparation under the microscope by saying *'You only see what you already know.'* The truth of these gentle words stayed with me through the early days of my homoeopathic studies, and they would come back to me whenever I was presumptuous enough to attempt to criticise the more obscure or apparently contradictory teachings of Hahnemann and his followers. We should always be open to the possibility that what seems on the surface to be an inconsistency may, in fact, be a profound truth which our intellect is unable to comprehend.

It was Dr Paschero's teaching and understanding of his subject which inspired me to more reflective consideration of our materia medica. As I gained more experience with repertory work I came to realise that within its pages lay a wealth of information which could, when used in conjunction with the existing symptom pictures, provide a useful contribution towards the task of forming the complete image of the remedy. Once I had acquired a basic understanding of the human being behind the symptoms, I was at last able to begin to recognise the importance of certain symptoms which I had repertorised in clinical practice.

In 1963 I thought I would try out the idea of studying remedies through Kent's *Repertory*, that great treasure which he bequeathed to our body of homoeopathic knowledge. I reasoned that, for example, the perfect Lycopodium patient should, in theory, have the 460 Lycopodium symptoms from A to Z appearing in due alphabetical order. I expected to find that several symptoms would simply confirm what I already knew from the materia medica, while some would be completely new, and that others would correspond to symptoms I had found in Lycopodium patients but had not associated with the remedy because they had not been included in the materia medica.

But no matter how many pieces of isolated information I acquired, I found that my understanding of the remedy was in no way enhanced. However, when I considered them all together as a unified whole, I was able to catch a glimpse of the main theme around which all the symptoms would obediently gather in a logical sequence, like subtle notes in some strange symphony. Now the meaning behind these words of Paschero became clear to me: 'The mental symptom is the antechamber of the clinical picture. The patient's mental disposition is the result of the many inter-related physiological and pathological factors which affect his life. The way that the individual deals with his particular problems, whether of an emotional or a physical nature, is revealed through his mental symptoms.'

It is my intention to supersede existing works of materia medica with their often unworkable approach to the memorisation of barely understood remedy pictures, with this new materia medica, which it is hoped will foster a clear understanding of symptoms through the comparative study of remedies. Every symptom has a meaning and a purpose, as I hope to demonstrate in the following chapters, and it is only through the dynamic relationships between symptoms that we will see the whole picture of the remedy.

Each chapter follows the same format: firstly, an image of the remedy as perceived through the pages of Kent's *Repertory*; secondly, a summary and synthesis of the symptomatology, albeit a rather lengthy one at times, to facilitate an understanding of the essence of the remedy; thirdly, a diagrammatic summary of those symptoms which are fundamental to the dynamic of the remedy. (This part has undoubtedly been one of the most challenging, and I must admit that I have relied heavily on similar works by Dr Paschero, whose impeccable authority I have followed with a fidelity bordering on plagiarism.) Finally, there is a study of the comparative materia medica, upon which the title of this work is based. Comparing remedies in this way helps the homoeopath to familiarise himself or herself with the similarities and differences between remedies, and to know them as living people, in their deepest and most intimate pain.

The remedies which are included in the comparative study are those which would come through a repertorisation of the thirty or forty symptoms taken from a typical remedy picture. From those symptoms I have extracted between five and ten which define the Minimum Characteristic Syndrome, and, for the purposes of repertorisation, I have included only those remedies which share at least 50 per cent of these symptoms, excluding any which fall below this – apart from a few exceptionally interesting remedies.

The terms 'minimum characteristic syndrome' and 'minimum syndrome of maximum value' may be unfamiliar to English-speaking readers, though they are well established among homoeopaths in Argentina through the work of Dr Paschero, who coined them to describe the small, closely-knit group of symptoms which provide a clear and characteristic definition of the remedy.

Throughout this study of the similarities and differences, symptomatology and possible causations of remedies, I have followed the guidance of the great masters in their descriptions of remedy pictures, and I have contributed some of the experience I have gained from treating patients with similar symptomatologies.

The reader will observe that symptoms have been classified neither according to their miasmatic background nor according to my own subjective opinions or preconceptions – I believe firmly that personal opinions are of secondary importance to the dynamic and integral self-expression of the patient as he lives each moment of his life. I do not look upon the results of this study as some absolute statement of truth; rather, it is my hope that it will help the homoeopath to face one of his most daunting tasks – that of translating the existential drama played out by the patient, with all his individuality and integrity, into the language of the materia medica which is, by its nature, a catalogue of generalisations and objective facts.

I feel a great sense of achievement now that this modest study, which has spanned more than thirty years of my medical career, is complete. I am greatly indebted to my friend and teacher, Dr Paschero, for his support, and I dedicate this work to him with great affection and respect. Many doctors at the Faculty gave me invaluable guidance throughout my homoeopathic training; and I must express my gratitude to Dr Hugo Ardiles, who so willingly took on the task of correcting the drafts and proofs of the original edition. Special thanks must go to Mr Edgardo Gil, colleague, friend and administrative secretary to the Faculty, who was responsible for the typing of the manuscript, and whose sustained enthusiasm and motivation carried me through to the completion of this work.

Hahnemann says in Paragraph 1 of his *Organon*: 'The physician's high and only mission is to restore the sick to health, to cure . . .' It is my sincere hope that this work will contribute towards the accomplishment of this aim.

Eugenio Federico Candegabe
Buenos Aires

Note

Repertory references are to Kent's *Repertory* unless otherwise stated. Gradings are given as follows:

low type: *1*
italics: 2
black type: *3*

Extracts attributed to Dr Paschero are all from his book *Homeopatía*, to be published in English by Beaconsfield Publishers in 1997.

1

Introduction

The study of materia medica and its clinical application is a difficult task. Although pure materia medica may provide an accurate description of the symptomatology, it makes no attempt to synthesise that information into what we know as the essential characteristics of the remedy. Clinical materia medica is the compilation of the writer's clinical experience and is, consequently, subjective and incomplete.

The repertories, including Barthel and Klunker's *Synthetic Repertory*, whether used manually or on computer, contain a vast wealth of information, but they, too, do not provide a complete image of the remedy.

After I had spent some years wrestling with this problem, and doing repeated repertorisations of each case, I decided to embark on a more detailed study of the repertory. I had observed that, with each repertorisation, there would be several remedies that had many symptoms in common with the simillimum of the case. Some were familiar to me, others were not, and there were still others that had not even been mentioned in works of clinical materia medica. Through the repertory, it was possible to learn a lot more about little-known aspects of remedies.

If a remedy is studied both in the materia medica and the repertory, a surprisingly complete image will emerge, defining and characterising the remedy in a highly typical manner.

With this typical picture, it becomes easy to see the connections between symptoms, which are more than just a collection of disparate facts; each symptom, with its modalities and actions, has a dynamic intention and result. Furthermore, the symptoms arrange themselves into levels of hierarchy, so that the essential characteristics of the remedy are clear.

A good caricature of a face will contain only those few outstanding features which are necessary to distinguish it from all other faces.

1

Similarly, with a remedy picture, between five and ten symptoms are all that is necessary to synthesise the information into the Minimum Characteristic Syndrome.

This small group of symptoms can then form the basis for repertorisation, and a comparison of similar remedies can be made using this somewhat mathematical process, whereby the essential similarities and differences between remedies will become self-evident.

The reader is recommended to take time over reading this book. It is the fruit of thirty years' experience, and I have done my best to ensure that everything in it is relevant and important. It will enable the practitioner to solve many seemingly intractable problems, and may even provide the inspiration for others to continue with this work.

PATHOGENESIS AND MEDICINE

Hahnemann says in Paragraph 9 of the *Organon*: 'In the healthy condition of man, the spiritual vital force ... rules with unbounded sway, and retains all the parts of the organism in admirable, harmonious, vital operation ... so that our indwelling, reason-gifted mind can freely employ this living healthy instrument for the higher purposes of our existence.' It should hardly be necessary to stress the importance of working according to the fundamental precepts of this well-known paragraph, which draws together all the factors present in a case – namely, the pathogenesis, miasm, symptoms, repertorisation, remedy and case history.

Once we have truly understood the significance of Paragraph 9, we should study the following extracts from Paragraph 3: '... what is to be cured ... in every individual case of disease ...', and from Paragraph 5: 'Useful to the physician in assisting him to cure ... are also the most significant points in the whole history of the chronic disease, to enable him to discover its *fundamental cause*, which is generally due to a chronic miasm ...', and from Paragraph 11: '... it is only this spiritual ... vital force ... that is primarily deranged by the dynamic influence upon it of a morbific agent inimical to life ... [which] by morbid symptoms, and in no other way can it make itself known.'

Thus if the cause of all disease (as expressed by its symptoms) is a chronic miasm, and if we accept that all human beings are diseased in one way or another, since the state of perfect health does not exist, then we must conclude that we all suffer from psora, with sycosis and syphilis to a greater or lesser degree. However, we should not conclude that every sign or symptom is a manifestation of psora, sycosis or syphilis, nor should we assume that everything about our unhealthy beings is simply the expression of a miasm.

Hahnemann, in his *Chronic Diseases*, says: '[Psora is a chronic miasm which has] ... gradually ultimated itself in the various bodily constitutions of individuals who differed from one another in their domiciles, their climatic peculiarities, their education, habits, occupations, modes of life and of diet, and was moulded by varying bodily and psychic relations. It is, therefore, not strange that one single and only medicine is insufficient to heal the entire Psora and all its forms.'

Hahnemann believed that psora is influenced by both internal and external factors, and he saw temperament and constitution as entirely separate from it, as borne out by the following statement: '... A choleric irritable disposition will lead to the development of a certain type of temperament as psora takes hold of the economy.' In other words, they may bear an influence on psora, but they are distinct from it.

Let us now reconsider Paragraph 9 from a miasmatic point of view. The miasms are obstacles to the realisation of our spiritual potential; therefore, the progress we make in that direction is a sign of health, or freedom from miasm. But these positive aspects of human behaviour on the path to self-realisation are also symptoms, signs or expressions of our being. The quality of the miasmatic symptom is dependence, whereas the essence of the non-miasmatic symptom is freedom; just as Hahnemann says – that the spirit may freely employ this living, healthy instrument for the higher purposes of our existence – freedom from ourselves, from our inner conflicts, from the chains of our miasms.

The study of pathogenesis is the main source of our materia medica, and Kent, in his commentary on Paragraph 105 of the *Organon*, talks about the basic criteria used in drug provings. He says, 'All the natural things of the prover are eliminated.' Before the experiment begins, the prover should take time to examine carefully '... all the symptoms that he or she is a victim of ... at the present time, and for many months back ...' He should then ... 'write down carefully all these symptoms and place them by themselves. This group of symptoms is recognised as the diseased state of that individual.' Further on he says, 'These few symptoms ... will go to make up the chronic effect of the remedy ...' (*Lectures on Homoeopathic Philosophy*, No. 28.)

Hahnemann sums it up in Paragraph 105: 'The second point of the business of a true physician ... [is] to be able to select from among [the medicines] one, from the list of whose symptoms an artificial disease may be constructed, as similar as possible to the totality of the principal symptoms of the natural disease sought to be cured.'

Hahnemann's aptly named 'artificial disease' is just that; while its pathogenetic symptoms may be fundamental to the heart of the remedy, they lack a history and are, therefore, of limited importance. A symptom becomes strange, rare and peculiar only in the context of the case history. It acquires a meaning, an intention and a result which are unique to the individual patient who experiences it. The pathogenesis of a remedy is what Kent calls a mirror image, and what Hahnemann calls the artificial disease – it is not the disease itself. It would be a violation of pathogenetic principles to attribute the profound experience of the prover to the pathogenetic effect of a medicine, when the symptom is, by definition, strange to him. One symptom taken out of context is irrelevant; it becomes significant only when it is considered in the light of the whole case history. For this reason, I do not hold with the categorising of pathogenetic symptoms under any framework, miasmatic or not, where the symptoms are divorced from the reality of the patient's suffering. In this way our unique experience of human existence is robbed of its life.

Our aim should be to instil in each patient a sense of the dynamic quality of life and medicine. In other words, a group of symptoms is not merely an accumulation of pieces of information extracted from each prover. Its therapeutic potential lies in its power to express its strange, rare and peculiar characteristics through the life of the patient, in all its harmonious glory.

In essence, each symptom is nothing more or less than the unique expression of the miasmatic background of the prover; its significance and its metaphor are as changeable as the meaning, intention and result of each individual patient.

THE SEARCH FOR THE PATIENT THROUGH THE REPERTORY

In homoeopathy, information on remedies comes from three different sources: pure materia medica, clinical materia medica and the repertories. The first gives a detailed account of the provings, and is valuable for its authenticity and impartiality; but we cannot rely on this alone, as it lacks cohesion and synthesis. In spite of a rigorous adhesion to observation, its greatest drawback is the inability to evaluate each symptom according to its dynamic qualities – its meaning, intention and result – unless all symptoms extracted from the provings are considered to have an existential relationship to the totality of symptoms.

The second source of knowledge is clinical materia medica. This offers the enormous benefit of the physician's clinical experience, however subjective this information may be. It is generally agreed that the writings of Kent, Tyler, Nash, Allen, Gallavardin, Clarke and Roberts, to name but a few, are extremely valuable aids in the search for the essence of the remedy – the mode of action, conditions and fundamental cause – that Hahnemann talks about in Paragraphs 3 and 5.

The characteristics of the remedy can be perceived through the way it lives, its attitudes and expectations, its reactions to circumstances and situations which affect it and influence its behaviour from birth to death.

The third source of knowledge comes from the repertories, the best being, in my opinion, those written by Kent and Barthel.

As we all know, the original purpose of the repertory was to classify symptoms in order to facilitate finding that remedy which would cover a given symptom picture. It is not appropriate here to pay tribute to the brilliance of the system which Kent devised for compiling and using the repertory. I will, instead, focus on another fundamental aspect, which I now believe to be the most important contribution that Kent made to homoeopathy.

It is often the case that the laborious and repetitive process of repertorisation actually improves our knowledge of the similarities and differences between remedies. My original plan was to repertorise remedies in order to make this vast wealth of information easier to absorb. As I embarked on this study, it gradually dawned on me that there was a basic characteristic theme, a group of symptoms around which all the others would obediently gather.

The selection of a remedy inevitably involves a process of comparing and differentiating between similar remedies. I would go so far as to say that every repertorisation is, in fact, a study of comparisons. We take the remedies which come through and compare them to one another and to the case before us.

I believe that this aspect of repertory work should be explored further, especially in the Mind section, and to this end I would like to make the following points:

1) The way that symptoms are rated according to Kent's system, i.e. black type, italics and low type, should vary according to how

symptoms compare with each other. For example, in 'Company, desire for, alone while, agg.', Lycopodium figures in italics, but the value would be higher in a differential diagnosis with the symptom 'Mood changeable, variable' where this appears in black type, simply because there are only sixteen remedies in the former rubric and more than one hundred in the latter.

2) The repertory is our only source of information about the relative value of a symptom. For example, it is only through the repertory that we will discover that China is the only remedy in 'Mirth on waking', or that only Nitricum Acidum and Staphysagria have 'Anxiety, walking rapidly, when', or that Argentum Nitricum is the only remedy in the rubric 'Anxiety, walking rapidly, when, which makes him walk faster'.

3) A remedy can be studied and analysed in great depth, using the repertory as a guide. To take Silicea as an example, there are some striking paradoxes in this remedy, which appears in 'Consolation aggravates' and 'Magnetised, desires to be', in 'Mildness', in 'Obstinate', in 'Timidity' and in 'Egotism', although this is all explicable in terms of his acute awareness of his mental weakness, which makes him both 'Conscientious about trifles' and 'Obstinate'.

Furthermore, Silicea does not appear in any of the rubrics which take a more active attitude towards life, such as hatred, resentment, grief, mortification, or sensitivity to offence, and he neither desires nor rejects company; the one exception is the aggravation while alone, because of his lack of stamina and strength. In other words, for him to accept consolation would be to undermine his strong sense of responsibility (conscientiousness) and his large ego (egotism), and his inbuilt timidity prevents him from looking for company, while his feelings of vulnerability prevent him from rejecting it. He is caught between the need to lean on other people and the desire to assert himself, and he believes his salvation lies in the silent all-knowing image of the father figure. This explains his desire to be magnetised and his aggravation when alone. For does he not cry as he relates his symptoms ('Weeping, telling of her sickness, when') (Candegabe) and, like Staphysagria, feel 'Dullness from conversation'? It is the modalities which link symptoms to each other, and point the way to what Hahnemann called the conditions and mode of action of the remedy.

4) The repertory clearly shows us that every symptom has a 'why' and a 'wherefore' in the context of other symptoms. A remedy is

characterised by the dynamic relationship between its symptoms and not by the symptoms alone. Lycopodium is not characterised just by his lack of self-confidence ('Confidence, want of self'), but by the way in which this characteristic symptom expresses itself through him; in other words, how the feeling permeates every cell of his body and pushes him on to win the fight and show the world how powerful he really is. With his 'Haughty' and 'Dictatorial' nature, his love of power ('Power, love of'), his sympathetic nature ('Sympathetic'), the occasional involuntary smile ('Smiling, involuntary'), the 'Jesting', the ability to laugh when things get serious ('Laughing, serious matters, over'), and his love of 'Theorizing', he tries to cover up his 'Cowardice', and his doubts ('Doubtful, soul's welfare, of'), his low self-esteem ('Confidence, want of self'), his tearfulness ('Weeping'), and his fear of being alone ('Fear, alone, of being'). Lycopodium is characterised first and foremost by the contradictions in his nature: pride and humility, the despot and the coward.

The many facets of Lycopodium all point to one central theme, his basic lack of self-confidence; but it is these facets which reveal the particular Lycopodium attitude to life and all its problems. It cannot be stressed too strongly that the patient is characterised, not by a group of isolated symptoms, but by his personality, and his personality is his way of being a dynamic and animating influence.

5) I have often observed the following to be true. When a rubric from the repertory contains only one or two remedies, then the symptom, whether it be a delusion, a sensation, a dream or a modality of a mental symptom, is central to the remedy. For example, the rubric 'Company, desire for' has the following sub-rubric: 'yet treats them outrageously', with Kali Carbonicum as the only remedy. The whole character of Kali Carbonicum can be summed up by this one rubric. He cannot be alone, he fears solitude, but he will rebuff rudely all attempts to come to his aid. Paschero says of this remedy: 'His bad temper and dis-contentment are reactions to the state of profound weakness which handicaps him both physically and intellectually, and which forces him to need other people.' This is precisely what is meant by the rubric. A victim of his mood swings ('Mood, changeable') and his 'Antagonism with himself', his fear of being alone ('Fear, alone, of being') and his 'Quarrelsome' nature make him 'Contrary', 'Obstinate' and 'Unobserving' of society's rules.

In the Delusions section, Kali Carbonicum is the only remedy under 'Delusions, neck is too large', and one of only three under 'Delusions, birds, sees', the other two being Lac Caninum and Belladonna. The former symptom symbolises his struggle for independence, where the head – the mind – is firmly attached to the body, helpless and passive as that of a newborn baby, by a large powerful neck – the umbilical cord. The latter symptom, a vision of birds, is also a symbol of his desire for freedom.

It is only through the repertory that we can discover which symptoms are exclusive to one or two remedies. The thirst for power ('Power, love of') and the fear that he will never arrive at his destination ('Fear, destination, of being unable to reach his') are unique to Lycopodium and together they characterise a nature which is essentially both dictatorial and insecure.

Baryta Carbonica is the only remedy who, as a child, thinks all visitors laugh at him and tries to hide behind the furniture. This child is painfully shy ('Timidity'), and afraid of strangers ('Fear, strangers, of'); he feels rejected ('Delusions, deserted, forsaken') and disapproved of ('Delusions, criticised, that he is'), and spends his time conscientiously fussing over trifles with great 'Dullness, sluggishness, difficulty of thinking and comprehending'. He lives in constant fear of being criticised, laughed at or abandoned, and he hides behind his fears, his mental dullness, his timidity and his perfectionism; from this it should be easy to understand the meaning of the strange delusion that he walks on his knees ('Delusions, knees, that he walks on'), one which is peculiar to the remedy. This is a clear example of the way in which the repertory helps to confirm and clarify our picture of the remedy.

6) Two similar remedies can be distinguished by the presence of a single characteristic symptom which is unique to one of the remedies. To take Nux Vomica and Nitricum Acidum as examples, they are both in the following rubrics: 'Irritability', 'Violent', 'Sensitive, external impressions, to all', 'Horrible things, sad stories, affect her profoundly', 'Anger over his mistakes', 'Sympathetic', 'Anxiety, conscience, of', 'Malicious', and so on. However, the symptom 'Hatred, persons of, who had offended, unmoved by apologies' is unique to Nitricum Acidum. This one symptom illustrates the essence of the remedy. He holds on to his hatred to such a degree that he is unmoved by apologies, and he allows his blind prejudice to shut him off from life. As Paschero has said, he is a 'violent and aggressive person whose faith in people and in life is totally destroyed'. He hopes for nothing, so he is neither offended easily, nor mortified, nor

intolerant of contradiction. He is consumed by rage, bitterness and despair, and the single symptom 'Hatred, persons of, who had offended, unmoved by apologies' says it all. By contrast, Nux Vomica does not hate; he fights, he complains, he tolerates neither contradiction nor injustice, he is positive, affectionate, sensitive to people's opinions and easily offended.

7) While the attributes of a remedy can be gathered from reading materia medica, the remedy can only be fully defined by what it does not have, and this information can only be found in the repertory. For example, Nux Vomica is the only remedy in the rubric 'Quiet disposition, wants to be, desires repose and tranquility', but it does *not* appear in the rubric 'Tranquility', meaning peacefulness or composure, nor does it appear in the rubric 'Slowness'. Hence, we may deduce that Nux Vomica desires repose and tranquility precisely because he does not have it, and that his impatient and fiery nature is constantly searching outside for something he will never find inside himself.

8) The meaning is completely dependent upon the character of the remedy. For example, the meaning of the symptom 'Well, says he is, when very sick' will vary according to the remedy. Arsenicum would say he is well because he despairs of his recovery ('Despair, recovery'), and believes that all medicines are useless; this would also account for his dislike of consolation ('Consolation agg.'), despite his fear of being alone ('Fear, alone, of being'). Pulsatilla, on the other hand, enjoys being comforted ('Consolation amel.'), in keeping with her great need for company and affection; in her, this affirmation reveals her wish to get well quickly, lest the people who care for her should tire themselves out worrying about her and go away ('Forsaken feeling'). This is what lies behind the silent grief ('Grief, silent'), the 'Indifference' and the tears when she talks about her sickness ('Weeping, telling of her sickness, when'). Hyoscyamus, to take another example, says he is well because he is 'Suspicious' and jealous ('Jealousy'), and suffers from a paranoid delusion that he has been poisoned ('Delusions, poisoned, thought he had been').

9) The comparative study of remedies through the repertory can also enhance our knowledge of lesser-known remedies which may come through on repertorisation. For example, Arnica has five of the ten symptoms which feature in the Minimum Characteristic Syndrome of Lachesis. The rubrics are 'Haughty', 'Malicious', 'Suspicious',

'Dictatorial' and 'Loquacity'. Arnica is oversensitive to all external impressions ('Sensitive, external impressions, to all') in that he finds all physical contact painful. His fear of being touched is as great as his fear of being approached ('Fear, approaching him, of others'). He feels vulnerable, so he withdraws into himself and avoids people; he resents the doctor, once a tried and trusted friend, now an unwelcome intruder, and sends him packing; he says he is well, when very sick, because, in a syphilitic case, he is utterly indifferent to everything ('Indifference, everything, to'), including the state of his health; in a sycotic case, he will say he is well because he refuses to answer ('Answers, refuses to'), is 'Suspicious', and dislikes consolation ('Consolation agg.'). We can amplify this picture with the symptoms 'Haughty', 'Quarrelsome', 'Repulsive mood', 'Censorious', 'Defiant' and 'Contradict, disposition to'. Arnica has all the makings of the perfect political leader. He is impervious to the pain and suffering of others, indifferent to everything, reserved yet extremely affable, and ready to fight when necessary.

Surprisingly, all the symptoms which make up the Minimum Characteristic Syndrome of Silicea are also found in Bryonia, Ignatia, Lycopodium and Nux Vomica: they are 'Confidence, want of self', 'Timidity', 'Anticipation, complaints from', 'Obstinate' and 'Conscientious about trifles'. In addition, they all have difficulty in thinking, but in Bryonia's case an unshakable determination to succeed, no matter what, ensures that he suffers no aggravation from mental exertion. Bryonia is characterised by the 'Irritability' provoked by his physical weakness, which is symbolised by 'Motion agg.' and 'Escape, attempts to'. He is 'Impetuous' and 'Industrious' and, in the heights of his delirium, talks and thinks of nothing but business. By contrast, Silicea is a nice, harmless person with a touchingly childlike need for support and comfort, prone to homesickness, aggravation while alone, and the desire to be magnetised. Bryonia is motivated by his fear of poverty ('Fear, poverty') and his feelings of inferiority to reach for perfection in his sycotic life. He attempts to overcome the psoric flaw in his character – 'Ailments from anticipation' – with his intolerance of contradiction and the persistence with which he doggedly pursues his aims.

The conflict between the psoric weakness and the sycotic impulses create enormous frustrations for him, which are exacerbated by the aggravation from motion; he becomes impetuous, capricious and thoughtless. Once again, the essence of the remedy is brought out by just three core symptoms: 'Quiet disposition, wants to be', 'Delusions, business, fancies he is doing' and 'Delirium, busy'.

The subject is endless. But, to my mind, it is far more beneficial for the student to take an active part in the process of learning, using these ideas as a springboard for new discoveries and observations, rather than studying a fixed set of theories. The repertory is a truly excellent tool for analysing and understanding the complex beings which inhabit its pages, beings which are inextricably linked to their disease patterns and who reveal themselves to our eyes in surprising and exciting ways.

I am sure that the reader will find much both to agree and to disagree with in this work; I hope that these ideas provide at least a small contribution to our understanding of the great truth of homoeopathy.

THE VALUE OF SYMPTOMS

Let the facts speak for themselves. Hahnemann says in Paragraph 110 of the *Organon*, 'I saw, moreover, that the morbid lesions which previous authors had observed to result from medicinal substances when taken into the stomach of healthy persons . . . in large doses . . . accorded very much with my own observations when experimenting with the same substances on myself and other healthy individuals . . . None of these observers ever dreamed that the symptoms they recorded merely as proofs of the noxious and poisonous character of these substances were sure revelations of the power of these drugs to extinguish curatively similar symptoms occuring in natural diseases . . .'

Hahnemann's teachings in the *Organon* and *Chronic Diseases* are based upon accurate observation of natural laws. With a perfect blending of philosophy and science, he substantiates his theories against what is known to be true. Other homoeopaths have followed in his footsteps: Kent in his observations about prognosis in *Lectures on Homoeopathic Philosophy*, Hering with his law of cure, Gathak and Allen with their comprehensive work on the miasms – all have maintained a strict adherence to concrete observable facts.

In the words of Paschero, 'Pathogenesis is purely and simply the manifestation of symptomatology which previously lay dormant in the person, whose particular susceptibilities to health and disease are governed by a far-reaching and profound influence on his constitutional predisposition, which Hahnemann called the miasm.'

This work is primarily concerned with the following aspects of homoeopathy: an in-depth study of materia medica; a repertory analysis of each remedy; a comparative study of materia medica; a miasmatic analysis of the remedies; and, finally, the clinical application of miasmatic theory – several different means to the same end, the prescription of the simillimum.

Hahnemann says in Paragraph 153, 'In this search for a homoeopathic specific remedy, the more striking, singular, uncommon and peculiar (characteristic) signs and symptoms of the case of disease are chiefly and most solely to be kept in view.' In other words, this is the one essential ingredient in any prescription, although the actual practice of homoeopathy involves a lot more than this.

It would seem to be the case, therefore, that if we could master the remedies, get to know them down to the smallest detail and from every possible angle, we would then be able to make a confident selection of the correct remedy. However, Kent warns us of the fallacy of this argument. 'The science of Homoeopathy treats of the knowledge . . . the application of that science . . . is the art of Homoeopathy . . . for all healing consists in making application of the science.' The artistic application of science demands an intuitive ability, a subconscious knowledge which is, like life itself, impenetrable to its very soul. The homoeopath may be skilled in the art of applying homoeopathic theory to clinical practice, but this does not in any way make him any better than other human beings. He should carry no illusions of superiority about himself until he has reached the pinnacle of perfection in his theoretical knowledge, his skilful practice and his total understanding of human psychology in all its facets. Thus, if the homoeopath puts aside his own human qualities, and uses only his theoretical knowledge and his techniques to deal with the total being of his patient, he will encounter doubt and uncertainty. He will meet the patient as a unique living individual only if he integrates his whole self, with all his emotions and life experience, into his work as a homoeopath. He must use his feelings and his intuition to penetrate to the deepest layers of the patient, with the sole and humble intention of helping him. This is what Hahnemann means when he talks about the unprejudiced observer who can perceive the feelings and emotions of the patient, thus making himself at once giver and receiver of the healing art.

Orthodox medicine has always believed that disease is caused by the malfunctioning of organs and tissues, but the homoeopath must always look beyond this purely materialistic view. Then he will see that the so-called clinical 'disease' is an indication of the underlying patho-logical tendencies and disease susceptibilities which are peculiar to the individual patient. Also, that the whole life history of the patient, his mental and emotional state, his desires, his frustrations, his achievements, his ambitions are of equal, if not more, significance. The patient's present persona is a combination of the most primitive childhood patterns of behaviour and the most exciting and wonderful expressions of life. The life history of the patient represents his attempt to adapt to his particular circumstances, on a mental and a physical level, and all pathology is both the expression and the ultimate result of that attempt at adaptation.

The task of finding the exact remedy is discussed in several paragraphs of the *Organon*, among them Paragraph 153, which says that the answer lies in 'the more striking, singular, uncommon and peculiar (characteristic) signs and symptoms . . .' In this study I hope to clarify what is meant by these four words. The paragraph continues, 'for it is more particularly these that very similar ones in the list of symptoms of the selected medicine must correspond to.'

Ever since the first repertories were introduced by Boenninghausen and Kent, those homoeopaths who have been able to choose the correct remedy by memorising all the characteristic symptoms of the materia medica have long been admired and respected. I believe that the repertories of Kent and, more recently, Barthel, are essential tools for this work, and that we should pay heed to the words of Kent in his preface to the *Repertory*, where he gives precise instructions for the use of the book. Once the repertory work is completed, he advises us to 'study the materia medica of such remedy or remedies as run through the symptoms of the case until there is no doubt about which is the most similar of all remedies'. This echoes Hahnemann's words in Paragraph 3, '. . . if he knows how to adapt it, as well in respect to the suitability of the medicine most appropriate according to its mode of action to the case before him . . ., this ability is the hallmark of a true physician.'

Hahnemann and Kent work from the fundamental principle that the essence of the remedy should be homoeopathically similar to the essence or mental and physical make-up of the patient. So what precisely is the similarity between the patient and the remedy? What does the often repeated yet rarely understood phrase 'essence of the remedy' actually mean? The 'essence' can be perceived through the mental and physical make-up, the way the person copes with the business of life, with its multifarious risks and dangers, the way he deals with his lot from birth to death. Hahnemann says in Paragraph 5, 'Useful to the physician in assisting him to cure are . . . the most significant points in the whole history of the chronic disease, to enable him to discover *its fundamental cause*, which is generally due to a chronic miasm. In these investigations ... his moral and intellectual character, his occupation, mode of living and habits etc. ... are to be taken into consideration.'

In other words, Kent and Hahnemann teach us – and I, too, subscribe to this view – that symptoms are not meaningful in themselves unless they form part of a clear and characteristic totality, where they acquire a significance which is relative to the totality. Like all living things, every symptom has a meaning, an intention and a result. The meaning is an original and intimate form of self-expression, the intention is an inner quest to find a personal solution to one's existential conflict through one's actions. However, a symptom must convey the mental attitudes which govern the way a person chooses to act, otherwise it will remain simply a collection of words from the repertory or a literary expression, as irrelevant as a dead language. It would be a serious mistake to assume that any group of symptoms will lead to an accurate prescription. As Kent once commented to a student, 'Indeed, you have collected a great many symptoms, but you have no case.' To have a case, the group of symptoms which leads to the selection of the remedy must act in the same way that the remedy acts.

Hahnemann says in Paragraph 18, 'The sum of all the symptoms and conditions in each individual case of disease must be the sole indication, the sole guide to direct us in the choice of a remedy.'

In other words, the 'conditions' in each individual case of disease will lead us to the selection of the remedy, according to its mode of action. The remedy is perceived not only by its characteristic symptoms but, more importantly, by its mode of action, which gives a particular significance and value to every remedy, and which we must observe and understand in each individual patient if we are to make a correct diagnosis. All the great masters of homoeopathy have adhered to this fundamental principle.

Diverse symptoms become logical when seen through the eyes of the person who suffers them. The great masters of homoeopathy were without doubt helped in their understanding of the essence of Pulsatilla by their many Pulsatilla cases. Dr Paschero laid great stress on this important point in his works on clinical materia medica and in his *Essential Components of the Remedy*. Hahnemann also emphasised this point in the footnote to Paragraph 213, 'Thus Aconite will seldom or never effect either a rapid or permanent cure in a patient of a quiet, calm, equable disposition; and just as little will Nux Vomica be serviceable where the disposition is mild and phlegmatic, Pulsatilla where it is happy, gay and obstinate, etc.' Thus can it be said that first-hand experience of the 'essence of the remedy' has been gained by those homoeopathic physicians who have supported their patients and shared in their lives.

If a remedy is studied simply by mechanical use of the repertory it may lose its dynamic quality of individual totality, making it difficult to distinguish between two similar remedies whose characteristic symptoms are almost identical. Let us compare, for example, Natrum Mur. and Lycopodium; they both have resentment, aversion to company and to consolation, mortification, need for affection and a continuous dwelling on the past – but 'essentially' they are not the same. Whereas the key symptoms of Natrum Mur. are resentment and frustration brought about by the suppression of his extreme irritability, the key symptom of Lycopodium is lack of self-confidence. Natrum Mur. feels resentful when he feels unloved, Lycopodium feels resentful if he is not consulted. Natrum Mur. avoids people out of spite, Lycopodium does so in order to hide his weakness. Natrum Mur. is averse to consolation because he wants to indulge his feelings of disappointed love. Lycopodium is averse to consolation because it hurts his pride. Natrum Mur. is blocked emotionally by the feelings of mortification and pain which he suffers in silence – he is stuck in the past and broods continually over his disappointments in love; in Lycopodium the elements of egotism, servility and aggression compete for dominance. The bitterness which underlies Natrum Mur.'s whole attitude to life can be heard in his voice; Lycopodium's voice is an echo of the feelings of weakness which lie behind that egotistical front, the weakness that brings tears to his eyes when he is thanked. It is obvious that Natrum Mur. and Lycopodium are quite separate remedies, with completely different reasons for their feelings of resentment and desire for solitude. If two roads happen to cross at some point, it does not necessarily mean that they are travelling in the same direction, and likewise we should never assume that two remedies are alike just because they have some symptoms in common.

Let us look at the remedy Calcarea Carbonica. Its Minimum Characteristic Syndrome of maximum importance is fear, apathy and obstinacy. This combination of symptoms reveals the slow, deliberate and calculating way that Calcarea deals with life's frustrations and disappointments; his free-floating fears are an expression of his inner feelings of hostility. Calcarea lives in his head, where he feels secure and confident; his fears live in some dark underworld – fear of loneliness, of the dark, of ghosts, of the future, of disease, fear that something may happen – all are projections of the hostility he feels inside. He gets terribly disturbed if he hears of bad news, of acts of cruelty or tragic stories, and he can talk about nothing but crimes, fire and rats.

These are the 'conditions' of the symptoms which show us the 'mode of action of the remedy' and which lead the physician 'to discover the *fundamental cause*, which is usually due to a chronic miasm'. Paragraphs 3, 5 and 18 teach us the importance of avoiding abstract speculations about the meaning of symptoms. Hahnemann says in Paragraph 83, 'This individualising examination of a case of disease ... demands of the physician nothing but freedom from prejudice and sound senses, attention in observing and fidelity in tracing the picture of the disease.' Similarly, in Paragraph 7, '... of this outwardly reflected picture of the internal essence of the disease, that is, of the affection of the vital force ...' He goes on to say, in Paragraph 98, '... so, certainly, on the other hand, in all diseases, but especially in the chronic ones, the investigation of the true, complete picture and its *peculiarities* demands especial circumspection, tact, knowledge of human nature, caution in conducting the inquiry and patience in an eminent degree.' And, as we said at the beginning, we should use our own emotional insights to help us achieve this level of knowledge of human nature.

THE MIASMATIC SIGNIFICANCE OF SYMPTOMS

As we discussed earlier in this chapter, the importance of individual symptoms is secondary to the ways and conditions in which the whole group of symptoms presents itself. Also, there is a fundamental causative factor, discernible through the case history of the patient, which has created a certain mental attitude, and which will guide us to the choice of the most exact prescription, according to its mode of action. As we have seen, the relative value of a symptom is determined by its meaning, intention and result. A symptom is an expression of a vital phenomenon, as dynamic and three-dimensional as the world we live in.

If we assume that every patient is basically tri-miasmatic, the labels 'psoric', 'sycotic' or 'syphilitic' will indicate nothing more than a certain tendency of the vital force. The patient's collection of symptoms will add a quality of dynamism and relativity to this tendency. This point is illustrated by the following example:

Lycopodium's aversion to company could be considered to be psoric when it reflects his feelings of incompetence, sycotic when seen as a way of hiding his weakness in order to muster his forces and win some victory, and decidedly syphilitic when coupled with a feeling of complete failure, total indifference to everything, and weariness of life.

One can equally consider the symptom 'Sympathetic', which denotes an exaggerated sense of compassion for other people's suffering. In Phosphorus, with his hypersensitivity to all external impressions and his feelings of universal love, this could be considered to be a psoric symptom. In Nitric Acid, whose hatred and resentment of those who have wronged him fuels a deep desire for revenge and destruction – which in turn is tempered by his guilty conscience – the symptom 'Sympathetic' could be regarded as both sycotic and syphilitic. The phagadenic ulcers with jagged margins are visible illustrations of this merging of the two miasms. In Lycopodium, the symptom could be seen as a sycotic reflection of his apparently overprotective nature, while his secret sense of pride and self-satisfaction remain hidden from view.

Ultimately, the miasmatic significance of the symptoms in a case will become apparent in the thread which runs through the patient's story. This will reveal the meaning of his life, his work and his quest, and the symptoms will acquire greater or lesser value according to the contribution they make to the meaning, intention and result. The human soul and psyche are by their nature fluid and will not fit neatly into any rigid framework.

It follows that a group of apparently sycotic symptoms, such as meticulous attention to detail, amelioration by occupation and intolerance of contradiction, will not by itself convey the picture of a remedy, unless the symptoms are expressed in terms of the fundamental cause – the origins of the remedy which will be homoeopathic according to its mode of action. Hence, we find that the sycotic Sepia has a syphilitic indifference to everything; the sycotic Silicea shows his tubercular roots through his severe lack of self-confidence, his timidity and his fear of failure; and the sycosis of Thuja is typified by his egotism, irritability and anxiety of conscience. Clearly, a differential diagnosis must be based on the medical history of the patient, which will indicate the fundamental cause and mode of action of the syphilitic indifference of Sepia, the psoric timidity and fear of Silicea and the sycotic abnormalities of Thuja.

In other words, whether we find that a certain case leans towards the psoric, sycotic or syphilitic will depend on the theme which runs through the meaning, the intention, and the quest. The medical history, with details of vaccinations, suppressive drug treatments, hereditary factors etc., will give an indication of the predominating miasms in the patient's past and present. But, more importantly, it is his mental attitude, his hopes, desires and ambitions, that will reveal the extent of the influence of a given miasm on his current state of health.

If we were, however, to stick rigidly to the miasmatic framework where every symptom is categorised as psoric, sycotic or syphilitic, without reference to the totality of symptoms nor to the human being who experiences them, we would ultimately fail in our responsibility towards our patients. We must always bear in mind that, while theoretical dogma is by its nature rigid, its practical application should be responsive to the ever-changing dynamic of symptoms which are working at all times to achieve and maintain balance within the organism.

We should therefore always base our examination of the active miasm on the fundamental cause of the case history, in order to arrive at a correct diagnosis. It is of course useful to study a remedy miasmatically or through the repertory, but even the best tools have their limitations, and the resulting information will be static unless it is brought to life by 'the Art' which Kent speaks about, the vital essence at the heart of the remedy. The human being is the highest form of life, is both the observer and the observed, and his or her essence is as dynamic and mysterious as life itself.

Nowadays the practice of homoeopathy presents us with many more problems than in Kent's time. When Hahnemann was practising, one-sided cases were very rarely seen, according to Paragraph 177; now we have to deal with cases where the use of allopathic drugs has deformed and silenced the natural language of the disease, where the systematic suppression of the symptoms of the defence mechanism and the increasing use of psychotropic drugs have reinforced the drug miasm to an unprecedented degree. In view of this, I would recommend the reader to study Paragraphs 171 to 185, where Hahnemann discusses the problem of one-sided cases and gives clear and concise guidelines for dealing with them. Nevertheless, the reader should bear in mind that the application of these guidelines would tax the skill of even the most experienced homoeopath, and he may well find that some of his questions remain unanswered.

We read in Paragraphs 9 and 11 that disease is not an accident, but rather the expression of a deranged vital force which inhibits our self-development. Cure, or the restoration of health, is not simply a matter of removing symptoms; it is the mobilising of the law of cure, from the centre to the periphery and from the mind to the organs. Cure involves the realisation of the duty which originated with the miracle of our birth, the duty we all share as unique human beings – the duty of self-fulfilment. Disease is disharmony, malfunction, fear, pride, aggression, overgrowth and decay. Health is harmony, inner freedom, joy in love, and the will to serve.

A state of absolute health is in fact unattainable, but as we strive we progress along the way, and the attainment becomes our lifelong objective.

If disease is the expression of a deranged vital force which inhibits the spirit from realising the higher purposes of its existence, then the initiation of the process of cure will be heralded by an inner sense of peace, as the spirit and the conscience become at one with each other.

If the attainment of perfect health were humanly possible, we would never get ill. Our state of ill health, which has been so from birth, is due to the disturbance and disruption created by the miasms on our defence mechanisms. Disease is but a frustrated attempt at cure. Disease and cure are different aspects of the same vital process.

If the symptoms of disease are miasmatic, the symptoms of cure are amiasmatic: they are an expression of the search for those higher purposes of our existence. The symptom may be the same, but its quality or essence is different; as I have already remarked, the quality of the miasmatic symptom is dependence, the essence of the amiasmatic symptom is freedom.

As Rilke said, disease is the organism's way of liberating itself from foreign matter. Our task is to help it to have its disease, fully and completely, until it comes to a head and erupts, and then moves on along the path of progress. I am talking here about progress in the universal sense of the origins and meaning of existence, which underlies all religious philosophy, Adler's concept of a common humanity, or Jung's concept of the collective unconscious.

Let us return to Paragraph 9 of the *Organon*, which says of this apparent anomaly '. . . so that our indwelling, reason-gifted mind can freely employ this living healthy instrument for the higher purposes of our existence'. If we can accept that disease is the organism's attempt to liberate itself from a miasm, we will then appreciate the true value of disease and perceive more clearly our part in the solution of the problem. Thus will spirit triumph over matter and humankind will progress towards self-realisation.

COMPARATIVE MATERIA MEDICA

2

Lycopodium Clavatum

DESCRIPTION

In Kent's *Repertory* ninety-five pages are devoted to the four hundred and sixty-odd symptoms of the Mind section.

Paschero has said that all human beings 'go through various stages of physical and intellectual development, and their psychological needs fluctuate between the desire for dependence, support and protection, and the desire for success and independence through self-assertion and competition with other people ... Lycopodium gives us the most perfect image of this constitutional duality, one which is shared by the whole human race, and which is responsible for all manner of mental anxieties, physical disease and pathology.'

Bernard, the great French constitutional homoeopath, says about this remedy: 'He is generally tall and thin, even emaciated, with a wrinkled old face and worried expression, dark hair, dark shining eyes ... similar to the Phosphoric type in his hypersensitivity, quick intelligence, artistic taste and refined intellect. His one outstanding feature is his huge stomach which is out of proportion to the rest of him; this is Lycopodium's centre of pathology.'

The attitude is classic: the stern demeanour, the harsh and imperious tone, the frowning expression. He stands with his arms folded over his stomach until he suddenly leans back, flaps his nostrils as if in need of air, and then holds forth to the person he is speaking to.

On a mental level the key to the Lycopodium personality is his lack of self-confidence, and on a physical level the centre of pathology is the liver malfunctioning. His feelings of inferiority affect him on all levels, physical and mental, and provoke in him feelings of aggression which are only held in check by his astuteness, the two being in constant conflict with each other. Nobody more than Lycopodium takes such great pains to show that he is better than anyone else. For him the world is one big battlefield; with his great lack of self-confidence ('Confidence, want of self': *2*) his goal is to win power ('Power, love of': *1*); his great fear is to be thrown out of the competition, unable to reach his destination ('Fear, destination, of being unable to reach his': *1*).

The duality of Lycopodium is expressed by each one of the symptoms which characterise his personality – it can in fact be said that he lives a lie. His need to be better than other people arises from his fear of being discovered; he is the proudest ('Haughty': *3*) coward ('Cowardice': *3*) of our whole materia medica. To achieve his ambitions nothing is left to chance; every step he takes is a leaden weight, taken with the most infinite care, with a meticulous attention to detail ('Conscientious about trifles': *2*). He has to fight against his basic anxiety before undertaking any commitment, the classic anticipatory anxiety ('Anticipation, complaints from': *3*). Lycopodium will prepare himself with exhaustive dedication before a test. The tension will bring on an attack of diarrhoea ('Diarrhoea, excitement': *1*) or fear in the stomach ('Fear, stomach, arising from': *2*); he trembles and shakes as he goes to take the exam, but as soon as he gets down to it he acquires increasingly more control of himself until he becomes the best, the most outstanding candidate, and in the end boasts of his success to the other participants with great self-satisfaction and conceit.

In Lycopodium the symptom of anticipation is high in the hierarchy of symptoms, as it portrays the patient's permanent state of tension in his dealings with the world. He senses that the people around him are constantly watching him and he must never fail and never lose. His personality centres around his attempt to resolve his lack of self-confidence, so that his life is one long exam where he continually puts himself to the test. For him leisure is a complete waste of time, and the illness which keeps him away from his work is a terrible calamity. Lycopodium cannot be idle for one minute; he is at the height of his power when he is engaged in activity, and he must excel at whatever he does ('Occupation, amel.': *1*).

His weakness and his cowardice are in direct contrast to his self-conceit; out of cowardice he suppresses his anger with silent grief ('Anger, ailments after with silent grief': *3*) and can bring himself to get angry only with people who are absent ('Irritability, absent persons, with': *1*), and the symptom 'Hard for inferiors and kind for superiors' shows us how intelligently he deals with his servile tendencies and his weak nature. He is haunted by the fear of making a mistake, being found to be at fault or being discredited, hence the anger he feels when contradicted ('Anger, contradiction, from': *3*, and 'Contradiction, intolerant of': *3*). This is the remedy of the mothers-in-law who put their noses into everybody's business and expect their children to follow their instructions to the letter, the overprotective parents who bring their children up under the shadow of their own insecurities and their own fear of what may happen ('Fear, happen, something will': *1*), the business manager who does not tolerate the slightest objection to his orders, because to be otherwise would mean coming up against his innermost feelings of incompetence, so to cover up his vulnerability he turns to despotism ('Dictatorial': *2*).

The cult of his personality ('Egotism, ailments from': *2*) puts him in a state of constant tension, for his daily contact with the world is a battle that he must always win. He becomes 'Defiant' (*2*), 'Presumptuous' (*1*), 'Morose' (*2*), 'Violent' (*2*), 'Quarrelsome' (*2*), with a habitual frown on his face ('Frown, disposed to': *1*); he complains ('Complaining': *2*) and he curses ('Cursing': *2*). He is the 'know-all' who rides roughshod over people with his insolence ('Insolent': *3*), 'Rudeness' (*3*), and repulsive behaviour ('Repulsive mood': *1*) by beating ('Striking': *2*), hurling insults ('Abusive': *1*) and enraged assaults ('Anger, violent': *2*, 'Rage': *3*). Lycopodium children are often brought for treatment by their parents because of their severely disturbed behaviour; these children are abusive to their parents ('Abusive, children insulting parents': *2*), and in their obstinate determination to be independent they become disobedient and inclined to contradict everything ('Disobedience': *2*, 'Contradict, disposition to': *2*).

These extreme feelings of aggression are reflected in the hypertonicity of the voluntary muscles which have a tendency to start ('Starting': *2*) at the least provocation ('Starting, trifles, at': *2*), on falling asleep ('Starting, sleep, on falling': *3*), during sleep ('Starting, sleep, during': *1*), and from sleep ('Starting, from sleep': *3*); any unexpected noises also make him start ('Starting, noise, from': *2*). The starting is both a reaction to fear and a muscular spasm which at its worst seems to rise up from his very feet ('Starting, feet, as if coming from the': *1*).

But the strategy of our patient's defence mechanism does not rely solely on periodical suppressions and outbursts; in fact these are the tools which Lycopodium uses least often in his dealings with the outside world. The prescriber will intuitively sense a subtle hint of self-worship in every gesture he makes, in every attitude he adopts, behind which he hides a profound lack of self-confidence and an equally profound fear that he will be found out. There is a constant duality between the two components – the lack of self-confidence and the arrogance – and it is by perceiving this duality that we gain an insight into this multi-faceted and changeable polychrest remedy. It explains why we may find that this same remedy is needed by all members of a family, even though each one has a completely different personality.

Lycopodium is gifted with a brilliant mind, he is often happy and jolly ('Cheerful': 2), even joyful ('Mirth': 2) and often 'too' nice ('Mildness': 2); he wins you with his *savoir faire*, his unconscious self-deprecating smile ('Smiling, involuntary': 1), his clever conversation which occasionally wanders off the point ('Speech, wandering': 3); he is always ready and willing to recognise his own mistakes ('Reproaches himself': 1) and, with his love of justice and truth, he loses himself in daydreams of a better world, as he sees it ('Theorizing': 1).

But this mild individual who skilfully adapts his behaviour to match the company he keeps ('Mood, changeable, variable': 3) is constantly on the lookout for other people's mistakes, which earn his scathing criticism ('Censorious': 2, 'Jesting': 1). The condescending gesture and the smug little laugh make his victim look like a complete fool ('Laughing': 2, 'Laughing, everything seems ludicrous': 1). The laughing over serious matters expresses his disdain for the problem if it is someone else's, and protects his own ego if the problem is his ('Laughing, serious matters, over': 1). Lycopodium laughs while he is asleep ('Laughing, sleep, during': 3), as if amused by the ideas in his subconscious mind, and even his anxiety makes him laugh ('Laughing, anxiety, during': 1). For Lycopodium everything that other people do, think, believe or hold dear to them is bad, and they become the object of his scorn ('Contemptuous': 2) and criticism ('Censorious': 2) and finally, true to his contrary nature, he becomes bored with them ('Contrary': 1).

As long as Lycopodium keeps his intellectual faculties intact, it is possible that no other symptomatology may appear, apart from that which I have already discussed, but as the strains and stresses of life gradually begin to take a toll of his mind and body, his basic anxieties will begin to surface. Our patient may 'sense' that he will never live up to his standards of perfection. Although this may not be objectively true, it is real enough when considered against the image of perfect and total power that he himself has constructed. His feeling of failure highlights his feelings of self-doubt. Whatever he undertakes, he is filled with doubts ('Irresolution': 2), even down to the most trivial actions ('Irresolution, acts, in': 1). His attention to detail becomes even more meticulous, especially between the hours of 4 and 8 p.m. ('Conscientious, about trifles, from 4 to 8 p.m.': 2). Any commitment or engagement fills him with dread, whether it is speaking in public or taking an exam; any delay makes him impatient ('Impatience': 2). He feels weak and dull ('Dullness': 3), except while walking in the open air ('Dullness, walking, while, in open air amel.': 3), from the increasing lack of oxygenation brought about by the flatulence that is characteristic of the remedy; the open air ameliorates not only his dullness but also his anxiety ('Anxiety, air, in open, amel': 2).

In this state of mind he is more likely to make mistakes in calculating ('Mistakes, in calculating': 2), speaking ('Mistakes, speaking': 2), and spelling ('Mistakes, spelling, in': 2); he puts words in the wrong place ('Mistakes, words, misplacing': 2), makes mistakes with syllables ('Mistakes, speaking, wrong syllables': 3); in his writing he confuses letters ('Mistakes, writing, confounding letters': 1), he omits letters ('Mistakes, writing, omitting letters': 2), and words ('Mistakes, writing, omitting words': 2), he transposes letters ('Mistakes, writing, transposing letters': 2) and above all he uses wrong words ('Mistakes, wrong words, using': 3). All this leads him to believe that his memory is failing ('Memory, weakness of': 3), especially for proper names ('Memory, weakness of, names, for proper': 2), for what he has read ('Memory, weakness, read, for what has': 2), for words ('Memory, weakness of, words, for': 2), until he finds it difficult to express himself ('Memory, weakness of, expressing one's self, for': 2). This person who could once boast of a great wealth of ideas and clarity of mind ('Ideas abundant, clearness of mind': 2) now feels totally undermined by his apparent inability to think ('Ideas, deficiency of': 3), which throws him into a state of bewilderment ('Confusion of mind': 2) which is aggravated by any mental effort whatsoever ('Confusion, mental exertion, from': 2). He is worse on waking ('Confusion, morning, waking, on': 2), after eating ('Confusion, eating, after': 2), and in a warm atmosphere ('Confusion, warm room, in': 3), and is ameliorated noticeably by walking in the open air ('Confusion, walking, while, open air, in, amel': 3).

As his feelings of insecurity grow, Lycopodium runs away. The fears of being found out, of suffering defeat, of being made to look foolish, are all projected into his fear of people ('Fear, people, of': 3) or, more specifically, his fear of men ('Fear, men, of': 3). The aversion to company that he feels ('Company, aversion to': 2) protects his need to hide, and is in apparent contradiction to his fear of being alone ('Fear, alone, of being': 3) and to the aggravation while alone

('Company, desire for, alone, while agg.': 2). Lycopodium wants to be alone in his room to avoid the sight of people but in no way wants to be alone in the house, because he feels vulnerable. This ambivalence or duality is to be found in all facets of his personality. For example, he fears women because of the diminution of his sexual potency. Loss of erection during intercourse is characteristic of our patient, and leads him to indulge in lascivious fantasies ('Fancies, exaltation of, lascivious': 2) or to mental disturbances resulting from sexual excesses ('Sexual excesses, mental symptoms from': 3), in an attempt to reassert his failing manhood.

Another characteristic of the remedy is a kind of mental hyperactivity, a state of excitability which increases while he is asleep ('Excitement, night, sleep, during': 1) or in the early hours of the afternoon ('Excitement, afternoon': 1), combined with a hyper-sensitivity to sensual impressions ('Sensitive, sensual impressions, to': 2), and to noise ('Sensitive, noise, to slightest': 2). His perceptions are sharpened as if preparing himself for an attack; he is frightened by the slightest thing ('Fear, trifles': 2), like the ringing of the doorbell ('Fear, noise at door': 2), announcing an unexpected visitor. He is frightened of the dark ('Fear, dark': 2), of the ghosts that haunt his nights ('Fear, ghosts, of': 2), of death ('Fear, death, of': 2) and all his fears are felt in his stomach ('Fear, stomach, arising from': 2), in his heart ('Fear, heart, arising from': 1), or they bring on diarrhoea ('Diarrhoea, excitement': 1). He is a bag of nerves ('Frightened easily': 3), convinced that something is going to happen to him ('Fear, happen, something will': 1). Battered and shaken, and realising his need for support ('Helplessness, feeling of': 1), he is frightened of being alone, but his distrust of people causes his fear of a crowd ('Fear, crowd, in a': 2) to develop into a fear of being approached by other people ('Fear, approaching him, of others': 2). By the same token, Lycopodium fears the approach of daylight; many of his symptoms are aggravated on waking, such as his fears ('Fear, on waking': 2), which manifest themselves as irritability. The irritability on waking that is so typical of Lycopodium ('Irritability, morning, waking, on': 3) is an aspect of his feelings of insecurity and anticipation.

Now we may see Lycopodium acting out the drama of his life like the actor standing before his audience; the flow of aggressive feelings which he projected on to his world in an attempt to impose his personality has turned against him. His constant state of disquiet ('Restlessness': 3) and anxiety ('Anxiety': 3) is an expression of the fear that his world is about to collapse. The rubrics which express this are: 'Anxiety, chagrin, after': *1*, 'Anxiety, vexation, after': *1*, 'Anxiety, crowd, in a': *1*, 'Anxiety, company, when in': *1*, 'Anxiety, house, in': *3* – feeling oppressed by being closed in – and 'Anxiety, air, in open, amel.': *2*. This last symptom is a symbol of freedom – an open space with no barriers which gives Lycopodium a feeling of great inner strength. For him, any form of rest – tranquillity, constriction or confinement – will only serve to increase his anxiety. From this it should be easy to understand why Lycopodium cannot tolerate tight-fitting or heavy clothing, for he fears confined spaces ('Fear, narrow place, in': *2*), is uneasy in a closed room ('Restlessness, room, in': *3*), and uneasy when he cannot move his legs ('Restlessness, sitting, while': *3*). The night, the unknown, the dark, all bring out his fears: that is why he is more anxious before going to sleep, before losing consciousness ('Anxiety, sleep, on going to': *2*) and his anxiety forces him out of bed ('Restlessness, bed, driving out of': *2*). The anxiety for his salvation ('Anxiety, salvation, about': *2*) is perhaps due to his feeling of having neglected his duty, of not having fulfilled his obligations. Anxiety, an essential component of psora, takes on a life expression in accordance with the individuality of the remedy.

Caught in his own trap, he avoids his responsibilities because he is afraid of facing up to them. He is bored by the work he once tackled with great energy ('Indolence': *2*, 'Work, aversion to mental': *2*), now that any effort whatsoever aggravates him ('Exertion, agg. from mental': *3*), to the point where he does not even want to think ('Thinking, aversion to': *2*) or talk ('Talk, indisposed to, desire to be silent': *2*), as he collapses into a state of real mental prostration ('Prostration of mind': *3*).

Now Lycopodium feels that he has been beaten. He believes that he is more unwell than he really is ('Delusions, sick, imagines himself': *2*). She feels indifferent towards everything around her ('Indifference': *2*), especially towards her children ('Indifference, relations, to her children': *2*). Kent says: 'The world may come to an end, the whole family may die or his house may burn down.' His feeling of complete apathy ('Indifference, external things, to': *2*) is accompanied by a profound depression ('Sadness': *3*), which he feels the more keenly on waking ('Sadness, waking, on': *1*) and in the evening ('Sadness, evening': *2*). As he sinks ever deeper into misanthropy ('Misanthropy': *2*), he seeks refuge in solitude ('Company, aversion to, amel. when alone': *2*), although paradoxically he feels depressed when he is alone ('Sadness, alone, when': *1*) and his thoughts turn to the unpleasant events in his past ('Dwells on past disagreeable occurrences': *1*). In this frame of mind he may fall prey to the feeling that he has neglected his responsibilities ('Delusions, neglected his duty, that he has': 2), and his anxiety for the salvation of his soul ('Anxiety, salvation, about': 2) makes him at times doubtful of its welfare ('Doubtful, soul's welfare, of': 1) and at other times throws him into complete despair ('Despair, religious, of salvation': 2). In a state of total collapse and exhaustion on both a mental and a physical level, he has a premonition that death is near ('Death, presentiment of': 2) and he welcomes it ('Loathing, life': 2), most markedly in the morning ('Loathing, life, morning': 3), the only time of day when his mind turns to thoughts of suicide ('Suicidal disposition, morning': 1), in keeping with the particular morning-time aggravation of this remedy.

Seated at the bedside of the Lycopodium patient who is now a broken man, totally disabled by his disease, we will hear his protesting ('Lamenting': 3), his constant worrying about the future ('Lamenting, future, about': 1) and his complaints that he has been abandoned, left without support ('Helplessness, feeling of': 1). His respiration will be laboured as he says all this, he will flare his nostrils anxiously, deprived as he is of air by his flatulence; he will mutter under his breath ('Muttering': 2) in his state of delirium and depression ('Delirium': 3, 'Delirium, sorrowful': 1), full of ravings, ramblings and moans, until he collapses into a stupor ('Stupefaction': 2), which happens mainly in the afternoon ('Stupor, afternoon': 1) or while reading ('Stupor, reading, on': 1), and from which it is very difficult to rouse him ('Stupor, rouses, with difficulty': 1). Lycopodium may suffer a loss of consciousness ('Unconsciousness': 2), which is a deeper level of insensibility than stupor, when the general modalities are present – in a warm atmosphere ('Unconsciousness, warm room': 2), while standing ('Unconsciousness, standing, while': 1), in a crowded room ('Unconsciousness, crowded room, in a': 2), after menstruation ('Unconsciousness, menses, after': 2), while talking ('Unconsciousness, talking, while': 1) and, on occasions, he is still able to function automatically while unconscious ('Unconsciousness, conduct, automatic': 1). The physiological basis for this Lycopodium symptom is the congestion to the head which is engendered by a sluggish venous circulation and hepatic portal vein involvement.

Returning to the theme of the Lycopodium lament, we find that he will always justify his complaints with very valid arguments so that his pride remains intact. His lament may be a protest or a complaint ('Complaining': 2) but it is rarely a moan. Lycopodium will only allow himself to moan while he is asleep ('Moaning, sleep, during': 2) or, in the case of the woman, during menstruation ('Moaning, menses, during': *1*), when she feels at a great disadvantage in relation to men. Rather than simply moan, Lycopodium will shout ('Shrieking': *3*) in annoyance, with rage, or to impose his authority, or during sleep ('Shrieking, sleep, during': *3*) or when he wakes ('Shrieking, waking, on': *2*) to release his subconscious tension. The classic brain cry ('Shrieking, brain cry': *2*) or the shrieking before convulsions ('Shrieking, convulsions, before': *2*) are due to a peculiar hypersensitivity of the cortex. The children shout to impose their wills ('Shrieking, children, in': *1*). The urine with red sand explains why the child shouts before urination ('Shrieking, urination, before': *3*), but the shouting is in itself a peculiar and characteristic expression of suffering.

We have seen that the desire to hide is the *modus operandi* of Lycopodium: when the competition gets hot, he runs away. He does not want to be with people, he rejects the company of strangers ('Company, aversion to, presence of strangers, to': *1*), but at the same time he does not want to be left alone. He does not want to be with people because he is afraid they will discover his secret lack of self-confidence which he takes such great pains to hide. So, on the surface it would appear that there is a contradiction between his need for people, on the one hand, and his rejection of them, on the other. But if we examine this more closely we see that he avoids people because he is afraid of defeat; when the patient does not want anyone near him it is because he would feel humiliated if people saw him as the invalid he has become. For this reason he will sharply reject any consolation offered him ('Consolation agg.': *1*): he feels degraded by people's pity. But, in his heart of hearts, he is extremely timid ('Timidity': *3*) and weak, in constant need of affection, which of course he does not get because of his tremendous aggressiveness.

He is a private person ('Reserved': *1*), fully aware of his own problems, wary ('Suspicious': *3*) that other people will find him out. He gets offended ('Offended, easily': *2*) by the slightest rebuff, real or imagined, by the slightest snub or lack of consideration from others ('Scorn, ailments from': *1*). He broods over the offences and emotional frustrations he has suffered at the hands of other people ('Malicious': *2*). He is 'Discontented': *2*, annoyed with himself ('Discontented, himself, with': *1*), irritable, and his bad temper can be sparked off by any situation he considers to be unjust or undeserved ('Mortification, ailments after': *3*). Mortification causes him profound grief and humiliation, and inflicts a permanent wound on his pride and self-esteem. His pride, his cowardice and his weakness of character combine to make him suffer his rage in silence ('Anger, ailments after, with silent grief': *3*) and suffer his grief intensely ('Grief': *2*, 'Grief, ailments from': *1*), inconsolably ('Inconsolable': *1*).

But this timid person is also highly sentimental ('Sentimental': *1*); he feels sympathy for other people's pain ('Sympathetic': *1*) because of his own need for affection. He is moved to tears by an altruistic deed, gentle music ('Sensitive, music, to': *2*), a family event, a farewell, a token of friendship; his sentimentality is the external manifestation of his desperate inner need for fatherly love. The weeping when thanked ('Weeping, thanked, when': *3*) encapsulates in one image the drama of his whole life. He wanted to be loved, but his total lack of self-confidence changed his feelings of inadequacy into feelings of pride and a need for power, so that if he could not be loved, he could at least demand respect and obedience. But when, beaten and battered, he reaches the end of his days, he realises that he really is loved for what he truly is, and not for what his love of power would have him be. He breaks down the barriers which his pride has built between him and other people and he collapses in floods of tears, weeping and wailing ('Weeping, aloud': *3*) as he comes face to face with reality. Aggression and weeping are the two opposing poles of Lycopodium. He weeps when he is told off ('Weeping, admonitions, cause': *2*), from 4 to 8 p.m. ('Weeping, 4 to 8 p.m.': *3*). The children weep at the least provocation ('Weeping, at the least worry, children': *1*), or on waking ('Weeping, waking, on': *1*). The women weep before menstruation ('Weeping, menses, before': *2*), during menstruation ('Weeping, menses, during': *1*) or after menstruation ('Weeping, menses, after': *1*), bearing witness to the female Lycopodium's eternal power struggles with men, which are intensified during the menstrual cycle.

To the uninitiated observer, it might seem extraordinary to find that this patient, who displays such overt masculinity, should also burst into tears so easily. But it is a discreet, controlled weeping, which may come upon him for no apparent reason ('Weeping, causeless': *2*), which may change into laughter ('Weeping, alternating with laughter': *2*) and which only happens at certain moments. His weeping also does him good ('Weeping, ameliorates symptoms': *2*) because it stirs up his emotional responses and brings him closer to the hearts of other people.

Clinical experience has shown that it would be a mistake to think of Lycopodium as a predominantly male remedy. The female Lycopodium presents us with the image of a self-important young woman who conceals her feelings of inadequacy behind her self-conceit. In the consulting room, she leans back in the chair, crosses her legs, rests her arms on the arms of the chair and lets her hands hang down. She is an intellectual who feels more at ease in a scientific discussion than in a fashion boutique, and she considers household chores to be beneath her. As we have already seen, she is generally worse before menses, but here the irritability ('Irritability, menses, before': 2) is highly characteristic, as this is the only remedy that is quite so harsh and bad-tempered at this time ('Morose, menses, before': 2). She considers her femininity to be a real handicap in her continual battle with the male sex; thus she feels aversion to her children, who chain her to the household chores ('Children, aversion to, flies from his own': 1), as if she were separated from them ('Estranged, flies from her own children': 1) and, in the end, she disowns and deserts her children ('Forsakes his own children': 1).

I tend to use these rubrics more for the female Lycopodium who dislikes her children ('Children, dislikes her own': 2) than for the male, who tends to manifest these symptoms more often. In his case, this negative attitude towards his children may stem from his feelings of being in competition with them, where he sees that they are as good as him, or even better, or where he perceives their lack of respect, consideration or support for him as he approaches the final years of his life. The basic causes here are his feelings of inadequacy and worthlessness. In the mother's case, while she may also compete with her children and sense their lack of support, her children symbolise all that stands in the way of her success – they are the products of her femininity.

I have left the sections on delusions, sensations and dreams to the end because, despite their comparative brevity, the rubrics contained in them paint a distinctive image of the remedy's mental picture.

Delusions and Sensations

The pathological tendencies of the remedy are reflected in the delusion that he is ill ('Delusions, sick, imagines himself': 2); his doubts and insecurities in the feeling that he has done wrong ('Delusions, wrong, fancies he has done': 1); the self-reproach, which stems from the excessively high standards he sets himself, in the delusion that he has neglected his duties ('Delusions, neglected his duty, that he has': 2); his fear of loss, of failure, in the sensation that everything will vanish ('Delusions, vanish, seems as if everything would': 1); his mental confusion and his duality in the sensation of being in different places

('Delusions, places, of being in different': *2*) or of being in two places at the same time ('Delusions, places, of being in two, at the same time': *2*). The fear of being found out, and the need for solitude, are both expressed by the delusion that his house is full of people ('Delusions, house is full of people': *1*) or that he sees people on entering a room ('Delusions, room, sees people on entering': *1*). His inner feelings of aggression project on to the external world as the delusion of seeing images and phantoms ('Delusions, images, phantoms, sees': *2*) in the afternoon ('Delusions, images sees, afternoon': *1*), which frighten him ('Delusions, images, frightful': *1*), during sleep ('Delusions, images frightful, during sleep': *1*) and which keep him awake ('Delusions, images, frightful, sleep, preventing': *1*). All these rubrics are almost uniquely found in Lycopodium.

The fear of aggression – another expression of his paranoia – is revealed in the feeling that people are going to attack him ('Delusions, injury, is about to receive': *1*), that they will kill him ('Delusions, murdered, that he would be': *1*) or that someone is present ('Delusions, present, someone is': *1*). Visions appear before him during the day ('Delusions, visions, daytime': *1*), horrible visions ('Delusions, visions horrible': *1*), when he closes his eyes ('Delusions, visions, closing the eyes, on': *1*).

Misfortune and unhappiness follow him to the end of his days; he feels that he is an unfortunate victim of circumstances ('Delusions, unfortunate, that he is': *1*). Searching for some peace of mind, he uses childish fantasies ('Delusions, child, childish fantasies, has': *1*) to protect himself from the responsibilities of adulthood. These fantasies, which are unique to Lycopodium, are the symbol of the true subconscious motivation behind the domineering egotistical exterior – a weak, lonely and frightened child who is desperately trying to recapture the forgotten lullaby. This may also be the meaning behind another symptom which is unique to Lycopodium – the delusion that in the evening he hears music that he heard in the daytime ('Delusions, music, fancies he hears, evening, hears the music heard in the day': *1*). Now, in the evening of his life, he notices the music he heard, but did not listen to, in the daytime of his life.

Dreams

His anxiety is reflected in his anxious dreams ('Dreams, anxious': *3*) and restless sleep ('Sleep, restless': *3*), especially when lying on the left side ('Sleep, restless, lying on left side': *1*). The vivid dreams

('Dreams, vivid': *3*), with the feeling that they carry on after he wakes up ('Dreams, continued after waking': *2*), may be an expression of his heavily suppressed emotions. The confused dreams ('Dreams, confused': *2*), about misfortunes ('Dreams, misfortune, of': *3*) or business ('Dreams, business, of': *2*), illustrate his lack of mental clarity, his fear of the unexpected and of failure. One curious symptom is that Lycopodium becomes drowsy soon after dinner ('Sleepiness, dinner, after': *3*), with frequent ineffectual yawning ('Yawning, dinner, after: *2*' and 'Yawning, ineffectual': *2*).

SUMMARY

Low Self-Esteem
The deep-seated feelings of inadequacy are the key to his personality. The starting point is the lack of self-confidence; the goal is to win power.

Related Rubrics
'Confidence, want of self': *2*.
'Power, love of': *1*.

Compensatory Pride
To achieve this end he adopts an attitude of haughtiness and pride. With abuse and effrontery he turns himself into a dictator.

Related Rubrics
'Cursing': *2*.
'Dictatorial': *2*.
'Haughty': *3*.
'Insolent': *3*.
'Rudeness': *3*.

Perfectionism
In order to achieve his success, he trains himself to be a meticulous perfectionist, using every moment God sends to achieve his end, from which he gets the anxiety that is ameliorated by occupation.

Related Rubrics
'Conscientious about trifles': *2*.
'Occupation, amel.': *1*.

Anticipatory Anxiety

His anxiety reappears with every undertaking. He anticipates everything with fear and anxiety, haunted by the vision of failure.

Related Rubric
'Anticipation, complaints from': *1*.

Contradiction

He allows no-one to come between him and his obsessive need for
perfection. His contradictory nature and his inability to allow others to
contradict him are his most effective verbal weapons.

Related Rubrics
'Contradict, disposition to': *2*.
'Contradiction, is intolerant of': *3*.

Irritability

With the anticipation, he feels an intolerable tension when he wakes up
at the start of a new day, at which makes him irritable.

Related Rubric
'Irritability, morning, waking, on': *3*.

Mortification

In his heart of hearts Lycopodium is a timid person, in constant need of
affection. His pride suffers from the injustices of daily life, large or
small, and he feels humiliated by the lack of consideration he imagines
he receives from other people. He expresses his wounded pride
through being easily offended, resentful and blaming others.

Related Rubrics
'Malicious': *2*.
'Mortification, ailments after': *3*.
'Offended, easily': *2*.
'Reproaches others': *2*.
'Timidity': *3*.

Paradoxical Emotional Problems

In no other remedy do we find the duality of success and failure, strength and weakness, so intricately interwoven; he feels vulnerable, lacking in support, and he does not want to be alone. At the same time he fears and avoids people. He is both worse and better for being alone. He desires and is averse to company. This is the subtle paradox of his emotional polarities.

Related Rubrics
'Company, aversion to': *2*.
'Company, aversion to, amel. when alone': *2*.
'Company, desire for': *3*.
'Company, desire for, alone, while agg.': *2*.
'Fear, people, of': *3*.
'Helplessness, feeling of': *1*.

Release of Tension

His weeping reveals his profound weakness, especially when his pride is touched by a sincere show of affection. It is a controlled weeping that seeps out, draining away his anxiety and tension. Thus Lycopodium weeps when thanked, and weeping ameliorates his symptoms. The drama of his internal conflict makes him weep and wail, his pride makes him weep from a telling-off and from consolation, and laughter alternates with the weeping, with a touch of hysterics at times. Sometimes he weeps for no reason at all, and at other times he weeps with anxiety about his future.

Related Rubrics
'Weeping, admonitions cause': *2*.
'Weeping, aloud': *3*.
'Weeping, alternating with laughter': *2*.
'Weeping, ameliorates symptoms': *2*.
'Weeping, causeless': *2*.
'Weeping, consolation agg.': *1*.
'Weeping, future, about the': *1*.
'Weeping, thanked, when': *3*.

Intellectual Deficiency

On the level of the intellect, the weakness of memory and the resulting mistakes he makes are evidence of his pathological tendencies. He forgets proper names, words, what he has read, he makes mistakes when reading, misplaces words when speaking, and misplaces letters or omits them when writing. He uses wrong words.

Related Rubrics
'Memory, weakness of': *3*.
'Memory, weakness, expressing one's self, for': *2*.
'Memory, weakness, names, for proper': *2*.
'Memory, weakness, read, for what has': *2*.
'Memory, weakness, words, for': *2*.
'Mistakes, reading': *2*.
'Mistakes, words, misplacing': *2*.
'Mistakes, words, writing, confounding letters': *1*.
'Mistakes, words, writing, omitting letters': *2*.
'Mistakes, words, wrong words, using': *3*.

Physical Congestion

The intellectual weakness has its correlation on a physical level in the congestion of the head, which causes a marked need for air, as evidenced in the flapping of the nostrils, and the amelioration of the congestion and mental confusion while walking in the open air.

Related Rubrics
'Confusion, walking, while, open air amel.': *3*.
'Dullness, walking, while, in open air amel.': *3*.
'Nose, motion of wings, fanlike': *3*.

Fears

He is plagued by fears and anxieties. With his fear of solitude, which reveals his emotional vulnerability, he journeys through life with the fear of being unable to reach his destination, because of the underlying lack of self-confidence. Lycopodium lives out his days in constant competition with other people: his fear of people, of others approaching him, of a crowd, all express his feelings of competitiveness, his cowardice and his wish to hide. His fear of men expresses this whole syndrome. With the fear of imaginary things, of darkness, of ghosts, of a knock at the door, he is also easily alarmed by the merest trifle, because of his suppressed feelings of aggression.

His fear of the unexpected becomes a specific fear that something will happen to him or to the people he loves, and his extreme overprotectiveness towards them hides the insecurity he feels. All this accumulation of worry and anxiety gives him a fear of undertaking anything at all, to the point where he does everything with fear. This may be the meaning behind his fear while walking, especially in the open air. Arising from the affinity with gastric-hepatic problems, he has the sensation that the fear rises from the stomach.

Related Rubrics
'Fear, alone, of being': *3*.
'Fear, stomach, arising from': *2*.
'Fear, imaginary things': *1*.
'Fear, noise at door': *2*.
'Fear, crowd, in a': *2*.
'Fear, dark': *2*.
'Fear, destination, of being unable to reach his': *3*.
'Fear, ghosts, of': *2*.
'Fear, men, of': *3*.
'Fear, people, of': *3*.
'Fear, approaching him, of others': *1*.
'Fear, trifles': *2*.
'Fear, happen, something will': *1*.
'Fear, undertaking anything': *2*.
'Fear, walking, while': *2*.
'Fear, walking, while, open air': *1*.

Nervous Reactions

Lycopodium lives in a permanent state of alarm, hence the overexcited nerve impulses and reflexes. He jumps at unexpected noises, with fear which seems to rise up from the feet, on falling asleep, during and from sleep, and from fright.

Related Rubrics
'Starting, anxious': *1*.
'Starting, feet, as if coming from the': *1*.
'Starting, sleep, during': *1*.
'Starting, fright, from': *2*.
'Starting, noise, from': *2*.
'Starting, from sleep': *1*.
'Starting, sleep, on falling': *3*.

Mental Deterioration

But as he nears the end of his days, he feels that he has lost the fight. In a state of real mental prostration, he imagines himself to be more unwell than he is, and is overcome by a deep feeling of indifference. It may be that he only thinks about the unpleasant things that have happened to him in his life, with a feeling that he has neglected his duty. The anxiety for the salvation of his soul – his last remaining refuge – oscillates between doubt about his soul's welfare and complete despair. In a state of total collapse, he has a premonition that death is near and he longs for it, especially in the mornings, the only time of day when his mind turns to thoughts of suicide.

Related Rubrics
'Anxiety, salvation, about': *2.*
'Death, presentiment of': *2.*
'Delusions, neglected his duty, that he has': *2.*
'Delusions, sick, imagines himself': *2.*
'Despair, religious (of salvation etc.)': *2.*
'Doubtful, soul's welfare, of': *1.*
'Dwells on past disagreeable occurrences': *1.*
'Indifference': *2.*
'Loathing, life': *2.*
'Loathing, life, morning': *3.*
'Prostration of mind': *3.*
'Suicidal disposition, morning': *1.*

SCHEMATIC DIAGRAM AND REPERTORISATION

We can now produce a schematic picture of Lycopodium (overleaf) as taken from Kent's *Repertory*. The Minimum Characteristic Syndrome of the remedy is represented by a circle. In the centre of the circle we place the low self-esteem, 'Confidence, want of self' (1). Above it, we put the rubrics concerned with pride, 'Haughty' (2), 'Dictatorial' (3) and 'Contradict, disposition to' (4), which go to make up the counterbalance of power. To the right, we place the rubrics concerned with perfectionism, 'Conscientious about trifles' (6) and 'Occupation, amel.' (7), the two symptoms which Lycopodium depends upon to achieve his success. Below this, we place the anticipatory anxiety, 'Anticipation, complaints from' (5), which affects him before any challenging situation. To the left, there is 'Contradiction, is intolerant of' (8), the negative attitude he brings to bear on any opposition whatsoever which would undermine his self-confidence. At the top left-hand corner, we have placed the paradoxical emotional problems,

SCHEMATIC DIAGRAM – LYCOPODIUM

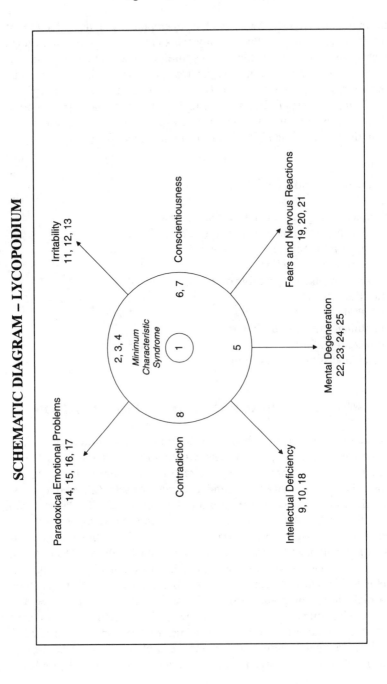

Irritability
11, 12, 13

Conscientiousness

Fears and Nervous Reactions
19, 20, 21

6, 7

2, 3, 4
*Minimum
Characteristic
Syndrome*

1

Mental Degeneration
22, 23, 24, 25

5

Paradoxical Emotional Problems
14, 15, 16, 17

8

Contradiction

Intellectual Deficiency
9, 10, 18

Minimum Characteristic Syndrome

1) Confidence, want of self
2) Haughty
3) Dictatorial
4) Contradict, disposition to
5) Anticipation, complaints from
6) Conscientious about trifles
7) Occupation, amel.
8) Contradiction, is intolerant of

Intellectual Deficiency

9) Memory, weakness of, names, for proper
10) Mistakes, wrong words, using

Irritability

11) Mortification, ailments after
12) Irritability, waking, on
13) Irritability, menses, before

Paradoxical Emotional Problems

14) Company, desire for
15) Company, aversion to

Release of Tension

16) Weeping, ameliorates symptoms
17) Weeping, thanked, when

Need for Freedom

18) Confusion, walking, while, open air amel.

Fears and Nervous Reactions

19) Fear, alone, of being
20) Fear, stomach, arising from
21) Starting, noise, from

Mental Degeneration

22) Prostration of mind
23) Dwells on past disagreeable occurrences
24) Anxiety, salvation, about
25) Loathing, life

REPERTORISATION – LYCOPODIUM

	1	2	3	4	5	6	7	8	9	10	11	12	13	14	15	16	17	18	19	20	21	22	23	24	25
Lyc.	2	3	2	2	1	2	1	3	2	3	3	3	2	3	2	2	3	3	3	2	2	3	1	2	2
Alum.	1	1	–	–	–	–	1	1	–	2	3	–	–	–	1	–	–	–	–	–	1	2	–	–	1
Anac.	3	1	–	1	–	–	–	1	2	–	–	1	–	–	3	2	–	–	–	–	–	2	–	–	3
Aur.	2	1	1	2	–	1	1	3	–	–	–	–	–	–	2	–	–	–	–	2	1	3	–	2	1
Bry.	2	–	–	–	–	1	1	2	–	–	2	1	–	1	2	–	–	1	1	1	1	3	–	2	3
Caust.	1	2	1	–	–	–	–	–	1	1	2	1	2	1	–	–	–	–	–	1	2	3	–	–	1
Chin.	2	1	–	2	–	1	1	–	3	3	–	1	–	–	2	–	–	–	–	–	–	2	2	–	3
Ferr.	–	1	1	1	–	1	2	2	–	–	–	–	–	–	–	–	–	–	3	–	–	–	–	–	1
Hyos.	1	2	–	1	–	1	–	–	–	–	–	–	–	3	2	–	–	–	–	–	–	3	–	1	1
Ign.	1	1	–	1	–	3	2	3	–	–	–	2	–	2	3	1	–	–	–	2	2	1	–	3	2
Lach.	1	2	2	1	–	–	–	1	1	–	1	–	–	1	2	1	–	–	1	–	3	3	1	–	3
Merc.	1	1	–	1	2	2	2	–	–	–	–	–	–	–	–	–	–	–	–	2	1	3	–	–	1
Natrum-c.	1	–	–	1	–	2	2	2	–	–	1	1	–	3	1	–	–	–	3	–	3	3	–	–	2
Nit-ac.	1	–	2	1	–	2	2	2	–	–	–	1	–	2	2	–	–	–	2	–	1	3	1	–	2
Nux-v.	1	1	–	1	–	2	2	2	1	–	1	1	2	2	3	1	–	–	1	–	3	3	–	–	2
Olnd.	1	–	–	2	–	–	–	–	1	–	1	–	–	3	1	1	–	3	3	–	–	3	2	–	3
Phos.	1	1	–	–	–	1	–	–	1	1	2	2	–	2	2	–	–	–	2	2	–	2	–	2	2
Puls.	2	1	–	–	–	1	3	3	–	–	1	1	–	2	1	1	–	3	2	–	–	3	2	2	2
Sep.	–	–	–	–	–	3	3	2	–	–	–	–	–	2	1	–	–	–	2	1	3	3	2	2	2
Sil.	2	2	–	–	–	2	1	1	–	1	1	1	–	2	1	1	–	–	2	–	–	3	–	2	1
Stram.	1	1	–	–	–	2	1	1	2	–	1	1	–	–	2	–	–	1	–	–	1	3	2	2	2
Sulph.	1	3	–	–	–	2	1	1	2	2	2	1	–	–	2	–	–	–	–	–	–	1	–	2	3
Thuj.	–	1	–	–	–	1	1	1	–	2	1	1	–	–	1	–	–	–	–	–	–	–	–	–	–
Ver-alb.	–	3	2	–	–	1	1	–	–	–	1	–	–	1	1	–	–	–	1	1	–	–	–	3	–

Minimum Characteristic Syndrome

1) Confidence, want of self
2) Haughty
3) Dictatorial
4) Contradict, disposition to
5) Anticipation, complaints from
6) Conscientious about trifles
7) Occupation, amel.
8) Contradiction, is intolerant of

Intellectual Deficiency

9) Memory, weakness of, names, for proper
10) Mistakes, wrong words, using

Irritability

11) Mortification, ailments after
12) Irritability, waking, on
13) Irritability, menses, before

Paradoxical Emotional Problems

14) Company, desire for
15) Company, aversion to

Release of Tension

16) Weeping, ameliorates symptoms
17) Weeping, thanked, when

Need for Freedom

18) Confusion, walking, while, open air amel.

Fears and Nervous Reactions

19) Fear, alone, of being
20) Fear, stomach, arising from
21) Starting, noise, from

Mental Degeneration

22) Prostration of mind
23) Dwells on past disagreeable occurrences
24) Anxiety, salvation, about
25) Loathing, life

'Company, desire for' (14) and 'Company, aversion to' (15). These symptoms symbolise his need for support and his fear of being found out. A good cry brings about the release of pent-up emotions, 'Weeping, ameliorates symptoms' (16) and 'Weeping, thanked, when' (17).

In the bottom left-hand corner we have placed the symptoms pertaining to his failing intellect, 'Memory, weakness of, names, for proper' (9), 'Mistakes, wrong words, using' (10), and 'Confusion, walking, while, open air amel.'(18) which illustrates the need for freedom on both a mental and a physical level: the need for open air, and the intolerance of tight clothing. At the top right-hand corner, the symptom 'Mortification, ailments after' (11) describes his intolerance of the injustices of life, large or small, while his 'Irritability, waking, on' (12) is the anger he feels in anticipation of the new day. In a woman, the 'Irritability, menses, before' (13) reminds us of her resentment and envy of men.

At the bottom right-hand corner, his 'Fear, alone, of being' (19), 'Fear, stomach, arising from' (20) and 'Starting, noise, from' (21) constitute the nervous reaction syndrome. Below the centre, we have grouped together four rubrics under the heading of mental degeneration, which form the final corollary of his life: 'Prostration of mind' (22), 'Dwells on past disagreeable occurrences' (23), 'Anxiety, salvation, about' (24), and finally, a complete apathy, 'Loathing, life' (25).

COMPARATIVE MATERIA MEDICA

Three remedies have seven symptoms from the Minimum Characteristic Syndrome of Lycopodium: Aurum, Ignatia and Nux Vomica.

Aurum

This remedy does not have the symptom 'Anticipation, complaints from' (5), which is typical of Lycopodium's anxiety for the outcome of any trying situation which may end in failure or defeat. Of primary importance in Aurum is the tremendous syphilitic aggression which overlays his basic lack of self-confidence and gives a particular significance to the rest of the symptoms in this group. The Aurum patient is obsessed by his destructive impulses, for which he hates himself and feels profoundly guilty. He feels completely wretched, to have failed in his duties and been deserted by his friends, and believes that his only hope lies in religion or suicide. This feeling of guilt, as if his conscience accuses him of a crime he has not committed, is fostered by a weak and aggressive nature which may suddenly explode with anger at the slightest offence or contradiction. These intense feelings of aggression may be unleashed by the loss of a loved one, a grief, an argument which has left him feeling angry, a humiliation or a slight which he suffers in silence until the suppression of his feelings produces the picture of anger, fear, anxiety, tremblings, angina, thoracic oppression, despair, weeping, depression and, finally, suicidal thoughts, with circulatory disturbances, flushes of heat, congestion to the head, desire for open air and aggravation at night.

The most typical case that I can recall is a patient who would wake up at two o'clock in the morning with palpitations, a feeling of anguish and a premonition of imminent death, the sensation of a great wave of heat sweeping through her chest – symptoms which were brought on by the nervous tension she suffered as a result of the interminable arguments with her husband.

In short, Aurum accepts his lack of self-confidence and does not try to compete with other people, as a more sycotic remedy would, and therefore he does not suffer from anticipation. His perfectionism, 'Conscientious about trifles' (6), is much less significant than his low self-esteem, 'Confidence, want of self' (1), with the accompanying feelings of guilt and abandonment. He does not suffer from a weak memory (sycosis) and the remaining symptoms in the first group have a definite syphilitic taint. It is easy to hurt Aurum, 'Mortification, ailments after' (11), because of his low self-image. He prefers solitude, 'Company, aversion to' (15), in order to indulge his guilt feelings, and of the remainder of the symptoms has only 'Fear, stomach, arising from' (20) and 'Starting, noise from' (21), both of which express his state of permanent circumspection brought about by his anxiety of conscience.

Ignatia

This remedy lacks the symptom, 'Dictatorial' (3), which is characteristic of the egocentric and arbitrary way in which Lycopodium tries to compensate for his basic lack of self-confidence. Ignatia is shallow, changeable, contradictory and extremely moody. Her disturbances are of a purely functional nature, unlike the pathological disturbances of Lycopodium. For this reason she also lacks symptoms 9 and 10, which relate to intellectual deficiency. She also lacks 'Irritability, waking, on' (12) and 'Irritability, menses, before' (13), which express Lycopodium's sycotic competitiveness in society. Ignatia does not share the fears and state of constant alarm in which Lycopodium lives, because Ignatia is a hysterical and hypersensitive person, and not an aggressively competitive one.

Nux Vomica

The characteristics of Nux Vomica are a great hypersensitivity to his surroundings, with irritability, coldness and antiperistaltic contractions of the digestive system.

Compared with the MCS of Lycopodium it lacks only symptom 3, 'Dictatorial'. Nux Vomica is brave and fearless, unlike the cowardly Lycopodium, and does not need to use despotism in order to impose his authority. Nux Vomica is a natural leader, a boss, the typical workaholic business executive. He is restless, hurried and sure of himself: 'What I say goes', and he orders his employees around angrily and impulsively, in a state of hyperstimulation. Nux Vomica does not have any complexes – he is an optimist, but the slightest hitch will spark off his temper, as it means that the completion of the task will be delayed, a situation which this impatient, fastidious perfectionist, 'Conscientious about trifles' (6), finds too much to tolerate. He feels better when he has something to do, 'Occupation, amel.' (7). He gets angry when people refuse to do what they are told, 'Contradiction, is intolerant of' (8), and he habitually goes against what people tell him he should do, because he knows best, and 'everyone else is a time-waster'.

This constant state of emotional stress, with the internal toxicity generated by his neurological imbalance and the external toxicity of self-abuse through the excessive consumption of alcohol, coffee and spices, explains his feelings of inadequacy, 'Confidence, want of self' (1), and his deficient memory – see symptoms 9 and 10). Symptoms 11, 12, 13 and 21 have already been explained. His sociability, 'Company, desire for' (14), is an aspect of his talent for public relations. His reactions are faster than other people's, so he finds others tedious, 'Company, aversion to' (15), and his lack of emotional susceptibility and fear account for the absence of the remaining rubrics.

Five remedies have six symptoms of the Minimum Characteristic Syndrome of Lycopodium: Mercurius, Natrum Carbonicum, Ferrum Metallicum, Stramonium and Veratrum Album.

Mercurius

Mercurius does not have the two symptoms which show the sycotic compensatory mechanism for dealing with a basic lack of self-confidence, namely 'Conscientious about trifles' (6) and 'Occupation, amel.' (7). As one would expect from a syphilitic remedy, he suffers from a marked mental deficiency, a sort of dullness, a slowness of reaction and regressively infantile behaviour. A weak character, dominated by his aggressive impulses, Mercurius is in a state of constant anxiety and restlessness, which is forever driving him to escape, to run away from home, pursued by the guilt of a past misdemeanour. The sight of a knife or other sharp instrument excites his aggressive feelings to the point where he would be capable of murder or suicide.

Paschero has said of this remedy that, in his state of paranoia, he projects his inner feelings of hostility onto the external world and sees everybody as his enemy: he is suspicious, trusts nobody, not even himself; he is afraid of being alone, he believes he is losing his reason, and he wants to kill the person who contradicts him. The Aurum patient's guilt becomes a hypochondriasis, a depression in which he blames himself for everything, and believes that other people have deserted him because he is no longer worthy of them, a depression which culminates finally in his suicide. Mercurius, on the other hand, has a criminal rather than a suicidal nature, and his peculiar mixture of guilt and aggression create a state of agitation and anxious haste which make him want to be forever fleeing, a fugitive from himself.

The Minimum Characteristic Syndrome of Mercurius has the following symptoms:

'Anxiety conscience of (as if guilty of a crime)': *2*.

'Excitement, evening, in bed': *2* – the clearest example of his night-time aggravations, when his aggressive impulses take over .

'Fear insanity, of': *1* – the fear that his aggressive impulses will start to control him,

'Homesickness': *2* – he recalls his paradise lost as he comes closer to the gates of Hell.

'Kill, desire to': *1* and 'Dictatorial': *2* – his ruthless desire for power.

'Death, presentiment of': *1*, 'Travel, desire to': *1* and 'Unobserving': *1* – his anarchic disrespect for all social norms, his desire to escape, and the persistent death wish.

Despite his general condition of intellectual deficiency, he does not have the specific Lycopodium symptom 'Mistakes, wrong words, using' (10). The remedy also lacks the 'Irritability, waking, on' (12) and 'Irritability, menses, before' (13), which express Lycopodium's annoyance with his personal failings. The lack of control over his feelings of aggression accounts for symptom 11, 'Mortification, ailments from', and his feeling of being at the mercy of his aggressive impulses explains his need for other people, 'Company, desire for' (14) and 'Fear, alone, of being' (19) – it is as if he needs other people to protect him from himself. His feeling of persecution by a hostile world explains the symptom 'Starting, noise, from' (21). He lacks the symptoms 'Company, aversion to' (15) and 'Weeping, thanked, when' (17), which express the Lycopodium desire to hide his exquisite sensitivity. He is, however, better for crying, 'Weeping, ameliorates symptoms' (16), because of his regressively infantile nature.

Five additional symptoms which complete the Mercurius picture are: a marked sensitivity to both heat and cold; a general aggravation at night; profuse perspiration, which aggravates the symptoms; fetid excoriating discharges; and tremblings.

Natrum Carbonicum

This remedy lacks the arrogance, 'Haughty' (2), and despotic disposition, 'Dictatorial' (3), which express the tremendous sycotic energy and astuteness with which Lycopodium defends himself from the outside world. Characteristic of Natrum Carbonicum is a profound depression, which surfaces with the decline of his physical and mental abilities. His flatulence and dyspepsia are aggravated by the sun, he is depressed, wants only peace and quiet, until his attention is distracted by an unexpected noise or gentle nostalgic music. He feels defeated and hard done by, his mental faculties have begun to fail him, he suffers confusion and vertigo from any mental effort.

He shares the remaining symptoms of the Minimum Characteristic Syndrome, but to a lesser degree. There is a general weakness of memory in Natrum Carbonicum, whereas in Lycopodium the memory deficiencies are selective. He wishes to escape from people, 'Company, aversion to' (15), and, like all the Natrums, is jumpy, 'Starting, noise, from' (21), and feels better when outdoors, 'Confusion, walking, while, open air amel.' (18).

In essence, the competitive and power-seeking Lycopodium is quite a different character from the withdrawn and misanthropic Natrum Carbonicum. In Allen's proving it says: 'She does not know what to do, on account of apprehensiveness and ennui, and thinks that she is quite lonely and forsaken, all day.' She cannot be bothered to eat, to work, or to be with her loved ones.

Ferrum Metallicum

This is one of those remedies which are mistakenly thought of as 'small remedies'. The truth is that the pathogenesis of the remedy has not been fully researched, and the little that is known about it is primarily pathological information. Generally, the Ferrum Met. patient is weak and incapable of any prolonged exertion. He has cold extremities and congestion in the head, or pallor with flushes of heat. There is great weakness with dyspnoea and a tendency to palpitations with fainting. This condition is usually brought on by the loss of vital fluids, especially blood loss. The pains are hammering and pulsating. The symptoms are aggravated by quick or violent movement. The weakness and prostration may ultimately lead to paralysis.

On a mental level he is confused and weak, with a profound sense of depression and dejection. He is a hypersensitive patient who suffers from extreme anxiety and is easily irritated by the slightest thing. He is quarrelsome and argumentative, impassioned and vehement; this can be caused by a sudden noise or the slightest contradiction, 'Contradiction, is intolerant of' (8), may unleash his fury. Kent tells us: 'Some of his symptoms are ameliorated by occupation, by doing something, however small, but his symptoms increase with rest.' Here, the meaning of the symptom 'Occupation, amel.' (7) is different from that of Lycopodium, where it is a reaction to his low opinion of himself. Ferrum Met. does not lack confidence, nor does he suffer from anticipatory anxiety, 'Anticipation, complaints from' (5), both of which underlie the Lycopodium symptomatology. Ferrum Met. has nothing more in common with Lycopodium, except for the desire for solitude, 'Company, aversion to' (15), which is a consequence of his weakness and depression. We may think of Ferrum Met. when presented with a patient who has a Lycopodium personality and who is suffering from circulatory disturbances such as congestions, irregular surgings and pulsations, with weakness and anaemia, flushed cheeks and pale lips; pseudo-plethoric patients with vertigo on rising, aggravation from rest and rapid movement, rheumatism of the deltoids – these are the keynote symptoms.

In essence, Ferrum Met. is a dogmatic dictator, 'Dictatorial' (3), in whom we find no self-doubt behind the mask of confidence; he has none of the cowardliness and emotional susceptibility of Lycopodium.

Stramonium

The following analysis of this polychrest is based on my clinical experience of approximately thirty cured Stramonium cases.

The differences between Stramonium and Lycopodium become clear when we look at the symptoms which are absent in the former remedy and present in the latter.

We have seen how Lycopodium tries to compensate for his lack of self-confidence by going for power and leadership, spurred on by his pride, ambition, industriousness, fastidiousness and anticipatory anxiety. He maintains tight control over his surroundings with his intolerance of contradiction, the imposition of his authority, and by using his mental agility to win arguments.

Stramonium, on the other hand, is neither power-hungry nor contradictory. He totally lacks the driving force of the Lycopodium ambition to be better than all the rest and, unlike Lycopodium, feels neither irritation at the prospect of another new day, nor annoyance at a woman's monthly indisposition.

Another point of difference is that Lycopodium needs to cry, 'Weeping, ameliorates symptoms' (16), to release the tension built up by his tortured pride and inhibition; the chink in the armour of his ambitious greed is the weeping when shown gratitude (17), as he perceives that those from whom he always demanded respect and obedience now show their affection for him. Furthermore, Stramonium does not suffer from Lycopodium's state of nervous excitability and does not figure, therefore, in symptoms 20 and 21. In addition, Stramonium is not inclined to brood over his past failures and how badly life has treated him, so he does not appear in symptom 23.

In the chapter on Lachesis I describe Stramonium as more victim than aggressor. His psoric tendency to turn in on himself creates feelings of unworthiness and helplessness – he feels like a piece of rubbish that has been left all alone in a desert, unloved and unwanted. This feeling of complete isolation is pure Stramonium, although Lycopodium can feel deserted by his loved ones. The three symptoms from the Minimum Characteristic Syndrome that are common to both remedies, 'Anticipation, complaints from' (5), 'Conscientious about trifles' (6) and 'Occupation amel.' (7), are all strategies that Stramonium uses to distract himself from his feelings of loneliness and rejection, by earning the approval of others, maybe the occasional hug or little present as a token of their esteem. His potential for extreme violence and his pride bring about the annoyance he feels when contradicted, 'Contradiction, is intolerant of' (8), although he has no real leanings towards power, hence the absence of symptoms 3 and 4.

Stramonium shares the Lycopodium deficiency of intellect and the feelings of mortification when he is hurt. In Lycopodium, the symptom 'Mortification, ailments after' (11) indicates his sensitivity to people's lack of respect, whereas in Stramonium it is a violent reaction to any opposition. Indeed, the keynotes of Stramonium, 'Rage, fury', and subsequent sub-rubrics, vividly convey his strongly syphilitic aggressive tendencies.

The need for company and affection has already been discussed. Basically, Stramonium feels totally isolated, and he rants and raves about this hostile world in which he feels 'completely trapped', as many patients have said. He inhabits a cruel underworld that torments him with nightmares and anxious dreams that wake him at night and force him once again to feel that terrible, frightening solitude. By contrast, Lycopodium will at times actually seek solitude, either from a sycotic desire to hide away, or from a syphilitic apathy and indifference to life, and he will seek company when he is feeling his usual vulnerable and insecure self.

Stramonium does not dwell on the past, whereas Lycopodium spends a lot of time picking at old wounds and trying to justify his past actions. Stramonium is present in the rubrics 'Prostration of mind' (22) and 'Loathing, life' (25). In his despair of religious salvation, his thoughts turn to suicide; he, who once claimed to be God, now believes himself to be a poor miserable sinner, the Devil incarnate, unclean and unfit for eternal glory. Lycopodium, on the other hand, will feel either anxiety about his salvation, or religious despair, in the belief that he has neglected his duty.

Veratrum Album

The Veratrum patient feels very unsure of himself in the world, but he is not interested in the power struggles of which Lycopodium is so fond, hence the absence of symptoms 4 and 5. Anxiety is the theme that runs through the Veratrum picture, a fearful anxiety that torments him at night, with great restlessness – he is 'Inconsolable over fancied misfortune' (only remedy). From Allen's provings we have: 'Sensation in his whole being as if he were gradually nearing his end.' The anxiety is aggravated by loss on a mental or physical level; this could be a love disappointment, loss of social position, financial loss, loss of vital fluids through a haemorrhage, diarrhoea or other discharge.

To protect himself from emotional loss, he throws himself into love affairs and work. In love, he is passionate and affectionate, kissing everyone he sees. Lycopodium on the other hand is more reserved in matters of love, less demonstrative of his affection and more protective of his vulnerability. If Veratrum suffers a love disappointment he will pine for his lover and refuse to be comforted. Lycopodium's ego will not permit such indulgences. Veratrum's emotional symptoms are mainly centred around his own needs and comforts: unlike Lycopodium, he is neither sentimental, nor compassionate nor protective towards other people. The irritability symptoms (12 and 13), which denote the anxious anticipation with which Lycopodium faces the new day, or the onset of menses, are absent in Veratrum. The need to communicate with people is much less important to Veratrum, hence the appearance in lower case in the rubrics 'Company, desire for' (14), 'Company, aversion to' (15), and 'Fear, alone, of being' (19). When Veratrum throws himself into his work, he is plagued by the fear of losing, whether it be his salary, his financial position, his social standing, his business deals or his dignity. Lycopodium fears none of this. To counteract his anxieties, Veratrum can be arrogant and recklessly extravagant. He is consumed by an overwhelming ambition to succeed, and will lie, cheat and bully his way to the top. He manages to conceal the true nature of his ambitions, using malice and rage to distract people's attention away from his real motives: he will maintain a low profile and keep his opinions to himself, for fear of being found out, hence the absence of symptom 4. At work, he is conscientious, 'Conscientious about trifles' (6), industrious and better for occupation, 'Occupation, amel.' (7).

Veratrum does not have the 'Prostration of mind' (22) that afflicts Lycopodium, when he is crushed and defeated by the failure of his lifelong efforts to achieve the power he so desperately sought, in his quest to overcome his profound lack of self-confidence. When Veratrum reaches his lowest point, he is convinced that he is nothing but a miserable sinner, unclean in body and soul, and that he is doomed, 'Anxiety, salvation, about' (24), to a life of Hell. He is riddled with guilt and obsessed by thoughts of religious persecution. He knows in his bones that something dreadful is about to happen, he feels that death is near, and the slightest loss will push him closer to the edge. Veratrum, who once turned his back on goodness and strayed a long way from the path, now wishes he could retrace his steps back to what might have been; he feels so utterly lost and abandoned that life has no meaning for him, 'Loathing, life' (25). God has no comfort to offer him and, at the point of total breakdown, he hurls himself out of the window in an attempt to end it all.

Three remedies have five symptoms of the Minimum Characteristic Syndrome of Lycopodium: Silicea, Thuja and Anacardium.

Silicea

While the competitive Lycopodium spends most of his time trying to be better than everyone, Silicea only wishes to be no worse than anyone else; hence the absence from symptoms 2, 3 and 4. Silicea feels totally inadequate and ill-equipped to deal with life. He is in a constant state of nervous tension, 'Starting, noise, from' (21) and in need of protection, 'Company, desire for' (14), with the sub-rubric, 'alone, while agg.'. In practice, it is more difficult to detect a Silicea than a Lycopodium. In repertorisation, Lycopodium covers nearly all the symptoms of Silicea, but not vice versa. Understandably then, Lycopodium has often mistakenly been prescribed for patients needing Silicea. A Silicea patient will be more easily discernible if we take into account his childhood temperament; a combination of timidity, diffidence, obstinacy, irritability and fastidiousness.

Thuja

Thuja is the essence of sycosis. He is a self-satisfied and complacent individual, hence his absence from symptom 1. He keeps his true nature concealed in order not to arouse suspicion, and would never openly contradict, or seek to impose his opinions; he is, therefore, not found in symptoms 3 or 4. His anticipatory anxiety is hidden from view, 'Anticipation, complaints from' (5), his perfectionism is an obsession, 'Conscientious about trifles' (6), and his fevered activity springs from a compulsive need to work, 'Occupation, amel.' (7), to palliate the anxiety of conscience which lies at the root of his emotional problems. Like Lycopodium, he has a large number of symptoms which relate to mental weakness: he forgets what he has done, what he was going to say and, more importantly, he makes mistakes while speaking or writing, omitting letters, syllables and words. In common with many sycotic remedies, he has the irritability on waking (12), and he keeps himself hidden with his aversion to company (15). He also shares the keynote 'Fear, stomach, arising from' (20).

Thuja differs fundamentally from Lycopodium in that he lacks the feelings of inadequacy, the sentimentality, the emotional suscep-tibilities, the tendency to mortification, the aversion to solitude, the need for company and the child-like need for paternal protection.

Anacardium

Anacardium is a depressed, indecisive character who is caught in an eternal conflict of wills, whose weak spirit can never decide between his desire and his duty. Typical of Anacardium is his sudden loss of memory and his ambivalent nature; he is in constant conflict with himself. It is this loss of memory that causes his panic attacks before taking an exam, 'Anticipation, complaints from' (5).

This remedy has changeability with mental slowness and dullness. Doubtful of everything, he does nothing. He is caught between the opposing forces of his instinctive aggression and his conscience. He has a cruel temper, is subject to fits of violent anger, and lacks all moral feeling; he has no confidence in himself, and is at the mercy of his whims and impulses to love and hate, to insult and curse, with the sensation of being double (Alumina, Thuja), or that his soul is escap-ing from his body (Thuja), or of living in a dream. His personality split is emotionally based whereas, in Alumina, the split is on an intellectual level. He has two keynote symptoms – the sensation of a plug in various places and the amelioration of all symptoms by eating. He shares with Lycopodium symptoms 1, 2, 4 and 5, but lacks the authoritarianism, perfectionism and amelioration from occupation. While Lycopodium judges himself against other people, Anacardium's conflict is with himself. He has no idea if he is good or bad. He is a lone wolf who relies on no-one but himself. The repertory substantiates this – he does not appear in symptoms 11, 12, 14 and 17, all of which express ways of interacting with the world. He shuns the company of people, 'Company, aversion to' (15), because of his need to focus on himself, and he releases emotional tension by weeping, 'Weeping, ameliorates symptoms' (16).

Seven remedies have four symptoms of the Minimum Characteristic Syndrome of Lycopodium: Alumina, Bryonia, Causticum, China, Hyoscyamus, Lachesis and Sepia.

Alumina

This remedy does not have symptoms 3, 4 and 6 of the Minimum Characteristic Syndrome, which together constitute the Lycopodium defence against his innermost feelings of inadequacy. Alumina suffers from great mental apathy and is unable to concentrate or follow through an idea. The main characteristic of this remedy is the state of confusion and unreality. The centres of perception are slow to function, and he has the delusion that another person is perceiving what he is seeing or hearing, or that someone else is performing his actions for him. The patient starts to doubt the reality of everything, even his own identity ('Confusion, identity, as to his': *3*). Like Mercurius, if he sees a sharp instrument, his aggressive impulses come to the fore and he trembles with the fear of committing murder or suicide. The surfacing of these feelings of aggression puts him into a state of hurried anxiety where nothing moves quickly enough, and he wants to run away and hide. He is depressed and grumbles about everything; he is irritable, full of apprehension and, when he thinks about his condition, believes he is going mad. The pathogenesis is rich in general symptoms – predominantly, there is dryness of all mucous membranes, with the exception of a profuse vaginal discharge, and there is the characteristic inactivity of the rectum with chronic constipation.

Because of his confused state, he makes mistakes in speaking. His difficulties with self-expression and his suppressed nervous tension explain the symptoms 'Weeping, ameliorates symptoms' (16) and 'Starting, noise, from' (21). The syphilitic taint of the remedy is revealed in the rubrics 'Haughty' (2) and 'Contradiction, is intolerant of' (8), which cover up his fundamentally low opinion of himself. In his state of emotional withdrawal, he looks for things to keep him busy, 'Occupation, amel.' (7), to palliate the feelings of guilt and confusion.

Bryonia

Bryonia has four of the eight symptoms of the Minimum Characteristic Syndrome of Lycopodium. This is another under-confident remedy, 'Confidence, want of self' (1), but without Lycopodium's keen competitive spirit and desire for success and power; hence he does not appear in symptoms 2, 3 or 4. With his basically psoric feelings of inadequacy and his aggravation from all movement, Bryonia avoids all competition. The way he uses his will-power to overcome his problems of movement is characteristic. He resolves his feelings of anxiety and uneasiness about the future, 'Anticipation, complaints from' (5), with a great attention to detail, 'Conscientious about trifles' (6), and single-mindedness, 'Contradiction, is intolerant of' (8). His impetuousness and industriousness – symptoms which do not appear in Lycopodium – are not competitive qualities, but contain an element of frustration and annoyance with his condition of physical weakness. Bryonia attempts to resolve his existential angst through his work – he talks of business, dreams of business and, when he is ill, his biggest concern is to get back to work.

He does not have the specific intellectual deficiency symptoms. His most obvious symptom is irritability. This is the result of the demands he makes on himself, the desire and the inability to do something, as expressed for example by the confusion that is aggravated while lying, and while walking, but is ameliorated in the open air. The combination of desire and disability is expressed by the desire to be always on the move, the anxious wish to keep moving, yet with the aggravation from motion and amelioration from rest. It is as if Bryonia were desperately fighting to escape from the prison of his impotence, only to be held back by his very weakness; this is why he desires things only to reject them later. The apparent contradiction between his psoric tendencies and the accumulated frustrations inherent in his sycotic way of life – the discrepancy between what he wishes to achieve and what it is possible to achieve – creates a moody individual, a slave to his whims and impulses. Even the act of eating has a touch of capriciousness about it – he has a large appetite but does not know what he wants to eat.

Bryonia is irritable when he wakes up, 'Irritability, waking, on' (12), because that is when he starts to move about. He easily feels slighted or snubbed by other people, and this is best expressed by the characteristic symptoms 'Mortification, ailments after' (11) and 'Anger, contradiction, from': 2. The female Bryonia, unlike Lycopodium, engages in no power struggles with men, hence the absence of symptom 13.

Bryonia both needs and shuns the company of people, 'Company, desire for' (14) and 'Company, aversion to' (15). He needs people and fears solitude, 'Fear, alone, of being' (19), because he despairs of his recovery and is frightened of disease and death. He wants to go back home to his people, and at the same time fearfully wishes to escape from home. The aversion to company, and the sycotic wish to hide, both express the wish not to be disturbed or touched. This avaricious individual with the coated tongue and bitter taste, thick skin and voracious appetite, is full of fears. He has fear in his stomach (20), fear of poverty, fear of the future, fear of strangers and fear of persecution.

Causticum

According to Kent, the most characteristic symptoms of this remedy are despair, anxiety and fear – this is the one remedy in our whole materia medica that is in greatest need of protection, 'Confidence, want of self' (1). A hopeless victim of the evils that beset him, he is in urgent need of sympathy and attention. He is quick to take on other people's pain and join with their suffering. Causticum is incapable of protecting himself from the world, so he does not have any defence strategies such as anticipatory anxiety or perfectionism. When angered, he becomes quarrelsome and contradictory. He is the typical dictator before his subordinate. When his feelings of aggression are aroused, he will pick an argument with anyone, 'Contradict, disposition to' (4), and his anarchic streak takes over as he disregards all social norms ('Unobserving': 2).

On a physical level, his lack of self-confidence and feelings of aggression are reflected in paralysis and muscular spasms. Because of his need for protection he is not intolerant of contradiction, and because of his feelings of inadequacy he does not feel better when occupied. Of the remaining symptoms, he has 'Mistakes, wrong words, using' (10), 'Company, desire for' (14) – because of his need for protection – and 'Starting, noise, from' (21), an expression of his fear of the world around him. His potential for aggression makes him feel guilty of a crime he has not committed, especially in the early evening, when he has a strong feeling that something dreadful is going to happen to him.

China

This remedy has four symptoms from the Minimum Characteristic Syndrome of Lycopodium. China produces the clinical picture of progressive anaemia, with pallor and debility, a picture that may be caused by the loss of vital fluids. There is a progressively increasing state of irritability and hypersensitivity, as if the nerves were permanently on edge. There is hypersensitivity to touch, motion, cold air, odours, with great weakness, emaciation and a tendency to dropsy. The face is wrinkled, pale and unhealthy. There is a state of neuromuscular excitability, with pinching, cramping pains, jerking and trembling, with paralytic weakness. There is a state of great debility, prostration and vertigo which is disproportionate to the amount of vital fluids or electrolytes lost.

The physical picture has its corresponding symptoms on the mental level. China is an irritable, weakened patient, a hypochondriac who is morally apathetic and insensitive. He protects himself from his debilitated state with his apathy, indifference and aversion to company (15). He feels unfortunate, unloved, forsaken, abused and persecuted. He continually blames other people for his own misfortunes. He finds fault with everything and everyone, and has a confirmed persecution mania. Just as he is unable to redress the balance after suffering losses on a physical level, so is he unable to recuperate from an emotional upset, and he becomes inconsolable. However, the outstandingly characteristic feature of China is his hyperactive brain, which remains unaffected by his weakened state and fills his fevered imagination with plans and theories about the dreams he will bring to fruition one day.

China has four symptoms of the Minimum Characteristic Syndrome of Lycopodium: 'Confidence, want of self' (1), 'Haughty' (2), 'Occupation, amel.' (7) and 'Company, aversion to' (15). His lack of self-confidence is a result of his debilitated condition. His arrogance is a defence mechanism which keeps people away, with his contemptuous, critical and reproachful attitude, and leads him to create those wonderful fantasies, castles in the air, in his bed at night, where all those fantasies are meticulously worked out, down to the last detail, 'Conscientious about trifles' (6). Consequently, if China can transform his dreams into reality, he will feel better for it, hence 'Occupation, amel.' (7).

It would seem from all this that China is something of a philosopher, like Sulphur, in whom he will confide his dreams. Unlike Sulphur, he will not shut himself away in his ivory tower; rather, he will bolster up his self-esteem by blaming others for his misfortunes. Furthermore, he does not have the symptoms which express the way Lycopodium deals with his real need for the love and respect of other people. In fact, China's aversion to company does precisely what it is intended to do, in that it keeps people at a distance. As far as his memory is concerned, he does not share Lycopodium's forgetfulness, but he does appear in all the rubrics denoting mistakes of memory – he makes mistakes with words, 'Mistakes, wrong words, using' (10), 'Mistakes, words, misplacing': 3, 'Mistakes, speaking': 2, 'Mistakes, writing, in': 2.

If we look at the group of symptoms from the Minimum Characteristic Syndrome in which China does not appear – 'Anticipation, complaints from' (5), 'Contradict, disposition to' (4), 'Contradiction, is intolerant of' (8), and 'Dictatorial' (3) – we can see that together they express the state of nervous expectation with which Lycopodium prepares to take on the world. Whereas in Lycopodium the symptoms 'Haughty' (2), 'Conscientious about trifles' (6) and 'Occupation, amel.' (7) are marks of a sycotic nature, in China these are predominantly signs of psora, and are indicative of his tendencies to fantasise, criticise and blame other people.

Hyoscyamus

This is a nervous, hysterical, emotional and sensitive patient. He is jealous, mistrustful, and frightened of being alone; he is loquacious, in a state of either great excitement or complete indifference, easily aroused sexually, and lascivious; he is given to outbursts of hysterical laughter and paroxysms of nervous hilarity. He may be a strong, robust individual, or an ageing alcoholic who suffers from muscular contractions, spasms, tics, convulsions and trembling. Hyoscyamus is a remedy of manic depression with its alternating states of manic excitement, characterised by violence and vehemence – where he will beat, break and bite everything in sight, taking off his clothes and exposing his genitals in a fit of erotic aggression – and passive depression, where he sits muttering to himself. As his pathology deepens, the periods of manic excitement become less frequent and the periods of depression become longer. In the chronic stage of his delirium his gestures become carphological, he watches the patterns on the walls and pushes away imaginary people at his bedside; his fingers act out the things he does every day.

Hyoscyamus is a jealous character, a victim of his own persecution complex; he, like Natrum Muriaticum, believes everyone has turned against him. He trusts no-one, believing that everyone has abandoned him ('Delusions, deserted, forsaken': *1*). Like Lachesis, he talks to himself or to the dead. The paroxysmal cough is aggravated while lying; the rectal incontinence and the aggravation from emotions, touch and restraint, all go to create the picture of a neurotic, hysterical remedy of the *Solanaceae* family, with his instability, changeability, suspiciousness, jealousy, erotic aggression, muscular spasms, tics, tremblings, convulsions and jerkings.

Hyoscyamus has four symptoms of the Minimum Characteristic Syndrome of Lycopodium: 'Confidence, want of self' (1), which comes from his feelings of confusion and unreality; 'Haughty' (2), arising from his state of mental excitement; 'Contradict, disposition to' (4), due to a confusion in his mind between what is real and what is unreal, which protects his feelings of inadequacy and gives him a different view of reality, a view that he tries to impose on other people; and 'Conscientious about trifles' (6) – he gives great importance to the smallest details, as when he spends hours looking at the tiny patterns on the walls of his room.

Hyoscyamus does not appear in symptoms 3, 5, 7 and 8, which reveal the unconscious strategies by which Lycopodium deals with his innate lack of confidence, preparing himself for all eventualities (5), imposing his indisputable authority (3), not tolerating any contradiction (8), and being constantly occupied at his work (7). The remaining symptoms provide the final distinctions between the two remedies. The deficiency of memory is an overall one, as one would expect in a remedy of the *Solanaceae* family: Hyoscyamus forgets everything he has heard, said, read, or thought, but he has no trouble with self-expression or in remembering words or names, and neither does he make general mistakes of writing or speaking. This suggests that his deficiency of memory comes about through his alternating states, and that it may also be subject to the same fluctuations. This same state of fluctuation may also account for the fact that sometimes he will need people, 'Company, desire for' (14), and fear solitude, 'Fear, alone, of being' (19), while at other times he will avoid company, 'Company, aversion to' (15). He does not appear in the remaining symptoms.

Hyoscyamus is a tri-miasmatic remedy, whose unstable and changeable disposition is a manifestation of the psoric component. While the presence of psora also accounts for his low self-esteem, the sycotic component contributes the elements of suspiciousness, jealousy, persecution mania, obsessions, memory disturbances and eroticism. The syphilitic component accounts for the loss of self-control over his feelings of aggression, which are highlighted during the manic phase of his delirium; he will attack people with his fists, teeth or a knife, smash the place up, expose his genitals, and make the kinds of gestures commonly seen in mentally handicapped children or elderly patients with senile dementia. The chronic Hyoscyamus patient will have other syphilitic symptoms, such as a sensation of being in a dream, a confusion about his internal and external reality, a delusion that his friends have deserted him, an avowedly contradictory disposition, a feeling of guilt at having committed some unforgiveable crime, a feeling of homesickness, and a sensation of being outside of himself, which is brought about by his general deficiency of memory.

Lachesis

Paschero says of this remedy: 'Lachesis is malicious, haughty, abusive, mistrustful and hypercritical.' Her intensely aggressive feelings find their outlet in a fear of death, which may come upon her during the night; she may wake up suffocating and feeling close to death, with oppressed respiration and menopausal flushes of heat. She defends herself by projecting on to the external world. She feels she is under the control of a superior force, and in this way simultaneously mitigates her guilt feelings and satisfies her aspirations – she has been singled out by superhuman beings.

This persecution complex is a projection of her internal feelings of hostility. She feels pursued by hostile people seeking to destroy her; she believes that she is being poisoned by the remedy and that she will surely die, that her family are even making arrangements for her funeral. Her total mistrust of people brings on a state of depression; she sighs deeply, trusts nobody, and accuses her husband of infidelities she would like to perpetrate herself. Her jealousy is a highly dramatic picture of condemnation, violent abuse, a torrent of bizarre and absurd accusations, wounding satirical remarks and ridicule. With her loquacity, aggression, sensuality and clairvoyant abilities, Lachesis conjures up the image of a witch possessed by the devil, or a medium in a trance.

Lachesis has four symptoms of the Minimum Characteristic Syndrome of Lycopodium. She has the basic lack of confidence, 'Confidence, want of self'(1), the arrogance, 'Haughty' (2), when her aggressive and erotic instincts are aroused, the domineering, 'Dictatorial' (3), and contradictory nature, 'Contradict, disposition to' (4). She does not figure in the four remaining rubrics, which express the permanent state of tension which afflicts Lycopodium, in his self-imposed compulsion to engage in battle, using his perfectionism, his sense of duty, his need to be productive and his intolerance of all opposition that would threaten to undermine his authority. By contrast, Lachesis is lively, sociable, garrulous, exuding arrogance and self-satisfaction, and projecting her own faults on to other people. Her state of hurried restlessness keeps her busy and hard at work, but she has not got the same compulsive need to work in order to feel better, as is the case with Lycopodium. She is warm-blooded, and her intolerance of tight clothing around the neck (where even a scarf is too tight) symbolises the strangulation which is a feature of *Lachesis Trigonocephalus*. On the level of generalities, she is aggravated by enclosed places and on waking, and ameliorated by the menstrual flow.

Sepia

Sepia does not have symptoms 1, 2, 3 and 5 of the Minimum Characteristic Syndrome, denoting the peculiar combination of low self-esteem with an enlarged ego that is peculiar to Lycopodium. The essence of Sepia is her emotional indifference, especially towards her husband, who brings out in her all the jealousy of the castrating female. Symptoms 4, 6, 7 and 8 reveal her sycotic nature, in the way she deals with her inability to love, and her battle with the opposite sex, which finds its symbolic expression in the irritability before menses, 'Irritability, menses, before' (13).

By using the Minimum Characteristic Syndrome to compare the two remedies, we will discover the essential differences between them. Lycopodium is an emotional cripple, who puts on a mask of arrogance or egocentric amiability. He is intelligent, quick-witted and aloof, and keeps himself constantly occupied; he does not tolerate contradiction because it threatens his position of superiority; he wins points by contradicting others, and he always needs to be doing things to stop himself falling prey to his deep feelings of inadequacy. Sepia, on the other hand, is truly self-confident, so she does not need the defences of arrogance or dominance, but her emotional indifference leads her into conflict with the opposite sex. She is the emasculating, castrating female – in a state of permanent antagonism with herself, she tolerates no contradiction from other people (8). Her perfectionism, 'Conscientious about trifles' (6), and amelioration by occupation (7), express her attempts to climb out of her apathy and indifference. She is the woman who has been left with all the housework to do, and she complains bitterly of her lot.

There is a general weakness of memory, which is aggravated by the mental and physical weariness and lethargy. She makes mistakes in speaking and writing, 'Mistakes, wrong words, using' (10), but to a lesser degree.

If we look at the other group of symptoms, we see that there are similarities where her emotional indifference is at odds with her conscience. Sepia can feel mortification when she blames external factors for her depressive states, 'Mortification, ailments after' (11). She may sometimes wish for company as an emotional release, 'Company, desire for' (14) – for example, she will complain all day that her husband is never there, but as soon as he gets home she will treat him badly if he puts a foot wrong – and, generally speaking, she feels better for being alone, 'Company, aversion to' (15). Nothing calms her nerves more than to be on her own, working feverishly at the housework, walking in the rain, or getting actively involved in a job that not only satisfies her compulsive need to compete with men, but also gives her a good excuse for being out of the house all day. The emasculating Sepia makes a successful boss, because she will never get emotionally involved; the crippled Lycopodium, haughty and disdainful, becomes a boss in order to 'fulfil herself' and compensate for her inferiority complex.

Sepia and Lycopodium are both bored by their children, the former because she does not love them, the latter because they proclaim her femininity, which she resents, and her subordination to her husband. Sepia is averse to her husband and will try to castrate and destroy him. Lycopodium looks up to her husband as a father-figure, looks after him like a son, loves him like a wife and fights him like a man.

Five remedies have three symptoms from the Minimum Characteristic Syndrome of Lycopodium: Oleander, Phosphorus, Pulsatilla, Sulphur and Nitricum Acidum.

Oleander

This is one of the so-called 'small' remedies, or rather a remedy about which too little is known. We are taught to pay special attention to a small remedy if it comes through in repertorising, even if it appears in lower case, and we should go to our materia medica for further information.

Oleander is a weak, pale individual, with deep-set, hollow eyes, whose limbs are weak, cold and numb, with a tendency to paralysis, and trembling in the knees when standing. He is subject to attacks of vertigo when he looks down, or when he looks fixedly at something. He has a large appetite, a tendency to dyspepsia and foul-smelling flatulence, a feeling of lassitude and emptiness in the stomach, which is relieved by alcohol. He has papular eruptions that ooze viscous secretions on the scalp and behind the ears, and that itch intensely when he takes off his clothes.

There is debility on the mental level of the remedy as well. Clarke says that he is a sad person who has no confidence, 'Confidence, want of self' (1). His intellect functions slowly, he has deficiency of understanding and memory, he is easily distracted, incapable of concentrating, especially while reading, to the point where he may lose the thread of what he is reading ('Dullness, reading, while': *1*). The slightest mental effort puts him into a state of stupefaction ('Dullness, mental exertion, from': 2) and heat pervades his entire body. The remedy has tubercular traits – great lethargy and aversion to mental effort on the one hand, bad temper and irritability on the other, with violent outbursts which are soon repented, as in the case of Sulphur. He is argumentative ('Quarrelsome': *1*, 'Violent': *1*) and has the same problems with contradiction as Lycopodium, 'Contradict, disposition to' (4) and 'Contradiction, is intolerant of' (8). He does not have the sycotic symptoms of the Minimum Characteristic Syndrome. The only other symptom he shares is the inability to remember proper names (9). It might be possible to confuse this remedy with Lycopodium in patients who present us with only a few symptoms, those so-called 'incomplete' cases, for whom, either out of habit or by mistake, we would prescribe Lycopodium on the basis of the two or three mental symptoms that agree.

In summary, Oleander is a slow and weak patient, on both a mental and a physical level. His limbs are cold, weak and numb, his knees shake while standing, and he has trembling. Guiding symptoms are: migraine headache that is better for looking sideways; a sensation as if his eyes are pulled backwards; canine hunger with trembling of the hands; rapid eating; dyspepsia and flatulence with foul-smelling wind; vomiting of food as soon as he has eaten, but does not lose his appetite; marked desire for alcohol, which ameliorates; incontinent diarrhoea containing undigested food; and viscous secretions.

Phosphorus

This is a tall, slim individual who suffers from nervous excitement, great debility and hypersensitivity of the senses. He is an emotional and vehement being who reacts with explosions of enthusiasm, temper or tears. Paschero says, 'It is the convulsive mode of response that heralds the onset of paralysis in the patient.' Phosphorus resembles Lycopodium when he is unwell: the drooping shoulders, the pigeon chest, the skinny arms and legs. Like Lycopodium, Phosphorus is hypersensitive and intelligent, with a refined intellect and artistic taste.

I make this brief comparison to demonstrate once again that the repertory is only a tool and not an end in itself; it is the deeply ingrained attitudes in each individual patient that bring about and give a special meaning to the symptoms, and which lead us to the definitive characteristics of the case. In common with Phosphorus, both Pulsatilla and Sulphur share only three symptoms of the Minimum Characteristic Syndrome, and yet in practice they are frequently confused with Lycopodium. The object of this study is to establish clear differences between remedies, so that there is a real understanding of the distinguishing features of groups of symptoms that may, superficially, appear to be similar.

Phosphorus shares symptoms 1, 2 and 5 of the Minimum Characteristic Syndrome of Lycopodium. As we mentioned earlier, Phosphorus and Nux Vomica are the two most hypersensitive remedies of our materia medica. An imbalance of phosphorus, one of the main components of the nerve cell, causes a state of overexcitability in the patient's contact with his environment. The lack of confidence, 'Confidence, want of self' (1), which is potentially present in all human beings, is intensified in Phosphorus by his emotional hypersensitivity and not by an exaggerated awareness of a real inadequacy, as is the case with Lycopodium. Similarly his arrogance, 'Haughty' (2), has a slightly different meaning: here it is a transient arrogance which comes to the fore during his fits of enthusiasm, passion, elation and euphoria that herald the onset of the destructive phase. In Lycopodium, arrogance forms an inherent part of his personality structure and can manifest itself as conceit, servility or egotism, according to the susceptibilities of the individual and the environment he lives in.

In the same way, the anticipatory anxiety, 'Anticipation, complaints from' (5), far from being a symbol of insecurity and competitive aggression, denotes in Phosphorus an exaggerated emotional hypersensitivity to a future event or commitment. I would place special emphasis on this point, as both remedies have 'Fear, stomach, arising from' (20), which may lead to confusion when accompanied by anticipation – our diagnosis may then be confirmed by the presence or absence of other symptoms in the Minimum Characteristic Syndrome that constitute the sycotic aspect of Lycopodium.

Phosphorus has a general weakness of memory, especially during his periods of depression, when he feels indifferent to everything around him, or when he is absent-minded – in a daydream, withdrawn – like Nux Moschata, who absent-mindedly forgets what he has read and makes mistakes in writing. Phosphorus is characteristically a tubercular remedy which does not have the irritability symptoms, 11, 12 and 13. His deep need for affection and human contact accounts for the desire for company, 'Company, desire for' (14), with its sub-rubric 'alone, while agg.' The desire for solitude, 'Company, aversion to' (15), comes about when he is emotionally drained (in a syphilitic case) or when in a state of ecstasy, in spiritual communication with the Almighty. The amelioration by weeping (16) is evidence of a highly emotional nature. Apart from the fear in the stomach, he also has the fear of being alone, 'Fear, alone, of being' (19), a fear which contains in it all the disparate fears to which Phosphorus is prone. He does not have the confusion symptom, 'Confusion, walking, while, open air amel.' (18), which, as has already been discussed, is the sycotic manifestation of Lycopodium's need for freedom. Phosphorus is hypersensitive to the slightest noise, hence the symptom 'Starting, noise from' (21) which, in Lycopodium, is a reaction emanating from fear.

Pulsatilla

The remedy is as frail and weak as the plant from which it is derived. She accepts her helplessness and tries to win the affection and support of other people, although she is afraid. She needs to feel that other people accept her, approve of her, and love her. She puts all her energy into achieving this security. She puts other people's needs first, she is meek and mild, a model of virtue, humility and love. The Pulsatilla daughter is the apple of her mother's eye, so gentle, so good-natured and so neat and tidy. Pulsatilla's self-protection is her submissiveness and meekness; it is in this way that she earns herself love and motherly caring, while protecting her basic lack of confidence, 'Confidence, want of self' (1) and her fear of being abandoned ('Forsaken feeling': 3). This explains why she wants to do everything really well, 'Conscientious about trifles' (6), so that nobody finds fault with her, and why she becomes anxious at new undertakings that put her to the test, 'Anticipation, complaints from' (5). In her role as housewife, Pulsatilla treats her home with the care and tenderness of a child ('Childish behaviour': *1* and 'Cares, full of, domestic affairs about': *2*).

The remedy may be clearly distinguished from Lycopodium by the remaining sycotic symptoms that can leave no doubt about the diagnosis if they are present. However, Pulsatilla may be confused with the psoric aspect of Lycopodium when she goes against all established norms of behaviour and becomes as 'Contrary': *2* as he can be; but Pulsatilla's contrariness will be changeable and capricious, with a childlike tenderness and an unconditional need of support. Lycopodium, by contrast, is always conditional about accepting the support offered to him; he will take it only as long as it does not compromise his deeply ingrained pride. It is rare to find a Lycopodium who does not suffer disturbances of memory or dysfunction of the liver. While Pulsatilla has the memory weakness symptom, 'Memory, weakness of, names, for proper' (9), Lycopodium's memory deficiency is much more clearly selective. Furthermore, Pulsatilla does not make mistakes with words.

The soft, affectionate, changeable and capricious nature of Pulsatilla is what differentiates her from Lycopodium, even when other symptoms agree. She desires company because it makes her feel better, 'Company, desire for' (14), and shuns company on occasions, 'Company, aversion to' (15), so as not to disturb other people – through her fear of being abandoned, and not through a wish to hide. However, Pulsatilla does not appear in symptom 17, 'Weeping, thanked, when', as, far from weeping when people show her gratitude, she smiles and dries her tears. Lycopodium, on the other hand, weeps because other people's gratitude breaks down his defences of arrogance and egotism. Pulsatilla smiles when she receives gratitude from other people because it gratifies her child-like need for affection. One last difference: Pulsatilla does not appear in the fear symptoms 20 and 21. She simply has nothing to hide. Her only defence is to submit meekly and only occasionally does she hide her grief ('Grief, silent': 2), to avoid hurting other people.

Sulphur

Like Pulsatilla and Lycopodium, Sulphur becomes aware of his inner feelings of inadequacy, 'Confidence, want of self' (1), when he exposes himself to the world around him. But whereas the first two remedies will go towards people – Pulsatilla to surrender herself and Lycopodium to engage in battle – Sulphur, who suffers from great debility and sluggishness of the circulatory system, will choose to take himself right away from people, to his ivory tower where nothing can touch him, rather than engage in a losing battle that will cost him a lot of effort. Safe behind the walls of his fortress, he watches the world with a critical and cynical eye, and congratulates himself on his escape; and his dirty offensive skin, with its itchy papular eruptions, is the symbolic manifestation of his separateness. With a self-sufficiency born of arrogance, 'Haughty' (2), he plans his life to suit himself, 'Conscientious about trifles' (6), and has no need for the compensatory strategies which Lycopodium uses to fight the world. It is rightly said that whereas Sulphur is dishonest with himself, Lycopodium is dishonest with other people. The independent and self-satisfied Sulphur is quite a different character from Lycopodium, with his sharp watchful eyes and deeply furrowed forehead. Sulphur shares

Lycopodium's weak memory for proper names (9), but for a different reason: in Lycopodium, it is the constant stress he lives under that weakens his memory, not only for names and words, but also for what he has just done, or read, and for expressing himself. In Sulphur, it is a consequence of his apathy and his lack of interest in communicating with the world: he forgets what he was about to do, what has happened, what he has said, what he was about to say, as if it were really of no importance to him to have any contact with the outside world at all.

He has the mortification symptom, 'Mortification, ailments after' (11), but the reason behind it is different. Lycopodium feels humiliated by any injustice, as it undermines his demand for respect and leadership: in Sulphur it wounds his ego. Sulphur nurtures his need to be a recluse, hence the aversion to company (15), although he may occasionally need people for his entertainment and amusement. But, unlike Lycopodium, he does not mind being alone; in fact, it makes him feel good. This same apathy and indifference to everything ('Indifference, everything to': *1*) accounts for the irritation he feels on waking (12), because a new day means socialising with people, and that means work. Lycopodium feels irritable when he wakes up because the new day puts him to the test once more, and tests unnerve him. The apathy also accounts for Sulphur's non-appearance in the remaining rubrics, except for 'Confusion, walking, while, open air amel.' (18), where Sulphur's sluggish circulation is ameliorated in the open air. Both Sulphur and Lycopodium have a great sense of independence – the former because he is an arrogant philosophising recluse, the latter because dependence implies submission and being less worthy than other people.

Nitricum Acidum

This remedy has very little in common with the remedy in question. This is an emaciated patient, with long-term chronic complaints, subject to recurrent colds, stubborn suppurations, diarrhoea, ulcerations, fistulae, cracked orifices and warty overgrowths – clearly a tri-miasmatic remedy. His basic feelings of inadequacy fill him with despair, he feels that the whole world is against him, and that he does not have a single friend. He has a big chip on his shoulder, intense feelings of aggression, he suffers great anguish and fear, and longs for death. His attitude to life is cynical, full of anger, hate and complete mistrust, especially of the person who has offended him – no matter how many apologies he receives, he will never forgive. Paschero comments: 'There is nothing cheerful, optimistic or pleasant about Nitricum Acidum. He is full of bitterness, anger and resentment towards his increasing physical disabilities, and he responds with rage, harshness, indifference or abuse. This state can be brought on by the loss of a loved one, or by the strain of caring for an invalid over a long period of time.'

He appears in only three symptoms of the Minimum Characteristic Syndrome of Lycopodium. The lack of confidence, 'Confidence, want of self' (1), is a result of his physical inadequacy, and his intense feelings of aggression and rage come out in his tendency to contradict everything and everyone, 'Contradict, disposition to' (4), and in the tense anticipatory anxiety, 'Anticipation, complaints from' (5), he feels while waiting for something to happen. Of the remaining symptoms, he only has symptom 17, 'Weeping, thanked, when', which acts as a safety valve for his perpetual feelings of rage; and symptom 21, 'Starting, noise, from', is an expression of his hypersensitivity to his environment – Nitricum Acidum is aggravated by noise, touch, being stroked, the creaking of floorboards, and the slightest difficulty. Symptom 14, 'Company, desire for', is not a significant symptom here.

This remedy is similar to Mercurius in its syphilitic component (salivation, offensive breath and perspiration, aggravation from changes in temperature), to Thuja in its sycotic component (irritability, warty growths) and to Nux Vomica in its psoric component (irritability, coldness, hypersensitivity). The syphilitic granular ulcerations and splinter-like pains are the ultimate manifestations of the Nit. Ac. pathology.

3

Silicea

DESCRIPTION

Silica plays a vital role in the structure of the human body, being an essential component of connective tissue, and yet the amount actually present in the body is very small – less than 0.001%.

In nature, rock, flint, grit and plant stem all owe their quality of resilience to the presence of the mineral silica, a quality that is reflected in the symptom picture of one of the deepest-acting remedies of our materia medica.

The reader should refer to Paragraphs 3, 7 and 153 of the *Organon*, as they are particularly relevant to the study of Silicea: 'If the physician clearly perceives what is to be cured ... the totality of the symptoms must be the principal, indeed the only thing the physician has to take note of in every case of disease and to remove by means of his art ... The more striking, singular, uncommon and peculiar (characteristic) signs and symptoms of the case of disease are chiefly and most solely to be kept in view.'

The homoeopath must not only be able to perceive what is to be cured in the patient, and what is curative in medicine, but he must also have a profound understanding of his duty as a physician if he is to make a correct prescription. With a coherent analysis of the case, a careful evaluation of the symptoms, and a clear understanding of the individual characteristics and idiosyncrasies of the patient, the indication for a particular remedy will become apparent.

The typical Silicea child is skinny, with a large head and pot belly. The fontanelles are slow to close, he is late learning to walk, and the glands are swollen and indurated. His sallow skin is cold to touch, he has profuse head sweats and offensive foot sweats, and his expression is both lively and longsuffering. The Silicea adult is timid, awkward and full of fear, and may present with a chronic tendency to suppurations, emaciation and a great sensitivity to cold.

Silicea is all too aware of his weaknesses. Like Lycopodium, the key to his character is a basic lack of self-confidence ('Confidence, want of self': *2*). He feels helpless and afraid. He is crippled by his fear of people ('Timidity': *2*), and imagines that people are constantly watching his every move, especially when he is among strangers ('Timidity, appearing in public': *3*).

The Silicea child will cling to his mother wherever he goes: in the consulting room or when faced with other children at school. It makes no difference where he is, he feels overwhelmed by the big wide world ('Cowardice': *2*) and tries to hide behind his mother, wishing he were back, safe and protected, inside her womb.

Silicea, paradoxically, is the most submissive and the most obstinate child of our whole materia medica. In an attempt to rise above his feelings of vulnerability and helplessness he can become extremely irritable and angry with his loved ones, but he cannot sustain his efforts to assert himself and, when he tries to suppress his negative feelings, he ends up feeling even more tense and anxious. He is trapped in a vicious circle from which there is no escape. Oddly enough, Silicea does not appear in the rubrics that express the aggressive side of human nature, such as 'Anger, violent', 'Quarrelsome' and 'Violent, vehement'. The reason is that the anger he feels is the defensive reaction of a distressed and powerless individual who must protect himself from a hostile world. Whereas Lycopodium is always on the offensive, Silicea is always on the defensive. While Silicea may share Lycopodium's intolerance of contradiction ('Contradiction, is intolerant of': *2*), he is, unlike Lycopodium, neither violent nor quarrelsome. Silicea can be intensely irritable and subject to bouts of rage, shouting and tears ('Irritability': *3*, 'Irritability, children, in': *2*), brought about by his feelings of impotence and frustration. But, despite his need for support, he will reject all attempts at consolation. The rebellious streak in his nature makes him rebuff even the gentlest treatment ('Irritability, consolation agg.': *3*, 'Weeping, consolation agg.': *3*, 'Obstinate': *2*, 'Obstinate, children, yet cry when kindly spoken to': *1*).

There is also a soft, gentle side to the remedy ('Mildness': *3*), a great capacity for soothing tenderness. He will always carry with him the memory of his mother's love and the special way she used to look at him ('Magnetized, desires to be': *3*).

As Silicea grows up, his inner conflicts become more pressing. He is caught between the need for security and support and the desire for independence and challenge. To feel good about himself, he needs to excel at everything he does, and to this end he pays great attention to the smallest detail, leaving nothing to chance. His books and toys are always neatly put away, his homework is meticulous – he is an exemplary student and a model of good behaviour.

The Silicea girl expresses this perfectionism in the way she takes such pride in keeping her bedroom clean and tidy ('Conscientious about trifles': 3). The Silicea boy compensates for his small stature ('Dwarfishness': 2) with an exaggerated sense of his own importance ('Egotism': 2). He hoards everything he can lay his hands on ('Avarice': 3, *Synthetic Repertory*, Vol. I (Barthel)) and guards it with his life.

He is plagued by self-doubt and insecurity, and any test of his ability completely throws him: he becomes clumsy and stupid ('Dullness': 3, 'Dullness, children': 2). In the days leading up to an exam, he is beside himself with worry ('Ailments from, anticipation': 3, Vol. I (Barthel)); he faces the test paper with terror, but once he gets down to it, he finds that he knows more than he realised, and does well. While Lycopodium tends to boast of knowledge he does not have, Silicea is prone to underestimate his real ability.

The Silicea patient is dominated by fear, although he does not appear in the specific fear rubrics, such as 'Fear, alone, of being', 'Fear, thunderstorm, of', 'Fear, ghosts, of' or 'Fear, dark'. He is overwhelmed and consumed by a terrible, vague sense of fear that keeps him in a perpetual state of nervous tension. Thus, he appears in rubrics such as 'Frightened easily': 2 and 'Fright, complaints from': 3. His imagination conjures up obscure, frightening fantasies ('Fancies, frightful': 2) rather than specific visions of ghosts and suchlike.

Silicea's tendency to turn his anger inwards on to himself comes out in the fear of pins ('Fear, pins, of': 2), and the delusion that he sees pins and needles ('Delusions, needles, sees': 2 and 'Delusion, pins, about': 2). He collects pins and needles and counts them. His fear of being robbed ('Fear, robbers, of': 1) comes from his basic feelings of insecurity, his avaricious nature and his fear of mental work.

Silicea falls easily into a state of profound dejection ('Discouraged': 1) and depression ('Sadness': 2); he is discontented ('Discontented': 2), sullen ('Morose': 3) and tearful ('Weeping, trifles, at': 1, 'Weeping, spoken to, when': 1 and 'Weeping, consolation agg.': 3); he wants to be left alone and undisturbed ('Conversation agg.': 2 and 'Touched, aversion to being': 2), and stoutly refuses to be cajoled out of it ('Jesting, averse to': 1). His mother will tell you that he is a worrier, and you will see for yourself the worry-lines starting to etch themselves on to his face; he looks totally preoccupied, lost in a world of his own ('Absent-minded': 2). This highly-strung child is jumpy and easily startled ('Starting, easily': 2). He will jump from fright ('Starting, fright, from': 2), at noises ('Starting, noise, from': 3), on falling asleep ('Starting, sleep, on falling': 2), during sleep ('Starting, sleep, during': 1) and from sleep ('Starting, from sleep': 2). He jumps when he is touched ('Starting, touched, when': 2) and at the slightest thing ('Starting, trifles, at': 2).

All human beings have the same apparently conflicting needs: on the one hand, for support and nurturing, and, on the other, for the freedom to fight for their rights and make their own way in the world. The Silicea patient is no exception. As a child, his basic feelings of insecurity are reinforced by the wealth of negative experiences that come his way. In this potentially hostile world, he is often at the receiving end of his family's coldness, indifference, intolerance and unfairness or, equally damaging, he is overprotected, controlled and dominated by them, and he soon learns that people are not to be trusted. He has to find a way to survive this grim reality and come to terms with the situation. According to his constitutional predisposition, he may choose to cling on to his family for protection, to rebel against them or to remove himself entirely from their grasp.

If he chooses protection, he will, like Pulsatilla, do his utmost to win their love and affection; paralysed by fear and helplessness, he depends on other people for support and reassurance. All his energy goes into making his world a safe place to live in. He submits meekly to the tyranny of others and allows no unkind thoughts to enter his head. Here we are not simply talking about obedience and self-sacrifice, but also the total repression of negative thoughts and feelings, betrayed only by the occasional outburst of temper or rage.

If he chooses rebellion, he will, like Lycopodium, confront and challenge the hostile world; to prove his strength and courage, he has to win the fight for supremacy and earn the respect of his opponents.

The third option open to him, that of withdrawing into his shell, comes into operation when his personal relationships become too problematic. He builds a wall between himself and the outside world, barricading himself in with his toys, dolls and books. He detaches himself emotionally, like Sulphur – the ragged philosopher – and becomes indifferent and apathetic. He lives in a world of his own where nothing can reach him. He is utterly oblivious to demands, entreaties and emotional ties. He feels completely self-sufficient, safe and superior, locked away inside the ivory tower of his own making.

Silicea's basic problems stay with him throughout his life. Like Lycopodium, the central issue is a basic lack of confidence and a weak, timid and indecisive nature that finds a compensatory outlet in the occasional fit of temper or rage. But whereas Lycopodium is a pedantic, overbearing, arrogant (or obsequious) egotist, Silicea alternates between two contrasting modes of behaviour: he can either be totally compliant and subservient, or stubbornly resistant to all attempts at manipulation. Self-repression is his *modus operandi*: at work, he does not dare open his mouth for fear of being laughed at, and he runs about at the beck and call of colleagues and superiors, trying to gain the approval of those he admires. His conduct is faultless: he is always punctual, and willingly works overtime whenever necessary. He has few friends, avoids all confrontations and never ventures his opinions.

But at home it is a different matter; if everything is not shipshape and orderly he will scold everybody for not taking their responsibilities as seriously as he does. He prides himself on his obsessive tidiness, a symptom of his fearful self-doubt, and takes great satisfaction in knowing that he is beyond reproach, that no-one will ever be able to accuse him of not coming up to scratch. He demands nothing less of himself than absolute perfection in everything he does and, if somebody should cast a doubt upon his work, or point out a mistake he has made, he will react violently, exploding with anger and refusing to listen to the person who has brought him face to face with his innermost feelings of worthlessness ('Anger, contradiction, from': 2, 'Contradiction, is intolerant of': 2). The sheer driving force of his will to succeed, and the firmness of his convictions may combine to create a natural leader, both in his personal and his public life. His personality is a strange mixture of obstinacy, fastidiousness and egotism; what distinguishes this remedy from its closest counterpart, Lycopodium, is the absence of pride and the timidity he feels when among strangers ('Timidity, appearing in public': 3).

When the pseudo-psoric traits of the remedy predominate, we have the picture of a nervous, frightened child hiding behind his mother. The fastidiousness is a compensatory reaction of the defence mechanism to the lack of love in his life, and an attempt to cover up his feelings of inadequacy. The fear of failure, which once lay dormant in his subconscious, now torments him to such a degree that it undermines his innate intelligence. Every decision he has to make creates a conflict ('Irresolution': 2) and, in the end, he is paralysed by fear ('Undertakes nothing, lest he fail': 1). When he tries to talk about it, he finds he is unable to explain the fear rationally ('Delusions, fail, everything will': 1).

Hence it is not surprising that he suffers from an incapacitating anxiety before every event ('Ailments from anticipation': *3* Barthel); he exhausts himself with all the worrying ('Exertion, agg. from mental': *3*); his memory begins to fail him ('Memory, weakness of': *2*), especially for mental work ('Memory, weakness of, labor, for mental': *2*). In common with Lycopodium, he makes mistakes while reading ('Mistakes, reading': *1*), misplaces words ('Mistakes, words, misplacing': *1*), finds it difficult to concentrate ('Concentration, difficult': *3*), feels confused on waking ('Confusion, waking, on': *2*), after meals ('Confusion, eating, after': *2*), when he tries to think ('Confusion, mental exertion, from': *2*), as if he were intoxicated ('Confusion, intoxicated, as if': *2*), and, a symptom that is unique to Silicea, his confusion increases with conversation ('Confusion, conversation agg.': *2*).

As mentioned earlier, Silicea dislikes being drawn into conversation ('Talk, indisposed to': *1*), because talking involves relating to people and the risk of showing oneself up ('Conversation agg.': *2*). As he grows older, his mind slows down ('Dullness': *3*), and the perfectionism becomes less of an obsession. He feels sluggish in the afternoon ('Dullness, afternoon': *2*), after mental work ('Dullness, mental exertion, from': *2*), and when he tries to write ('Dullness, writing, while': *2*). In the end, it becomes impossible for him to work ('Work, aversion to mental': *2*) as it is now something to be feared ('Fear, work, dread of': *2*), particularly when writing is involved ('Fear, work, literary, of': *2*).

From here, it is but one short step to the point of total deterioration ('Prostration of mind': *3*), where he is capable of neither reading ('Prostration of mind, reading, from': *2*) nor writing ('Prostration of mind, writing, after': *2*).

He knows he is beaten and he sinks down, overcome with weakness and despair. The tears start to fall ('Weeping, tearful mood': *1*), in the afternoon ('Weeping, afternoon': *2*), when he is spoken to ('Weeping, spoken to': *1*), while he is asleep ('Weeping, sleep, in': *2*), at the slightest thing ('Weeping, trifles, at': *1*) and when people misguidedly try to comfort him ('Weeping, consolation agg.': *3*). Life is a heavy burden ('Loathing, life': *2*) that he no longer wants to carry ('Weary of life': *2*). He wishes he were dead ('Death, desires': *2*) and thinks about how to end it all ('Suicidal disposition': *1*) by drowning ('Suicidal disposition, drowning, by': *2*) – a symbolic manifestation of his wish to return to the pre-natal state. He will, on occasions, carry out his threat to throw himself into the river ('Jumping, impulse to jump into the river': *1*). At whatever stage we meet him, we are sure to find a patient full of conflicts and uncertainties, with a peculiar combination of fastidiousness and irritability, neediness and submissiveness.

A person who is buffeted about by the conflicting desires to serve others and to assert the self can never be at peace; his anxiety becomes a full-blown guilt complex at the shame he feels for harbouring malice ('Anxiety, conscience, of, as if guilty of a crime': *2*). He will say that he is a bad person who has committed unforgivable sins. He is plagued by remorse ('Remorse': *2*) for the smallest wrongdoing ('Remorse, trifles, about': *2*).

His general state of fearfulness and vulnerability is expressed by symptoms such as anxiety from noises ('Anxiety, noise, from': *3*) and from the slightest thing ('Anxiety, trifles, about': *2*), his acute sensitivity ('Sensitive': *3*) to noise ('Sensitive, noise, to': *3*), however slight ('Sensitive, noise, to slightest': *3*), and his sensitivity to the sound of voices ('Sensitive, noise, to voices': *2*). His nerves are so on edge that it takes nothing to make him jump ('Starting, startled': *2*, 'Starting, easily': *2*). He jumps from fright ('Starting, fright, from': *2*), at noises ('Starting, noise, from': 3l, p.), if someone touches him ('Starting, touched, when': *2*), on falling asleep ('Starting, sleep, on falling': *2*), while he is asleep ('Starting, sleep, during': *1*) and from sleep ('Starting, from sleep': *2*).

His state of health may become the primary focus of his free-floating anxieties ('Anxiety, health, about': *1*), to the point where he may even lose all hope of recovery ('Despair, recovery': *1*), and the female Silicea may worry unduly during menstruation ('Anxiety, menses, during': *3*). Silicea spends most of his waking hours on the defensive, protecting his vulnerable inner self, and his fear allows him no rest ('Anxiety, lying, while': *2*); if he tries to relax at night, he is beset with anxiety ('Anxiety, evening': *1*, 'Anxiety, bed, in': *1*, 'Anxiety, sleep, before': *1*, 'Anxiety, midnight, before': *1*) that will only lift if he gets up and starts to move about ('Anxiety, motion amel.': *1*, 'Anxiety, midnight, before, on waking, amel. on rising': *1*).

He is filled with a restless uneasiness ('Restlessness': *3*) that never ceases, even at night ('Restlessness, bed, driving out of': 1). In the consulting room, he will fidget about on his chair ('Restlessness, sitting, while': *2*); he wakes up in the morning feeling agitated ('Restlessness, waking, on': *2*), confused ('Confusion, waking, on': *2*) and afraid ('Fear, waking, on': *2*).

As his moods swing between stubbornness and submissiveness, refusing to cooperate one minute, then eager and willing the next, so his feelings for others tend to wax and wane. However, it should be noted that this remedy does not appear in rubrics such as the desire for or aversion to company, affectionate, malicious, offended easily, mortification, ailments from grief, ailments after anger with silent grief, violent anger and ailments from suppressed anger. These rubrics apply to those who have an intense relationship with their environment. The written word is always open to interpretation, and its meaning should come from an understanding of the whole spirit of the person. Every dynamic disturbance of mind or body influences our attitudes, thoughts and feelings: as Hahnemann says in Paragraph 83 of the *Organon*, it is the task of the homoeopath, through precise and unprejudiced observation of the symptoms, to distinguish between what is normal and explicable, and what is strange, rare and peculiar in the case.

The symptoms of Silicea are deeply ingrained in the psyche of the patient who needs this remedy. He is unable to fend for himself in the world and, in his self-effacing way, tries to draw on the strength and support of those around him. He feels weak, depressed and vulnerable when alone ('Sadness, alone, when': *1*), but when he is in company he feels too self-conscious to speak. However, if someone should take pity on him and try to offer him consolation, he will react with tears of humiliation and anger; but he surrenders himself with child-like innocence to the person who offers him help and protection ('Magnetized, desires to be': *3*). At times he feels so destitute that, if he has to travel away from home for some reason, he gets ill with homesickness ('Homesickness': *2*).

Restrained and repressed all day long, his true nature comes to the fore during his hours of rest, in symptoms rich in symbolism. His sleep is restless ('Sleep, restless': *3*), he sleepwalks ('Somnambulism': *2*) and talks in his sleep ('Talking, sleep, in': *2*). His dreams give an interesting insight into his personality. In keeping with his day-time state of high anxiety and tension, the dreams that come to him are frightful ('Dreams, frightful': *3*) nightmares ('Dreams, nightmare': *2*) of murder ('Dreams, murder': *2*), robbers ('Dreams, robbers': *2*), ghosts ('Dreams, ghosts': *2*) and dogs ('Dreams, dogs': *2*) that pursue him ('Dreams, dogs, large dog following him': *1*); he has anxious dreams ('Dreams, anxious': *3*) that continue after waking ('Dreams, awake, while': *2*). While Silicea does not appear in the rubric 'Fear, thunderstorm, of', he dreams of storms ('Dreams, storms': *2*) and suffers an aggravation of his mental symptoms during stormy weather ('Thunderstorm, during': *2*). He is one of the few asthmatic children who are affected by thunderstorms ('Respiration, asthmatic, thunderstorm, during': *2*), and the remedy appears under Generalities in the rubrics 'Storm, approach of a': 1, and 'Storm, during': 2.

His dreams are vivid reflections ('Dreams, vivid': *3*) of the hostility he experiences in life, symbolised by the image of pins ('Delusions, pins, about': *2*). He has horrible visions ('Delusions, visions': 2, 'Delusions, visions, horrible': *1*) of criminals ('Delusions, criminals, about': *1*) and dogs ('Delusions, dogs, sees': *1*) and, like Calcarea Carbonica, when he closes his eyes he sees images and phantoms ('Delusions, images, phantoms, sees, closing the eyes, on': *1*) everywhere ('Delusions, images, closing the eyes, sees, all over': *2*). Like Cenchris and Lycopodium, he has the impression that he is in two places at the same time ('Delusions, places, of being in two at the same time': *2*). The conflicting needs for protection and independence create such inner turmoil that Silicea feels literally torn apart inside, divided in two ('Delusions, divided into two parts': *1*), and that her left half does not belong to her ('Delusions, halves, left half does not belong to her': *1*, 'Delusions, side, that she did not own her left': *1*).

He dreams of flooding water ('Dreams, water, flood': *2*) and still water ('Dreams, water': *2*), symbolising the wish to return to the safety of his mother's womb. The travelling he does in his dreams allows him to escape for a while from the distresses and terrors of real life ('Dreams, journey': *2*); he turns away from the present and travels back to a time when he felt sheltered and secure. Silicea is the only black type remedy in the rubrics 'Dreams, events, previous' and 'Dreams, events, long past').

He keeps waking up ('Sleep, waking, frequent': *2*) during the long, restless nights and he wakes up too early in the morning ('Sleep, waking, early': *2*), feeling that he has had no rest ('Sleep, unrefreshing': *2*). He cannot get to sleep ('Sleeplessness': *3*) for the thoughts buzzing around in his head ('Sleeplessness, thoughts, activity of mind, from': *2*); if he wakes in the middle of the night he cannot get back to sleep again ('Sleeplessness, waking, after': *3*). He has trouble going to sleep before midnight ('Sleeplessness, midnight, before': *3*) and after midnight ('Sleeplessness, midnight, after': *3*), and at times he cannot get to sleep before daybreak ('Sleeplessness, until morning': *1*). The insomnia can be accompanied by waves of heat and rushes of blood ('Sleeplessness, orgasm of blood': *3*) or pulsating sensations ('Sleeplessness, pulsation of body and particularly in the abdomen': *2*).

SUMMARY

Weakness and inhibition are the overriding features of this remedy. He feels impotent and inadequate, and his typically psoric fears and anxieties form a protective screen between him and the outside world.

Lack of Self-Confidence

His lack of self-confidence causes him great embarrassment in social situations. His lack of courage and decisiveness prevents him from ever trying anything new.

Related Rubrics
'Confidence, want of self': 2.
'Cowardice': 2.
'Timidity, appearing in public': 3.
'Undertakes nothing, lest he fail': 1.

Anticipatory Anxiety

Any extra stress, such as a test or exam, brings on an attack of anticipatory anxiety.

Related Rubric
'Ailments from: anticipation': 3 (Barthel).

Perfectionism

He sets himself impossibly high standards of perfection in the belief that therein lies his security.

Related Rubric
'Conscientious about trifles': 3.

Weakness of Intellect

He is unable to concentrate on anything for long, his mind is sluggish, dull and confused when he tries to read, write or talk.

Related Rubrics
'Concentration, difficult': 3.
'Confusion of mind': 3.
'Conversation agg.': 2.
'Dullness, mental exertion, from': 2.
'Prostration of mind': 3.
'Prostration, reading, from': 2.
'Prostration, writing, after': 2.

The Inner Child

He will never become a self-reliant individual while the meek and mild child within him needs so much reassurance and support. His reluctance to leave the past behind him is illustrated by the homesickness, the aggravation when alone, and the desire to surrender himself to another person's control.

Related Rubrics
'Company, desire for, alone, while agg.': *1.*
'Homesickness': *2.*
'Magnetized, desires to be': *3.*
'Mildness': *3.*

Frustration

The conflict aroused by the desire for independence and the need for protection infuriates him; he takes his frustration out on other people with his irritability, intolerance of contradiction, stubbornness and aversion to consolation. He then guiltily regrets his behaviour.

Related Rubrics
'Anxiety, conscience, of': *2.*
'Consolation agg.': *3.*
'Contradiction, is intolerant of': *2.*
'Irritability, children, in': *2.*
'Obstinate': *2.*

Hypersensitivity

His nerves are in a state of hypersensitivity. He jumps at the slightest noise, gets ill with fright, and his internalised anger comes out in the symbolic fear of pins.

Related Rubrics
'Delusions, pins, about': *2.*
'Fear, pins, of': *2.*
'Fright, complaints from': *3.*
'Frightened easily': *2.*
'Sensitive, noise, slightest, to': *3* (Barthel).
'Starting, noise, from': *3.*

SCHEMATIC DIAGRAM AND REPERTORISATION

In the centre of the diagram overleaf we have the MCS – that group of highly characteristic symptoms which identify the remedy and distinguish it from all others. Central to this core group is symptom 1, 'Confidence, want of self', an essential component of the remedy. To the left, we have symptom 2, the need for maternal love and reassurance. Below this we have symptom 4, 'Ailments from: anticipation', the paralysing fear when faced with a challenge. This symptom is a combination of psoric anxiety and timidity and tubercular inadequacy. Symptoms 3 and 5, 'Obstinate' and 'Conscientious about trifles', are sycotic attempts to compensate for his failings.

In the bottom left-hand corner are symptoms 6–9, concerned with weakness of intellect: 'Concentration, difficult', 'Dullness, mental exertion, from', 'Confusion of mind' and 'Prostration of mind'.

In the top left-hand corner, we have the symptoms of the inner child: 'Mildness' (10), 'Homesickness' (11), 'Magnetized, desires to be' (12) and 'Company, desire for, alone, while agg.' (13).

In the top right-hand corner, we have the symptoms that result from his frustrating inner conflicts: 'Consolation agg.' (14), 'Contradiction, is intolerant of' (15) and 'Irritability, children, in' (16).

His underlying feelings of guilt and self-reproach ('Anxiety, conscience, of', 17) make him tense, overwrought and acutely sensitive ('Sensitive, noise, slightest, to', 18); hence the starting from noise (19), the fearfulness (20) and the ailments from fright (21).

Silicea is a moody, unstable and defensive individual who goes through life trying to please, wanting to be perfect and needing to be mothered.

Certain paradoxical symptoms bring out the polarities in his nature. For example, we have symptoms, such as homesickness, dreams of water and dreams of past events, that express a deep nostalgia for the days of his childhood, when he enjoyed his mother's unconditional love: in contrast to this, we also know that Silicea is one of the remedies that can reject his mother's milk.

His emotional conflicts tear him apart and he imagines that he is divided in two parts, like Baptisia.

The denial of the needy inner child creates the illusion that the left side of his body does not belong to him.

He has fantasies of murdering his mother in a fit of temper, and suffers great remorse for his sinful thoughts; this translates into symptoms that express shame, guilt and the fear of punishment, such as the fear of pins, a phallic symbol of his father's wrath, and the sudden impulse to drown himself in the river, a symbol of his wish to return to the womb.

SCHEMATIC DIAGRAM – SILICEA

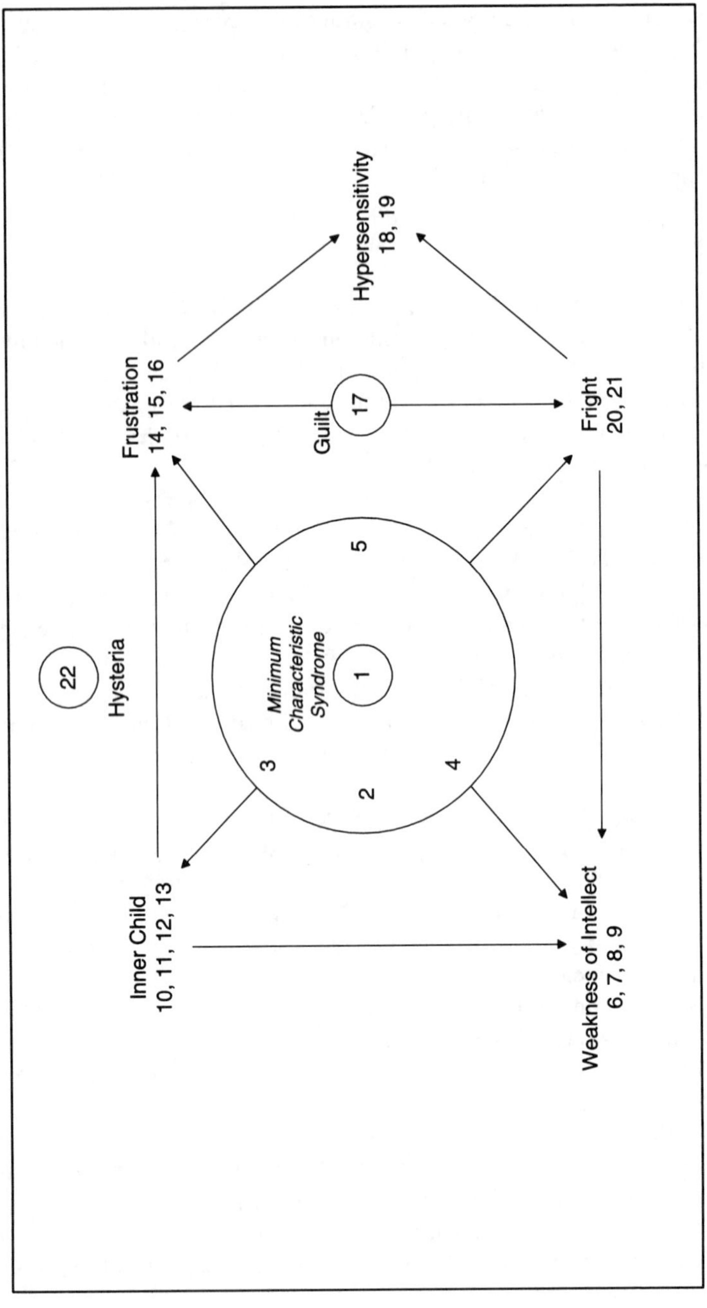

Hysteria
22

Frustration
14, 15, 16

Hypersensitivity
18, 19

Guilt
17

Fright
20, 21

Minimum
Characteristic
Syndrome
1

5

3

2

4

Inner Child
10, 11, 12, 13

Weakness of Intellect
6, 7, 8, 9

Minimum Characteristic Syndrome

1) Confidence, want of self
2) Timidity
3) Obstinate
4) Ailments from: anticipation
5) Conscientious about trifles

Weakness of Intellect

6) Concentration, difficult
7) Dullness, mental exertion, from
8) Confusion of mind
9) Prostration of mind

The Inner Child

10) Mildness
11) Homesickness
12) Magnetized, desires to be
13) Company, desire for, alone, while agg.

Frustration

14) Consolation agg.
15) Contradiction, is intolerant of
16) Irritability, children, in

Guilt

17) Anxiety, conscience, of

Hypersensitivity

18) Sensitive, noise, slightest, so
19) Starting, noise, from

Fright

20) Frightened easily
21) Fright, complaints from
   Fear, pins, of
   Delusion, pins, about

Hysteria

22) Hysteria
   *Delusions: Divided into two parts
   Side, that she did not own her left
   *Dreams: Water, flood
   Water
   Events, long past

Asterisked symptoms have not been repertorised. They are included here in order to provide a complete picture of the remedy.

REPERTORISATION – SILICEA

	1	2	3	4	5	6	7	8	9	10	11	12	13	14	15	16	17	18	19	20	21	22
Sil.	1	2	2	3	3	3	2	3	3	3	2	3	1	3	2	2	2	3	3	2	3	3
Ars.	–	2	2	3	2	1	–	2	1	3	–	–	3	2	1	1	3	–	1	3	1	2
Aur.	2	2	1	–	1	–	1	2	3	1	2	–	–	–	3	–	3	–	1	1	2	3
Bar-c.	2	3	–	2	2	3	1	2	2	–	–	–	–	–	–	–	–	1	2	3	–	2
Bry.	2	1	1	1	1	1	–	3	2	–	–	–	–	–	2	–	–	–	–	2	1	3
Calc.	1	3	3	3	–	–	1	3	2	2	–	3	1	1	–	–	–	–	2	2	1	2
Caust.	1	2	1	2	–	3	1	1	–	1	2	–	–	–	–	–	2	–	2	2	2	3
Chin.	2	2	2	1	1	1	–	2	–	–	–	–	–	1	–	–	–	–	–	–	–	–
Hep.	–	–	2	–	1	–	1	1	2	–	–	–	–	–	–	–	–	–	–	–	–	–
Hyos.	1	1	–	1	1	2	–	2	–	2	1	–	–	–	–	–	2	–	–	2	2	2
Ign.	1	1	2	3	3	1	1	1	–	1	2	–	–	3	3	–	2	–	–	2	3	3
Kali-c.	2	2	2	1	–	2	–	2	3	2	–	–	2	1	–	–	–	–	3	2	–	2
Lyc.	2	3	1	1	2	3	1	2	3	1	–	1	2	1	3	1	–	2	2	3	3	2
Nat-c.	1	3	–	2	2	2	3	2	2	3	–	–	–	–	1	–	–	–	3	3	1	2
Nat-m.	1	2	3	1	–	2	1	3	3	–	2	3	–	3	–	–	2	3	3	2	3	3
Nux-v.	1	2	1	1	2	3	2	3	3	2	–	–	3	1	2	–	2	2	3	2	2	3
Phos.	1	3	–	3	–	3	–	2	2	3	–	–	–	–	–	1	1	–	–	2	3	3
Puls.	2	2	2	3	1	2	1	2	2	2	1	–	–	–	–	–	1	–	–	2	3	2
Sulph.	1	3	1	–	2	2	2	2	3	2	–	–	–	–	–	–	2	–	1	2	–	3
Thuj.	–	–	–	1	2	2	–	2	1	2	–	–	–	1	1	–	2	–	–	–	–	–

Minimum Characteristic Syndrome

1) Confidence, want of self
2) Timidity
3) Obstinate
4) Ailments from: anticipation
5) Conscientious about trifles

Weakness of Intellect

6) Concentration, difficult
7) Dullness, mental exertion, from
8) Confusion of mind
9) Prostration of mind

The Inner Child

10) Mildness
11) Homesickness
12) Magnetized, desires to be
13) Company, desire for, alone, while agg.

Frustration

14) Consolation agg.
15) Contradiction, is intolerant of
16) Irritability, children, in

Guilt

17) Anxiety, conscience, of

Hypersensitivity

18) Sensitive, noise, slightest, so
19) Starting, noise, from

Fright

20) Frightened easily
21) Fright, complaints from
    Fear, pins, of
    Delusion, pins, about

Hysteria

22) Hysteria
    *Delusions: Divided into two
        parts
        Side, that she did
        not own her left
    *Dreams: Water, flood
        Water
        Events, long past

Asterisked symptoms have not been repertorised. They are included here in order to provide a complete picture of the remedy.

COMPARATIVE MATERIA MEDICA

From a miasmatic point of view, a tubercular case of Silicea would present a picture of emaciation, chilliness, timidity and tearfulness, and a sycotic case would have obesity with a distended abdomen, oedematous swellings, obstinacy, irritability and fastidiousness.

Four remedies have all the symptoms of the Minimum Characteristic Syndrome of Silicea: they are Lycopodium, Ignatia, Nux Vomica and Bryonia.

Lycopodium

The Lycopodium patient tries to compensate for his lack of confidence by putting himself first and treating others with arrogant disdain. He is argumentative and aggressive. Silicea, by contrast, is a passive by-stander in life who merely dislikes being told that he is wrong. Behind the mask of obsequiousness, Lycopodium is a proud egotist who will reject his loved ones when he is ill. His pride will not permit him such indulgences as 'Homesickness' (11), 'Anxiety, conscience, of' (17), or 'Magnetized, desires to be' (12).

Ignatia

Ignatia shares the hysterical and obsessive characteristics of Silicea, although here the nature of the disturbance is more functional than systemic. Ignatia is characterised by extreme changeability, contra-dictory mental and physical effects, and a sensitive, excitable disposition. If the emotions are suppressed, the nervous system will be affected and the patient will suffer a range of hysterically based physical symptoms. Ignatia has a highly emotional, volatile and erratic disposition.

This remedy does not have six of the repertorised symptoms, namely 'Prostration of mind' (9), the cause of Silicea's mental confusion and difficulty in comprehending; 'Magnetized, desires to be' (12) and 'Company, desire for, alone, while agg.' (13), rubrics that speak of Silicea's lack of self-reliance; 'Irritability, children, in' (16), 'Sensitive, noise, to slightest'(18) and 'Starting, noise, from' (19), rubrics that describe Silicea's highly wrought state. Both Ignatia and Silicea lack self-confidence – in the former it stems from an emotional instability, whereas in the latter it denotes a deeply ingrained and fundamental weakness.

84

Nux Vomica

Here the missing symptoms are those that express the need for support and maternal love, namely 'Mildness' (10), 'Homesickness' (11), 'Magnetized, desires to be' (12) and 'Company, desire for, alone, while agg.' (13). Hypersensitivity is one of the keynotes of this remedy, on both mental and physical levels. The Nux Vomica patient is irritable, impatient and hurried, constantly feeling the stress of his rather chaotic lifestyle and prone to impulsive and violent behaviour. Like Ignatia, his mental instability causes his lack of self-confidence. Other keynotes of this angry, fiery remedy are chilliness and digestive disturbances and spasms.

Bryonia

Bryonia has all the symptoms of the Minimum Characteristic Syndrome of Silicea. It does not have symptom 7, 'Dullness, mental exertion, from', which comes as a result of Silicea's untiring efforts to gain recognition. He is timid, but not especially so, when appearing in public. He is a most difficult patient, with the characteristic irritability and bad temper that comes from feeling trapped inside an ailing body that cannot tolerate the slightest motion. He wants to move, but he is stuck. In his dreams and deliriums he thinks of only one thing – his work. He does not have symptoms 10, 11, 12 or 13, which focus on the needy, child-like side of Silicea. Bryonia is intolerant of contradiction (15) because he finds all challenge stimulating to his sycotic energy, while the tubercular Silicea withdraws into his shell at the first sign of opposition. The symptoms that are common to both Silicea and Bryonia serve completely different functions in each remedy: in the former, they are the fierce attempts of the defence mechanism to shield from view his deepest feelings of worthlessness and, in the latter, they help to distract him from his worst nightmares – the fear of poverty and of the future.

Ten remedies have four symptoms of the Minimum Characteristic Syndrome of Silicea: Arsenicum, Aurum, Calcarea Carbonica, Causticum, China, Hyoscyamus, Natrum Carbonicum, Phosphorus, Pulsatilla and Sulphur.

Arsenicum

The essential characteristic of Arsenicum is a fearful anxiety which is at its most intense between the hours of 2 and 3 a.m., and which forces him out of bed in a desperate bid to escape from imminent death. He is prone to violent and destructive impulses, fits of anger with anxiety and chilliness, and bouts of anguished restlessness that drive him from place to place. The fear of being alone, for fear of dying, and the despair of recovery with the conviction that he is beyond help, are marks of the syphilitic miasm, with its attendant urges to violence and destruction. Arsenicum is a forceful personality who, when crossed, shows his displeasure with scathing criticism, abusive language and violent anger. His obsession with order and cleanliness ('Conscientious about trifles', 5) is a compensatory reaction to a deep-seated guilt complex ('Anxiety of conscience', 17).

Although Arsenicum has seventeen symptoms in common with Silicea, those that it lacks are crucial to our understanding of the differences between them. For example, Arsenicum shares none of Silicea's intellectual and emotional weakness, hence his absence from symptom 1, 'Confidence, want of self', and symptom 7, 'Dullness, mental exertion, from'. He does not appear in symptom 11, 'Homesickness', or symptom 12, 'Magnetized, desires to be', which represent Silicea's unwillingness to break away from the past. Arsenicum dismisses other people's concern for his health ('Consolation agg.', 14) because he believes his condition to be incurable. Silicea is averse to consolation because it makes him realise his own inadequacies. They are both fearful remedies; Arsenicum's major fear is of dying in solitude, while Silicea is obsessed with the fear of failure. Arsenicum's fears centre around the theme of self-destruction and decay. Silicea is more concerned with the feelings of vulnerability that inhibit his desperate desire for freedom.

Aurum

The reader should refer to the description of Aurum in the comparative materia medica section of Lycopodium (pages 42–3). Paschero says: 'Of all the syphilitic remedies, Aurum suffers the most intense anguish, depression and despair. He is consumed by feelings of guilt and self-condemnation that are exacerbated by explosions of rage and violent hysteria. The underlying source of his aggressive feelings is guilt in all its various aspects: anxiety of conscience, remorse, despair of religious salvation, self-reproach and suicidal impulses – his sole means of escape from this inner torment.'

Aurum does not have symptom 4, 'Ailments from: anticipation'; indeed, he has such a low opinion of himself that he avoids all competitive or challenging situations. He has symptom 10, 'Mildness', and symptom 11, 'Homesickness', but his basic distrust of people leads him to prefer his own company, hence his absence from symptoms 12 and 13, 'Magnetized, desires to be' and 'Company, desire for, alone, while agg.'.

Calcarea Carbonica

This remedy has none of the sycotic compensatory symptoms, such as 'Conscientious about trifles' (5). In health, Calcarea is calm and collected, self-reliant and effective, and a little on the chubby side. In sickness, he is an obstinate, apathetic lump, whose mounting frustrations and resentments culminate in an animal-like gut feeling of fear of divine punishment, ghosts, darkness and cruelty, and an over-sensitivity to news of horrible or tragic events.

Causticum

The Causticum patient is severely depressed, full of anxious forebodings, oversympathetic and overprotective. He lacks both the will and the energy to assert himself, hence his absence from symptom 5, 'Conscientious about trifles'. His life is beset by problems but he is too despondent to deal with them, too devoid of hope to attempt to cover up his feelings of worthlessness. He does not have symptoms 12, 13, 14 and 15. Although at times he can be quarrelsome and difficult, he is basically a sensitive soul who takes on other people's pain in a masochistic attempt to hurt himself. He is just one of life's unfortunates who deserves all the punishment he gets. He has the typical mentality of a dictator: an inferiority complex with an aggressive streak. Paralysis and muscular spasm are the physical expressions of this. He has a general mental sluggishness and prostration, not specifically after mental exertion.

China

The reader should refer to the description of China in the comparative materia medica section of Lycopodium (pages 55–7). In China, the absence of symptom 4, 'Ailments from: anticipation', brings to light a significant difference between the two remedies. Silicea can never allow himself to relax or unwind while he pursues his lifelong quest for personal validation, whereas China covers up his lack of self-confidence with indifference and insensitivity, and by blaming others for his own shortcomings and misfortunes. His propensity for contemptuous criticism and arrogant accusation may develop into a full-blown paranoia, where he feels abused and abandoned by his friends and despised and persecuted by his enemies. His debilitated condition accounts for symptom 6, 'Concentration, difficult'; symptom 7, 'Confusion of mind', comes from the wanderings of his fevered mind that cannot distinguish fact from fiction.

Although China shares four of the symptoms of the Minimum Characteristic Syndrome of Silicea, there are fundamental differences between them – Silicea uses his qualities of appealing helplessness and dogged persistence to gain acceptance and approval, while China, arrogantly and contemptuously, blames everyone but himself for his problems.

Hyoscyamus

The reader should refer to the description of Hyoscyamus in the comparative materia medica section of Lycopodium (pages 57–8). Like China, Hyoscyamus does not have Silicea's anticipatory anxiety. As discussed in the previous chapter, the Hyoscyamus patient is highly emotional, excitable, and subject to attacks of hysteria, jealousy and suspicion. His sense of unreality and disorientation ('Confusion of mind', 8) brings about the lack of self-confidence (1) and timidity (2). It also accounts for the arrogance and argumentativeness that are behind symptoms 3, 'Obstinate', and 5, 'Conscientious about trifles', and for the heartfelt longing to be with his own people again ('Homesickness', 11). He does not suffer from anticipatory anxiety (4), dullness from mental exertion (7) or mental prostration (9), and he shares none of Silicea's irritability, nervousness and feelings of inadequacy.

Natrum Carbonicum

This remedy is characterised by great debility and relaxation. On a mental level, he is timid (2), anxious ('Ailments from: anticipation', 4) and conscientious ('Conscientious about trifles', 5), although his natural inclination to work is hindered by a mind that is sluggish (7), confused (8) and easily distracted ('Concentration, difficult', 6). The slightest mental effort makes him dizzy and exhausted ('Prostration of mind', 9), hence the lack of obstinacy ('Obstinate', 3) which implies a strength of will he simply cannot muster. In the depths of his depression, he withdraws into himself and rejects everyone, even his nearest and dearest – consequently, 'Homesickness' (11) is not something that affects this solitary and paradoxical being, who is also frightened of being alone. He is 'Frightened easily' (20) and suffers from fright (21) and noise ('Starting, noise, from', 19). He trembles with pain as he turns to the spiritual world for help, with a desire to be magnetised (12) and a marked sensitivity to music.

Phosphorus

The key symptoms of Phosphorus are anxiety, prostration and hypersensitivity. His shyness (2) and lack of confidence (1) are the products of an acutely sensitive nature that does not resort to fastidiousness ('Conscientious about trifles', 5) by way of compensation. Phosphorus is one of the most affectionate of remedies, troubled neither by consolation (14), contradiction (15) nor loud voices ('Starting, noise, from', 19). There is no irritability in the Phosphorus child (16), but there is great sensitivity to slight noise.

Pulsatilla

As delicate and fragile as the windflower, Pulsatilla acknowledges her frailty and tentatively pleads for the love and approval of everyone she meets: her security depends on it. Her eyes shine with goodness and humility as she surrenders herself meekly to her protectors. She loves being caressed and stroked, but is not attracted to magnetism (12). Unlike Silicea, she would rather be alone than be a nuisance (13), she enjoys consolation (14) and avoids arguments (15) for the sake of peace. Furthermore, there is not a trace of stubbornness about her (3) and she has none of Silicea's fear symptoms (19, 20, 21). Any mother would be proud to have a gentle, loving Pulsatilla daughter.

Sulphur

The reader should refer to the description of Sulphur in the comparative materia medica section of Lycopodium (pages 65–6). This remedy shares four of the symptoms of the Minimum Characteristic Syndrome of Silicea, the missing symptom being number 4. In our previous discussion about Sulphur, we described him as someone who watches the world from his ivory tower and remains largely unaffected by what he sees. In his arrogant and selfish way, he spends long, lazy hours lost in thought, setting the world to right and congratulating himself on his great wisdom. His egotism is held in check only by his feelings of guilt ('Anxiety, conscience, of', 17). He feels guilty about those he knows

('Anxiety, friends at home, about': 2,) and about those he does not know ('Anxiety, others, for': 2), but he manages to hide his concern behind a smile ('Mildness', 10). On a physical level, he is prone to circulatory disturbances and sluggishness.

Four remedies have three symptoms of the Minimum Characteristic Syndrome of Silicea: Baryta Carbonica, Kali Carbonicum, Natrum Muriaticum and Thuja.

Baryta Carbonica

Here, the mental faculties are so severely impaired that he cannot cope with any social contact whatsoever. His obsession with detail is evidence of childishness, rather than a sycotic nature, and his fears are only to be expected in one so disabled.

Kali Carbonicum

The Kali Carbonicum patient is bad-tempered, impatient and impossible to please; he is moody, changeable and never at peace with himself. As his mind is too feeble and unreliable to be of any use, he is obliged to depend on other people for help, and this infuriates him. He is a strange mixture of anxiety, vulnerability, peevishness and exasperation.

Silicea's characteristic symptoms of self-affirmation and mental weakness (4, 5, 7 and 9) are missing in Kali Carbonicum.

Unlike Silicea, he does not search for parental approval, hence his absence from symptoms 10, 11 and 13. The outstanding characteristic of this remedy is an expression of tremendous frustration and discontentment, namely the fear of being alone, while treating those around him outrageously ('Company, desire for, yet treats them outrageously': 2). Both remedies share an aversion to consolation (14), but for different reasons: Silicea feels belittled by it and Kali Carbonicum feels trapped. Silicea cannot bear contradiction (15) for similar reasons, although Kali Carbonicum does not make a fuss, presumably because he is so afraid of being abandoned.

Like Silicea, Kali Carbonicum is easily startled (20), especially when he is touched. Silicea's fear of hostility is projected outwards on to the fear of pins, while Kali Carbonicum feels anxiety in the stomach ('Stomach, anxiety': 2). Silicea's guilt feelings ('Anxiety, conscience, of', 17) stem from his unpredictable behaviour, at times acquiescent and submissive, at others aggressive and assertive. Kali Carbonicum has no time for guilt; he imposes his will with a stubborn disregard for other people's feelings.

Natrum Muriaticum

This is an introverted, repressed individual who broods on the past and worries about the future. He has none of Silicea's compensatory reactions to a lack of confidence. The cravings for salt and large quantities of water are indications of a disturbance that is both metabolic and emotional; he dreams of finding the perfect love of a mother for her child while, in the real world, his love affairs end in heartbreak and disillusionment.

Thuja

Thuja has none of Silicea's basic insecurities, such as a lack of confidence (1) or timidity (2). As befits an essentially sycotic remedy, Thuja is characterised by an enlarged ego, a strong sense of guilt and an extreme excitability. This is a shrewd, suspicious character, with a troubled conscience and a marked predilection for perverse, immoral behaviour. His difficulty in concentrating ('Concentration, difficult', 6) encompasses an inability to comprehend anything outside the confines of his own little world.

Behind the mask of amiability ('Mildness', 10), he hides a complete indifference, hence his absence from symptoms 11, 12 and 13. He hates consolation (14) because it shows him up; he dislikes being contradicted (15) because it gets in his way. Silicea, by contrast, detests consolation and contradiction because they serve only to increase his doubts and insecurities.

Thuja's sense of guilt ('Anxiety, conscience, of', 17) arises in response to his devious and corrupt ways; in Silicea, it is a form of self-punishment for indulging in evil thoughts about his oppressors. The thought of breaking free from his chains and launching himself on to the world fills him with terror (18 to 21). Thuja, by contrast, fears being caught in the act and exposed to view, hence the fear of strangers approaching or touching him ('Fear, approaching him of others': *2*, 'Fear, strangers, of': *2*, 'Fear, touch, of': *1*, Barthel).

4

Thuja Occidentalis

DESCRIPTION

In health, the natural impulse of human beings is to work for their own spiritual progress, concentrating less on personal concerns and more on the good of society, working from the inner to the outer, according to Hering's law of cure, developing qualities of altruism and co-operation and reaching for the higher purposes of existence. The sycotic miasm blocks this process and perverts the natural course of things.

According to Gathak, the predominating feature of the sycotic mentality is the tendency to make a secret of everything. A sycotic individual will use cunning and guile to cover up all traces of his degenerate behaviour and unhealthy appetites. He is dishonest and deceitful and thinks that others are also of the same mentality. He is destitute of all love and affection for others, and believes that people are out to get him; he is suspicious of everyone, friends and colleagues alike, and changes doctors frequently because he has no faith in any of them ('Suspicious': *1*).

The other fundamental aspect of all sycotic remedies is a dull and sluggish mind ('Dullness, sluggishness, difficulty of thinking and comprehending': *2*). Here, the term 'comprehending' means more than mere intellectual activity: it is the ability to perceive the higher meaning of life and the reason for living. In Thuja this symptom means the inability to understand anything that falls outside his rigid, analytical framework where the same old questions and doubts keep circulating in his head.

The Thuja child is emotionally immature and adopts a rational approach to everything. His constant questioning becomes a neurotic search for answers ('Religious affections, fanaticism': *1*). He does not understand the concepts of morality and cultural restraint; if his insatiable desires are thwarted, he will either try to divert his frustration into ritualistic, repetitive acts, such as checking over and over again that he has locked the door or turned off the gas, or he will suddenly explode in a frenzy of rage.

Thuja's innate self-distrust is reinforced by a characteristic mental confusion and weakness of memory. He is, consequently, painstaking in his work ('Conscientious about trifles': 2) to the point of fanaticism.

The vital force of the Thuja patient is so deranged that he is tormented by feelings of guilt ('Anxiety, conscience, of': 2), restless uneasiness and hostility towards a world whose abundant goodness and love he cannot feel. He is torn between the desires of his lust and the dictates of his conscience, between the satisfaction of bodily needs and the nurturing of the spirit. This brief outline of the Thuja psychology will, it is hoped, shed some light on the nature of his pathology.

Thuja is incapable of reaching out emotionally to other people, so he cannot progress and develop according to Hering's Law of Cure. His sense of himself as an isolated being produces almost all of the symptoms of delusions and hallucinations. His inner conflicts tear him apart, literally divide him in two ('Delusions, divided into two parts': *1*, with the sub-rubric 'and could not tell of which part he had possession on waking': *1* – only remedy); he feels that his soul is separated from his body ('Delusions, soul, fancied body was too small for, or that it was separated from': *1*) and, during asthmatic attacks, he feels that the soul is trying to escape from the body, with chest pains, flushes of heat and feelings of suffocation. His ideas become fixed and obsessive ('Thoughts, persistent': 2, with the sub-rubric 'thinks mind and body are separated': *1*).

The delusion of being double ('Delusions, double, of being': *1*) and confusion of identity ('Delusion, identity, errors of personal': *1*) illustrate the sycotic tendency for proliferation. This centres around the stomach region from where Thuja, like Lycopodium, feels rising fear ('Fear, stomach, arising from': *1*) and other, stranger sensations of animals in the abdomen ('Delusions, animals of, abdomen, are in': *2* – only remedy), movements like the fist of a foetus ('Abdomen, movements, fist of a foetus, like': *3*) and others associated with pregnancy ('Delusions, pregnant, thought herself': *1*).

His defence mechanism uses subtle strategies to divert attention away from his secret vices; he believes that his body is as fragile ('Delusions, body, delicate': *2* – only remedy, 'Delusions, body, brittle is': *1* – only remedy) and as breakable as glass ('Delusions, glass, that she is made of': *1* – only remedy). From this it follows that he is afraid of being approached ('Fear, approaching him, of others': 2) and touched ('Touched, aversion to being': 2).

This last symptom is also found in the Thuja picture of insanity, where the patient recoils from touch ('Insanity, touched, will not be': 2 – only remedy). His feelings of fragility are further reinforced by the delusion that he is thin ('Delusions, thin, body is': *1* – only remedy), emaciated ('Delusions, emaciation': 2) and lighter than air ('Delusions, body, lighter than air': *1*).

The other side of this basically hydrogenoid constitution is one of slowness, lethargy and clumsiness; he feels heavy ('Delusions, heavy, is': *1*) and as hard as stone ('Delusions, building stones, appearance of': *1* – only remedy).

The guilty conscience that underlies his ambivalent attitude to good and evil leads him to believe that he has done something terribly wrong ('Delusions, wrong, fancies he has done': *1*), and he is haunted by visions of ghosts and phantoms, especially at night ('Delusions, images, phantoms, sees': 2, with the sub-rubrics 'at night': 2, and 'closing the eyes, on': 2). As his guilt feelings become more entrenched, they are projected on to the external world as a powerful, malign force that seeks to control him ('Delusions, super-human control, under is': 2); strange people come to invade his inner world ('Delusions, strangers seemed to be in the room': 2): he sees them ('Delusions, strangers, thinks he sees': 2), talks with them ('Delusions, people, sees, converses, with absent': *1*) and hears them calling him ('Delusions, calls, someone': *1*). He feels like a hunted criminal, with fear and anguish in his stomach ('Fear, stomach, arising from': *1*.)

His fear of being caught or found out is expressed by the fear of strangers ('Fear, strangers, of': 2), of being approached ('Fear, approaching him, of others': 2) and of being touched ('Insanity, touched, will not be': 2); he fears that his life is threatened by a serious disease ('Fear, disease, of impending': *1*) or an attack of apoplexy ('Fear, apoplexy, of': *1*) and that he is about to die ('Delusions, die, thought he was about to': 2 and 'Delusions, die, time has come to': *1*).

The delusions that are apparent in the psychological make-up of the remedy are fundamentally connected to the sycotic miasm. For example, the delusion of being under superhuman control is a graphic portrayal of the sycotic conviction that he is 'the son of God, the chosen one, the omnipotent one'; he is not to be held responsible for his licentious behaviour because 'it is not I who acted but He who ordered me'. In the delusion of being under superhuman control we see two basic elements of sycosis – deceitfulness and an inflated ego. The Thuja patient will return to this theme in the final stages of his disease, when he will become infected by a religious fanaticism and despair for his salvation. It is of interest to recall that the first unwitting prover of Thuja was, in fact, a priest who developed a urethral discharge after chewing the twigs of the *Thuja occidentalis* in his garden.

The unifying themes that run through a remedy are easily discernible by means of the repertory, whereas they remain hidden in the pages of a book of materia medica.

The combination of a rational, analytical mind, devoid of emotional warmth and love, and a penchant for mischief and misdeeds, creates an aggressive, dishonest individual who will cheat and manipulate people until he gets what he wants.

Sooner or later, we are bound to meet a Thuja patient in the consulting room, although the indication for the remedy may escape us as there are relatively few mental symptoms to go on. If we take a mechanical approach to case-taking, and merely list all the symptoms, we may fall into the trap that Kent warned about and use symptoms that are irrelevant to the central problem. The repertory is an effective tool, but we must always remember that it is only a tool. Of equal importance is our observation of the patient's gestures, attitudes and expressions as he speaks.

At times, the patient's appearance may lead us to the remedy. Thuja has a greasy, shiny face that is covered with pimples and blackheads, especially around the nasal folds. There can be polypi and warty excrescences on the shiny cheeks that are netted with spider-like veins, and on the forehead and bridge of the nose there may be an eczematous eruption that takes off the edge of the eyebrows; hard swellings in the alae nasi; an unhealthy, pitted skin; lips striated with vertical, white creases that look like milk. The perspiration smells sweet and honey-like, or fetid like garlic. A penetrating, acrid smell emanating from the genitals can be sweetish, offensive or like burnt sponge.

The Thuja child is tall and hefty, untidy, undisciplined, irritable, hyperactive, bossy, mentally rigid and totally undemonstrative. He laughs when he is reprimanded, and thinks it is a joke when his parents tell the doctor how difficult he is to live with. He may have been expelled or suspended from school because of his wild, unruly behaviour ('Chaotic': 2).

The Thuja adult, however, is so enigmatic and secretive that it is impossible to know what he is thinking. He is driven by restless-ness ('Restlessness': 2) and a compulsive need to keep himself busy ('Occupation, amel.': *1*), to assuage the inner turmoil and anxiety. Like Nux Vomica, Lycopodium and Sulphur, when Thuja is healthy he devotes his whole life to his work with great enthusiasm and dedication. Although he is not at his best in the morning, as the day goes on he can be pleasant company ('Mildness': 2), especially in the afternoon ('Cheerful, afternoon': *1*). Despite his poor memory, he is self-assured, self-sufficient and quick-witted. Unlike Lycopodium, Pulsatilla and Silicea, his self-esteem is not at the mercy of his emotions: like the bad workman, he will always blame his tools rather than himself when things go wrong. He distrusts his memory to such an extent that he has to make endless, detailed lists of what he has to do ('Conscientious about trifles': 2). He is quick to anger ('Anger': 2) when contradicted ('Anger, ailments, contradiction, from': 2) and will tolerate no opposing viewpoints ('Contradiction, is intolerant of': *1*) that threaten his rigid attitudes and preconceptions; any new, unknown territory worries him ('Ailments from: anticipation': *1*, Barthel). The strain of guarding the secrets of his private life while struggling with his conscience tells on him and explains why he is always so irritable ('Irritability': *3*). He is so intent upon the selfish gratification of his desires that all sense of co-operation and humanitarianism escapes him. If he does not get what he wants, he becomes stubborn ('Obstinate': *1*) and aggressive; if he cannot win with guile, he will win with brute force ('Quarrelsome': 2). He engineers cunning schemes in disregard of all social rules ('Unobserving': *1*), and with total disrespect for the wishes of other people ('Contrary': 2).

Thuja is the only remedy in italics in the rubric 'Fanaticism', a symptom that conveys his tenacious adherence to a fixed idea or prejudice, the inability to encompass change, the need for a strict routine, and an excessive zeal or fervour; all of which is completely foreign to the typically tubercular ebb and flow of attraction and repulsion.

Thuja's compensatory defence against the slowness and stagnation of sycosis is an energetic haste and agitated excitement ('Excitement': 2) that can come on during the night ('Excitement, night, waking, on': *1*); the female Thuja experiences a similar sensation before the menses ('Excitement, menses, before': *1*). Thuja is hurried in thought, movement, work and while walking ('Hurry': 2, with the sub-rubrics 'mental work, in': 2, 'movements, in': 2, 'occupation, in': 2, 'walking, while': 2). He feels that time passes too quickly ('Time, passes too quickly': *1*) because his sluggish mind can process only a few ideas or images at a time ('Slowness': *1*) and, as his memory tries to bring these ideas back to reality, he has the illusory sensation that time passes too quickly. It is rather like a film that has been shot in slow motion with very few images per second – when projected on to the screen (that is, the memory) it gives the impression that things are happening quickly. Conversely, Medorrhinum is like a film shot at high speed that, when projected on to the screen, gives the opposite illusion, that everything is happening slowly. A Thuja patient once told me that she had to be quick when she did her sewing because she felt that her mind and her arms were clumsy and slow and she was sure that she would not be able to finish on time. The Thuja haste is an attempt to counteract the feelings of stiffness and clumsiness.

As pathology advances, the mental faculties become weaker and he begins to lose his memory ('Memory, weakness, of': 2). He becomes absent-minded, especially in the morning ('Forgetful, morning, in': 2, with the sub-rubric 'waking, on': 2). His lapses of memory are selective; his work suffers ('Memory, weakness of, labor, for mental': 1), he forgets what he has just done ('Memory, weakness of, done, for what has just': 1), what he is about to say ('Memory, weakness of, say, for what is about to': 1 and 'Memory, weakness of, words, for': 1) and has difficulty expressing himself ('Memory, weakness of, expressing oneself, for': 1). He makes mistakes in speaking and writing, misplaces words, omits letters, syllables and words, and uses the wrong words ('Mistakes' with the sub-rubrics 'speaking': 2, 'words, misplacing': 1, 'writing, in': 3, 'writing, in, omitting letters': 2, 'writing, in, omitting syllables': 2, 'writing, words': 2, 'wrong words, using': 2).

His mind is distracted by all the fixed ideas ('Thoughts, persistent': 2) that go round and round in his head, and he finds it impossible to concentrate on anything for very long ('Concentration, difficult': 2). His perception of reality is distorted by circling thoughts and his degenerate emotions are in turmoil; he feels completely cut off from the world, in a state of chaos and confusion ('Confusion of mind': 2, with the modalities 'morning': 2, 'waking, on': 1, 'evening': 1 and 'dinner, after': 1). He has no sense of who or where he is, it all feels like a dream ('Confusion, dream, as if in': 1).

Thuja's personality is divided in two by the conflicting demands of his aggressive egocentricity and his guilty conscience. His basic duality is expressed by the belief that his mind and body are separated ('Thoughts, persistent, thinks mind and body are separated': 1), and by the confusion he feels about who he is ('Confusion, identity, as to his': 1). His confusion is so great that he even gets lost in familiar places ('Confusion, loses his way in well-known streets': 1), and does not know where he is ('Stupefaction, knows not where he is': 1). When he wakes in the morning he is unable to collect his thoughts; he feels stupefied, drugged and bewildered, incapable of getting dressed or remembering even the simplest things ('Stupefaction': 2, with the sub-rubrics 'morning': 2, 'morning, rising, after': 2 and 'motion, from': 1).

In the final stages of pathology he becomes increasingly less articulate ('Confusion, talking, while': 2), losing the thread of the conversation and the train of his thoughts ('Thoughts, vanishing of, speaking, while': 2). He overcompensates for this by trying to speak so rapidly ('Speech, hasty': 2) that he exhausts himself ('Conversation agg.': 1). Then he decides to avoid all conversation ('Talk, indisposed to': 2), especially on waking ('Talk, indisposed to, morning, waking, on': 1); if he has to speak, he answers slowly ('Answers, slowly': 2), and in monosyllables ('Speech, monosyllabic': 2). This is similar to the rubric 'Dullness, sluggishness, difficulty of thinking and comprehending': 2, with the curious sub-rubric 'dullness, perspiration, during': 1.

A far cry now from the hyperactivity and energetic productivity of his early years, his mind no longer serves him well ('Work, aversion to mental': 2). Dejected and hopeless, he fears for the future ('Anxiety, future, about': 1) with an inexplicable, indescribable anguish that torments him day and night and makes him morbid and introspective. He becomes disillusioned with the life he has led ('Loathing, life': 3), and bored with the eternal secrecy and subterfuge; and he begins to hate himself ('Reproaches, himself': 2) for all the lies and manipulative strategies he has used in the pursuit of his pleasures. He feels so depressed about himself and his life that he wants to shut everybody out and hide, even from people he does not know ('Company, aversion to': 2, with the sub-rubrics 'avoids the sight of people': 2 and 'presence of strangers, to': 2). He develops a distinct aversion to strangers ('Stranger, presence of, agg.': 2 and 'Fear, strangers, of': 2). In the depths of his depression, he loses all interest in everything ('Aversion, everything, to': 1 and 'Indifference': 2). He lets no-one comfort him; kind words only add to his unhappiness ('Consolation agg.: 1 and 'Weeping, consolation agg.: 1). He cares for nothing and nobody, especially the company of women ('Indifference, opposite sex, to': 1 – only remedy), a symptom that covers up his sexual inhibitions and indicates his potential homosexuality. Music is the only thing that rouses him ('Sensitive, music, to': 1), although it exacerbates the depression ('Sadness, music, from': 1 and 'Weeping, music, from': 2) and makes his feet tremble ('Trembling, foot, music, from': 1 – only remedy) – the symbolic crumbling of the idol with feet of clay.

Thuja controls his tears and lets them out only occasionally; gestures of consolation make him feel wretchedly guilty or exposed and vulnerable and the tears well up ('Weeping, consolation agg.: 1); he may weep in his sleep ('Weeping, sleep, in': *1*) when his guard is down; and the female may weep during the menses ('Weeping, menses, during': *194*). For the most part, however, he keeps his vulnerability well hidden and his tears in check: 'Lachrymation, especially in left eye, when walking in open air (the tears do not run off, but remain standing in the eye)' (J. H. Clarke *Materia Medica*, Vol. 3, p. 1429).

By now, he has reached the limits of his endurance and his problems weigh heavily upon him ('Sadness': *3* with the sub-rubric 'walking, while': *1*). As conscience wrestles with desire, his anxiety level increases ('Anxiety, sudden': *1* and 'Anxiety, 4 to 5 p.m.': *1* – only remedy). He is tormented by uncertainty and guilt, convinced that he is to be condemned to all eternity for his sins ('Anxiety, salvation, about': *2*), and turns to God with a desperate prayer for the salvation of his soul ('Despair, religious': *2*). In the final stages of his decline, his 'folie de doute' pushes him ever nearer to the brink of suicide ('Suicidal disposition': *1*, 'Suicidal thoughts': *1* and 'Kill, desire to, sudden impulse to, herself': *1*).

Dreams

It is always rewarding to study the dreams of a remedy. These are often rich in symbolism, and form an integral part of the psychological and morbid dynamic.

As we have already noted in our discussion of the delusions, once our patient drops his guard and closes his eyes, the spectre of guilt raises its head and he is plagued by visions of ghosts, spirits and faces ('Sleep, disturbed, visions, by': *1* with the sub-rubric 'closing the eyes, on': *2*). In sleep, his hostile nature continues to wage war against life in dreams of battles ('Dreams, battles': *1*), accidents ('Dreams, accidents': *1*) and murder ('Dreams, murder': *1*). Just as chaos reigns over his waking life, so are the dream images confused and blurred ('Dreams, confused': *1*). He has dreams of devastation and destruction ('Dreams, dead, of the': *3* and 'Dreams, dead bodies': *2*), especially when he sleeps on the left side. By comparison, Lachesis dreams not of the dead but of death itself; in her paranoia of persecution she fantasises that she is dead and that preparations are being made for her funeral.

Thuja's dreams are anxious ('Dreams, anxious': *3* with the sub-rubric 'lying on left side': *2*) and full of danger ('Dreams, danger': *1* with the sub-rubric 'lying on left side': *1* – only remedy). He dreams of death as the solution to all his problems ('Dreams, death, dying, of': *2*).

Awake or asleep, he is consumed with guilt and tormented by his addiction to sinful pleasure. The female Thuja, in rebellion against the constraints imposed by her sex, tends to have more anxious dreams during the menses ('Dreams, anxious, menses, during': *1*) and nightmares after the menses ('Dreams, nightmare, menses, after': *1* – only remedy).

Like Nux Vomica, Thuja has dreams of things that have happened ('Dreams, events, previous': *1*), work he has done ('Dreams, mental exertion': *2*) and intellectual achievement ('Dreams, excelling in mental work': *2*). He may appear to be confident and self-possessed when you see him seated at his desk at work, but his true, insecure self surfaces in his sleep. If he can keep his wits about him, he will stay out of harm's way; but, with the decline of his health, his mind begins to lose its grip and he dreams of failure and calamity ('Dreams, misfortune, of': *3*), especially at his morning-time aggravation of 3 a.m. He will wake up shouting and crying out ('Dreams, calling out': *1*), just like the Thuja child who wakes up in distress, calling for his mother. During his waking hours he can successfully cover up all traces of guilt and anxiety, but sleep plunges him into a deep, subconscious fear of life and divine punishment ('Dreams, mind, affecting the': *1*).

His nights are filled with dreams ('Dreams, many': *1*) both lascivious ('Dreams, amorous': *2*) and ridiculous ('Dreams, absurd': *1*). Some serve as an outlet for his libidinous fantasies, and others point an accusing finger at his mean and selfish behaviour. There is one dream, however, that expresses in a nutshell the whole picture of the Thuja mentality: I refer, of course, to the dreams of falling from a height – be it from a plane, mountain or building ('Dreams, falling, of': *3*, with the sub-rubric 'from high places': *3*). This dream alludes both to the downfall of the great idol with feet of clay, already mentioned in the symptom 'Trembling, foot, music, from', and to the transformation of his high sex drive into homosexuality, discussed previously in the symptom 'Indifference, opposite sex, to'. Thuja is the only remedy in both these rubrics.

He is restless all night long ('Sleep, restless': *2*). He lies awake into the night ('Sleeplessness, midnight, before': *2*) often until 1 a.m. ('Sleeplessness, until 1 a.m.': *1*). If he manages to fall asleep before midnight, he will wake up soon after ('Sleeplessness, midnight, after': *2*, with the sub-rubrics 'after 2 a.m.': *1* and 'after 3 a.m.': *2*). If he has stayed awake all night, he will drift into a deep sleep by dawn ('Sleep, deep, morning': *1* and 'Sleeplessness, midnight, until 4 a.m.': *1*). Thuja has, therefore, two time modalities for his insomnia: if he goes to sleep early and sleeps well, he will wake in a bewildered daze ('Waking, early': *2*) at around 3 a.m. ('Night, midnight, after, 3 a.m.': *2*); but if he does not get off to sleep as soon as he lies down, he will have to wait until morning before falling into a deep, heavy sleep ('Sleep, heavy, morning': *1* and 'Sleep, deep, morning': *1*). The result is that, one way or another, Thuja is tired, dull and sluggish on waking ('Sleep, waking, difficult, morning': *1*).

The reader may feel that this somewhat overdetailed description has itself been infected with the tinge of sycosis. I will now complete the picture of the Thuja insomnia with a list of the factors that aggravate it: anxiety, cold, heat, the products of his fertile imagination and lying on the left side ('Sleeplessness': *3* with the sub-rubrics 'anxiety, from': *1*, 'heat, during'; *1*, 'coldness, from': *1*, 'illusions of fancy': *1* and 'lying, side, on left, agg.': *2*). His favourite sleep positions are with his arms over his head, like Pulsatilla ('Sleep, position, arms over head': *1*), and on his back ('Lying, back, on, amel.': *2*).

The General Picture

To supplement the description of Thuja that the reader may find in any materia medica, I include below a summary of the typical symptoms that are encountered frequently in clinical practice:

- The characteristic facial features described earlier.
- A sycotic medical history: rheumatism, diabetes, cancer and gonor-rhoea. A history of vaccinations, the suppression of discharges, the cauterisation of warts, and allopathic treatment of venereal disease. Chronic infection of any kind. (The removal of warts or a discharge can activate the sycotic miasm because it suppresses the normal mechanisms of cure. In the same way, vaccination can cause sycosis by blocking the organism's vital reactivity to illness and thereby hindering the body's attempt to cure itself.)
- Respiratory or genital infections with yellowy-green, sticky, offensive discharges that smell of sweet honey, burnt feathers or garlic, and sensations of heat.
- Aggravation from damp.
- Split urinary stream with cutting pains.
- Aggravation at 3 a.m. and 3 p.m.
- Aggravation from rest.
- Aggravation from tea, onions and fatty foods.

- Desire for tea, onions and fatty foods.
- Headache on vertex as if pierced by a nail.
- Foul, profuse perspiration with sweetish or garlicky smell, on genitals and covered parts.
- Eruptions only on covered parts.
- Left side affected.
- Neuralgia with the pains extending along the nerves.
- Soft, pediculated warts, cauliflower excrescences that bleed easily, condylomata, polypi, genital and nasal warts.
- Ovarian tumours and fibroids.
- Inflammatory conditions such as arthritis and rheumatism, and uterine infections in women.

SUMMARY

The following twelve points summarise the picture of Thuja.

Secrecy

The ability to disguise his corrupt and antisocial behaviour and to manipulate circumstances to serve his perverted and selfish needs.

Mistrust

He is unable either to give or to receive love, because he distrusts people's motives and believes others to be as dishonest and self-seeking as he is.

Related Rubric
'Suspicious': *1*.

Ritualistic Behaviour

He experiences society as a hostile, repressive force whose values of co-operation and consideration for others are totally alien to him. With his failing mental faculties, poor memory and crippled emotions, he protects himself from the demands of other people with a defensive perfectionism, the neurotic, compulsive repetition of every action and thought.

Related Rubrics
'Conscientious about trifles': *2*.
'Dullness, sluggishness, difficulty of thinking and comprehending': *2*.
'Irritability': *3*.
'Memory, weakness of': *2*.

Guilty Conscience

Despite aggressive resistance, his conscience tries to guide him along the path of truth.

Related Rubric
'Anxiety, conscience, of': *2*.

Inner Duality

The delusions of the remedy illustrate the psychological conflict between the aggressive demands of his lower self and the moral constraints imposed by his higher self.

Related Rubric
'Delusions, imaginations, hallucinations': *1*.

a) The sensation that his body is divided into two parts, or that his body is too small for his soul, illustrates the primary split in his personality between his lower and his higher selves.

Related Rubrics
'Delusions, divided into two parts': *1*.
'Delusions, soul, fancied body was too small for': *1*.

b) Overgrowth and proliferation is expressed by the sensation of being double, or that something is moving in his abdomen; the illusion of being pregnant.

Related Rubrics
'Delusions, animals of, abdomen, are in': *2*.
'Delusions, double, of being': *1*.

c) His feelings of vulnerability and fragility are expressed by the sensation that his body is brittle, delicate or made of glass.

Related Rubrics
'Delusions, body, brittle, is': *1.*
'Delusions, body, delicate': *2.*
'Delusions, glass, that she is made of': *1.*

d) The hydrogenoid element, slow and heavy, as if made of stone, is transformed literally into the delusion that he is heavy, or made of stone.

Related Rubrics
'Delusions, building stones, appearance of': *1.*
'Delusions, heavy, is': *1.*

e) Delusions that express his fear of strangers, of being approached or touched, disclose his underlying fear of exposure.

Related Rubrics
'Fear, approaching him, of others': *2.*
'Fear, strangers, of': *2.*
'Touched, aversion to being': *2.*

f) The guilty fear that he will be divinely punished for his sins provokes the feeling that he is about to die.

Related Rubrics
'Delusions, wrong, fancies he has done': *1.*
'Delusions, die, thought he was about to': *2.*
'Delusions, die, time has come to': *1.*

g) Self-conceit and hidden motives lie beneath the delusion that his actions are controlled by a superior being: 'I am the chosen one, it is not I who acts but another who commands'.

Related Rubric
'Delusions, superhuman control, under is': *2.*

Positive Aggression
To prove his superiority, he competes aggressively with other people and strives for perfection in his work.

Related Rubrics
'Conscientious about trifles': *2.*
'Excitement, excitable': *2.*
'Hurry': *2.*
'Occupation, amel.': *1.*
'Restlessness': *2.*

Negative Aggression

He seeks to boost his ego by undermining others with his intolerance, belligerence, fanaticism and offensive behaviour.

Related Rubrics
'Contradiction, is intolerant of': *1.*
'Contrary': *2.*
'Fanaticism': *2.*
'Quarrelsome': *2.*
'Repulsive mood': *1.*

Mental Deterioration

Although the intelligence remains unaffected by the ravages of the sycotic miasm, there is a gradual decline in the powers of reasoning and memory. In the initial stages, weakness of memory causes difficulty of self-expression and he finds that he starts to use the wrong words, to make mistakes in writing and to forget words.

Related Rubrics
'Memory, weakness of': *2.*
'Memory, weakness of, expressing one's self, for': *1.*
'Memory, weakness of, words, for': *1.*
'Mistakes, writing, in': *3.*
'Mistakes, wrong words, using': *2.*

As the illness progresses, there is great difficulty in concentrating.

Related Rubric
'Concentration, difficult': *2.*

In the final stages this leads to sheer chaos and confusion, as he no longer knows who he is or where he is going. His internal conflicts have torn him apart and he is left with a bewildered, disorientated feeling that he is dreaming, that his soul has come away from his body, and that he has no identity.

Related Rubrics
'Chaotic': *1*.
'Confusion, dream, as if in': *1*.
'Confusion, identity, as to his': *1*.
'Confusion, loses his way in well-known streets': *1*.
'Thoughts, persistent, thinks mind and body are separated': *1*.
'Time, passes too quickly': *1*.

Turning Inwards

He gives up the fight, but still manages to hold on to his secrets by withdrawing into himself and refusing to speak. He rejects his work, his friends and the comfort they offer; he becomes apathetic, weary of living and afraid of what the future holds.

Related Rubrics
'Anxiety, future, about': *1*.
'Company, aversion to': *2*.
'Consolation agg.': *1*.
'Indifference, opposite sex, to': *1*.
'Loathing, life': *3*.
'Talk, indisposed to': *2*.

Sensitivity to Music

In the throes of his depression, he is deeply affected by music – it makes him weep and tremble with grief as he recalls his lost paradise.

Related Rubrics
'Sadness, walking, while': *1*.
'Trembling, foot, music, from': *1*.
'Weeping, music, from': *2*.

Suicidal Despair

The only way out of his tormenting anxiety, despair and self-condemnation is suicide.

Related Rubrics
'Anxiety, salvation, about': *2*.
'Despair, religious (of salvation etc.): *2*.

106

'Kill, sudden impulse to, herself': *1*.
'Suicidal disposition': *1*.

Dreams

Guilt, fear and destruction feature strongly in his dreams. Visions of phantoms, spectres and strange faces come to haunt his sleep, and his aggressively hostile nature conjures up dreams of accidents, battles and murder.

Related Rubrics
'Dreams, accidents': *1*.
'Dreams, battles': *1*.
'Dreams, calling out': *1*.
'Dreams, dying, of': *2*.
'Dreams, falling, of, from high places': *3*.
'Dreams, misfortune, of': *3*.
'Dreams, murder': *1*.

SCHEMATIC DIAGRAM AND REPERTORISATION

While sycosis may push a man to depravity and sin, it also instils in him a strong sense of guilt, as both Medorrhinum and Thuja will testify. But, whereas the former is an under-confident and fearful pseudo-psoric remedy, the latter is an aggressively egocentric one, and therein lies the fundamental difference between the two. In Medorrhinum, the feelings of guilt seem to intensify his fear and lack of confidence, whereas in Thuja they bring out his irritability and selfishness.

It seems to me that the definitive symptom of Thuja is mental sluggishness – 'Dullness' (13), a rubric whose significance reaches far beyond a mere lack of intellectual reasoning power, to signify an inability to comprehend the higher purposes of our existence (see Paragraph 9 of the *Organon*).

There is a school of philosophy that measures an individual's powers of understanding and reasoning, not by the brain's capacity for logical analysis but by the ability to perceive the connection between an object and its symbol. Our rational mind is so bound up with the gross, material manifestations of life that it would take a lifetime to train it to perceive the transcendental and the non-material, where God

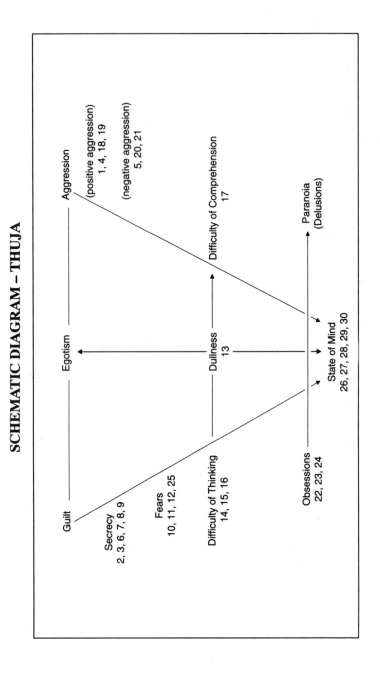

SCHEMATIC DIAGRAM – THUJA

Aggression

(positive aggression)
1, 4, 18, 19

(negative aggression)
5, 20, 21

Difficulty of Comprehension
17

Paranoia
(Delusions)

Egotism

Dullness
13

State of Mind
26, 27, 28, 29, 30

Guilt

Secrecy
2, 3, 6, 7, 8, 9

Fears
10, 11, 12, 25

Difficulty of Thinking
14, 15, 16

Obsessions
22, 23, 24

Minimum Characteristic

Syndrome

1) Conscientious about trifles
2) Company, aversion to
3) Suspicious
4) Occupation, amel.
5) Contradiction, is intolerant of
6) Anxiety, conscience, of
7) Anxiety, future, about

Secrecy

8) Consolation agg.
9) Talk, indisposed to

Fears

10) Fear, approaching him, of others
11) Fear, strangers, of
12) Fear, disease, of impending

Dullness

13) Dullness, sluggishness, difficulty of thinking and comprehending

Difficulty of Thinking

14) Memory, weakness of, words, for
15) Memory, weakness of, expressing one's self, for
16) Mistakes, writing, in

Difficulty of Comprehension

17) Confusion, dream, as if in
18) Excitement, night
19) Hurry
20) Quarrelsome
21) Contrary

Paranoia, Delusions, Obsessions

22) Thoughts, persistent
23) Reproaches himself
24) Thinking, complaints, of, agg.
25) Stomach, apprehension in

State of Mind

26) Chaotic
27) Loathing, life
28) Weeping, music, from
29) Suicidal disposition
30) Despair, religious (of salvation etc.)

REPERTORISATION – THUJA

	1	2	3	4	5	6	7	8	9	10	11	12	13	14	15	16	17	18	19	20	21	22	23	24	25	26	27	28	29	30
Thuj.	2	2	1	1	1	3	1	1	2	2	2	1	2	1	1	3	1	1	2	2	2	2	2	1	1	1	3	2	1	2
Ars.	2	–	3	–	1	3	–	2	2	–	–	1	1	–	–	1	–	–	2	2	1	2	2	1	–	2	3	–	2	3
Aur.	1	2	2	1	3	3	–	–	3	–	–	1	1	–	–	1	–	–	1	3	1	2	2	1	2	–	3	–	3	3
Bar-cb.	2	3	3	1	2	–	2	–	2	–	2	–	3	3	–	–	–	–	2	1	1	–	–	2	1	–	–	–	–	–
Bry.	1	2	3	–	–	–	3	–	1	–	–	1	3	–	–	–	1	–	2	2	–	1	–	2	1	–	–	–	–	–
Cham.	1	3	1	1	2	–	1	1	1	–	–	–	2	1	–	2	1	–	–	1	–	1	–	1	1	–	1	–	1	1
Ferr.	1	2	2	2	2	2	–	–	2	2	–	–	–	–	–	–	–	2	–	1	–	1	2	–	–	–	1	–	2	–
Hyos.	1	2	2	–	–	–	–	–	2	–	–	–	3	–	–	1	1	2	1	2	–	1	2	–	–	–	–	–	2	–
Ign.	3	3	–	2	3	2	–	3	2	2	–	–	1	–	–	1	1	1	2	1	1	1	2	–	–	1	1	–	1	1
Lyc.	2	2	3	2	3	2	2	1	2	2	–	–	3	2	2	3	–	–	2	3	1	2	1	–	2	2	2	2	1	2
Chin.	1	2	1	1	–	–	2	1	1	–	–	2	2	–	–	2	1	1	1	1	1	–	–	–	–	3	3	2	–	–
Nat-c.	2	2	2	2	1	2	2	1	2	–	–	2	3	2	2	1	–	2	2	2	2	2	–	–	–	1	1	1	2	2
Nux-v.	2	3	2	2	2	1	2	–	2	–	–	–	2	1	–	1	–	2	2	3	2	2	2	–	–	2	2	–	2	2
Puls.	1	2	3	–	–	1	2	–	3	–	–	–	3	–	–	1	–	1	1	–	1	1	2	–	–	2	2	–	2	2
Sep.	1	2	2	3	3	–	–	3	1	2	–	2	3	–	–	1	–	–	2	2	–	2	–	–	–	1	2	2	2	2
Sil.	3	3	1	1	2	2	1	3	1	–	1	–	3	–	–	1	–	–	1	2	1	–	–	–	–	–	2	–	2	2
Stram.	2	2	3	1	1	–	1	–	2	2	1	2	2	–	–	1	1	1	2	2	2	1	1	1	–	1	1	–	1	1
Staph.	–	–	1	–	–	–	2	1	2	–	–	–	3	–	–	1	–	–	–	1	–	–	–	–	–	1	1	–	–	–
Sulph.	2	2	3	–	–	2	1	–	3	–	–	1	3	2	1	1	1	2	2	2	2	2	2	–	–	2	2	–	1	2
Verat.	1	1	2	1	–	2	1	–	3	–	–	–	2	–	–	–	–	–	1	2	–	–	–	–	–	–	–	–	1	3

Minimum Characteristic Syndrome

1) Conscientious about trifles
2) Company, aversion to
3) Suspicious
4) Occupation, amel.
5) Contradiction, is intolerant of
6) Anxiety, conscience, of
7) Anxiety, future, about

Secrecy

8) Consolation agg.
9) Talk, indisposed to

Fears

10) Fear, approaching him, of others
11) Fear, strangers, of
12) Fear, disease, of impending

Dullness

13) Dullness, sluggishness, difficulty of thinking and comprehending

Difficulty of Thinking

14) Memory, weakness of, words, for
15) Memory, weakness of, expressing one's self, for
16) Mistakes, writing, in

Difficulty of Comprehension

17) Confusion, dream, as if in
18) Excitement, night
19) Hurry
20) Quarrelsome
21) Contrary

Paranoia, Delusions, Obsessions

22) Thoughts, persistent
23) Reproaches himself
24) Thinking, complaints, of, agg.
25) Stomach, apprehension in

State of Mind

26) Chaotic
27) Loathing, life
28) Weeping, music, from
29) Suicidal disposition
30) Despair, religious (of salvation etc.)

111

illuminates our spirits with shining examples of spiritual truth, beauty and love.

Man's quest for spiritual truth is hindered and, ultimately, blocked by the effects of the sycotic miasm. I feel therefore that the all-pervasive symptom 'Dullness' should rightly occupy a key position in the schematic portrait of Thuja. However, contradictory though it may seem, I have not included 'Dullness' in the Minimum Characteristic Syndrome of the remedy. This is because it is such a large rubric. When choosing MCS rubrics I seek out those with more than twenty remedies and fewer than one hundred. This results after the repertorisation in a good number, but not an excess, of remedies for the purposes of comparison.

To the left of centre, we can place the symptoms that describe the difficulties of thinking, 'Memory, weakness of, words, for' (14), 'Memory, weakness of, expressing oneself, for' (15) and 'Mistakes, writing, in' (16). To the right of centre, we can place the symptom concerned with difficulty of comprehension and consequent evasion of reality, 'Confusion, dream, as if in' (17).

Above the centre, we can place another essential characteristic, not only of Thuja but of all sycotic remedies – egotism, with its corresponding manifestations of positive and negative aggression to the right, with two arrows that are indicative of the connections between the elements of egotism, lack of comprehension and constructive/destructive aggression and, to the left, the other side of egotism, i.e. guilt, secrecy and fear.

In the bottom right-hand corner, under the heading Paranoia, we can place the symptoms of delusion that are caused by the basic conflicts between his sense of right and wrong and his aggressive competitiveness. In the bottom left-hand corner, under the heading Obsessions, we can place the symptoms concerned with the typically sycotic fixed ideas. At the bottom, under the heading State of mind, we can place those symptoms that reinforce his depression and feed his guilt.

COMPARATIVE MATERIA MEDICA

Nux Vomica

The reader should refer to the chapter on Lycopodium for a fuller discussion of this remedy.

Nux Vomica is the only remedy with all seven symptoms of the Minimum Characteristic Syndrome of Thuja. Here we have a perfectionist ('Conscientious about trifles', 1) who wastes not a moment of his precious time in the company of idle people ('Company, aversion to', 2), especially when he needs peace and quiet to unwind and recuperate from the effects of his toxic diet. He is hypersensitive to the opinions of others and readily takes offence. He is single-minded in his ambitions ('Contradiction, is intolerant of', 5) and refuses to take a break from work ('Occupation, amel.', 4), because he knows that 'time and tide wait for no man' and he fears the future ('Anxiety, future, about', 7). Like Edgar Allan Poe, he has no faith in his ability to succeed ('Succeeds, never': *1*) nor in the people around him ('Suspicious', 3). To relieve his state of perpetual nervous tension and to avoid all external stimuli (notably from noise, smells, cold and pain), he longs for a tranquil haven where no-one will talk to him ('Talk, indisposed to', 9) or try to interfere in his life ('Consolation agg.', 8). The combination of sycotic disruption and psoric hypersensitivity brings about feelings of guilt ('Anxiety, conscience, of', 6).

Whereas Thuja deals with his problems by withdrawing into himself, Nux Vomica finds it all intensely irritating. Nux has no fear of strangers (11), nor does he mind being approached (10). Nux Vomica's mind ceases to function ('Dullness', 13) when he is exhausted, Thuja's when he is confused; Nux Vomica becomes confused after a meal, whereas Thuja's confusion has a dreamlike quality. Neither remedy can understand the true meaning of life: Nux Vomica is too involved in his oversensitive reactions, and Thuja in his obsessions. Whereas Thuja is acutely conscious of his own mistakes, Nux Vomica has no such self-awareness, and while he may know what guilt is ('Anxiety, conscience, of', 6), he will always blame other people rather than himself (23).

Eventually, exhaustion and depression take their toll and Nux Vomica starts to hate life ('Loathing, life', 27); he toys with the idea of committing suicide but, like China, lacks the courage to do so. Thuja's self-destructive urges are held in check only by his fanatical religious beliefs; and, should these start to waver, he may find suddenly that he can no longer live with the utter confusion and despair. To sum up: while Nux Vomica may have many sycotic features in common with Thuja, it can be easily distinguished by such symptoms as the impulsiveness, the sensitivity to the feelings and opinions of others and the psoric sense of righteousness.

Aurum, China, Natrum Carbonicum and Stramonium all have six symptoms of the Minimum Characteristic Syndrome of Thuja.

Aurum

The following comparative study is a good example of the importance of considering a symptom, or series of symptoms, in the context of the whole life experience of the patient, rather than categorising symptoms automatically into miasmatic groups. Aurum, one of our great syphilitic remedies, has six out of seven symptoms of the Minimum Characteristic Syndrome of Thuja, a great sycotic remedy. As discussed in previous chapters, Aurum's essential characteristics are syphilitic destructiveness and low self-esteem. Compared with the self-sufficient Thuja, he feels a complete failure; he can neither do what is expected of him ('Anxiety, conscience, of', 6) nor keep his friends. Although he feels guilty about neglecting his duty, he does not have the fear of the wrath of God that engenders, in Thuja, the anxiety about the future (7).

He will explode with uncontrollable rage when contradicted ('Contradiction, is intolerant of', 5), humiliated or hurt. The force of his destructive feelings worries him: the attacks of angina pectoris with thoracic oppression serve as early warning signals of a suicidal nature. He blames himself for everything ('Reproaches himself', 23) and believes ('Suspicious', 3) that he has lost the trust of his friends. Basically, he is an introvert who prefers his own company ('Company, aversion to', 2), to brood on the object of his unrequited passion and wallow in his feelings of isolation and resentment of those who have deserted him.

To compensate for his inferiority complex, he devotes himself to the pursuit of perfection ('Conscientious about trifles', 1) in his work ('Occupation, amel.', 4).

At times he is too depressed to speak (9), but finds reassurance in consolation (hence his absence from symptom 8) as it contradicts his fear of abandonment. Unlike Thuja, he does not make a great secret of everything, and therefore has no reason to fear strangers (11) or being approached (10).

Although he has a dull mind and a poor memory (13), he does not feature in any of the specific weaknesses (14, 15 and 16). His ambitious and insecure nature shows itself in the peremptory way in which he deals with people ('Hurry', 19, 'Quarrelsome', 20 and 'Contrary', 21).

In true syphilitic style, Aurum gets confused when he tries to use his mind ('Confusion, mental exertion, from': 2), whereas Thuja's confusion is more typical of sycosis, focusing as it does on his identity and his position. He loses his way in familiar streets, has no idea who he is, and feels as if he is in a dream.

Aurum does not adhere to sycotic fixed ideas (22). He is consumed with guilt and remorse (23), and the more he thinks about how bad and worthless he is, the worse he feels (24) and his stomach tightens with fear (25). In Thuja, guilt has a modifying effect upon his egocentric and libertine character. The absence of symptoms 26 and 28 is not significant here.

Both remedies, under the influence of sycosis and syphilis respectively, are intent on self-destruction. Eventually they reach a point where they have had enough ('Loathing, life', 27), they can find no solace in religion (30) and they long to put an end to it all ('Suicidal disposition', 29). But the sycotic suicide, enacted by Thuja, would be an ostentatious performance, designed to disturb the maximum number of people – an act of religious devotion in obedience to a command from a superhuman power. The syphilitic suicide, personified in Aurum, would be a desperate response to the enormous guilt he feels for neglecting his duties. Through suicide, Thuja frees himself from the chains of guilt, cheats on death and finds immortality. Aurum's final wish is to reject the life that has rejected him and to silence, once and for all, the voices that urge him on to his death.

China (*See also* pages 55–7)

China has the first nine symptoms of Thuja, with the exception of symptom 5. He has a great dislike of people ('Company, aversion to', 2) whom he suspects ('Suspicious', 3) of being to blame for his misfortune, and whose kind words of sympathy and attempts at conversation he rejects ('Consolation agg.', 8 and 'Talk, indisposed to', 9). Thuja, on the other hand, is the complete master of himself and uninterested in others, so long as they do not interfere in his licentious and nefarious activities.

Thuja's fear of the future is tied up with his obsessive guilt, whereas to China the future represents the unattainable ('Anxiety, future, about', 7). Guilt, in Thuja, transforms into a pattern of compulsive, ritualistic behaviour, whereas in China it explains his characteristic fear of dogs and his persecution complex ('Anxiety, conscience, of', 6). Unlike Thuja, China has nothing to hide from the gaze of other people

(11 and 12). The absence of symptom 5 emphasises a significant difference between the two remedies: for Thuja, any expression of opposition threatens to expose his duplicity or to put a stop to his immoral ways; China, by contrast, has a streak of near anarchic rebelliousness that is calculated to destroy anyone who ventures near and, what is more, he lets everyone know about his predilection for violence.

But let us not forget the other side of China, the philosopher, the nocturnal architect of a thousand castles in the air who diligently ('Occupation, amel.', 4) weaves countless, detailed ('Conscientious about trifles', 1) plans, locked away in his ivory tower where he can safely heap all the blame for his problems on other people and nurture the chip on his shoulder ('Quarrelsome', 20).

Understandably, he suffers from the same dream-like confusion as Thuja (17) but his memory remains intact. He is neither 'Contrary', (21) nor hasty ('Hurry', 19). He does, however, suffer from fixed ideas (22) and a weariness of life (27) that may push him to the thought of suicide (29), particularly at night, during a fever, or when he feels run down, but it never comes to anything because he lacks the courage to go through with it.

Natrum Carbonicum

Decline of physical strength and impairment of the nervous system combine in this remedy to create a profoundly depressed and melancholic individual. Kent says of Natrum Carbonicum: 'Estrangement from family and friends. Aversion to mankind and to society; to relatives, to strangers' (*Lectures on Homoeopathic Materia Medica*, p. 708). Like Thuja and Sepia, the feeling that a great void separates him from others is exacerbated when he is in their company ('Company, aversion to', 2), and he just wants to be left alone in peace ('Talk, indisposed to', 9). He suffers from flatulence and acid dyspepsia which are aggravated by the sun; he has great sensitivity to noise, pain and emotion, and the sound of gentle music fills him with nostalgia and makes him weep and tremble (28).

With a remedy that is so dissimilar to Thuja, it may surprise the reader to know that China has seven of the first nine symptoms. It is worth reiterating here that a collection of isolated symptoms is meaningless if it has no reference to the whole character of the remedy.

Natrum Carbonicum is a timid, insecure and lonely person who has no faith in himself; he sees himself as a failure who can do nothing right. In a half-hearted attempt to counter his feelings of insecurity, he reacts angrily to contradiction ('Contradiction, is intolerant of', 5) and strives for perfection ('Conscientious about trifles', 1) in his work ('Occupation, amel.', 4). Above all, he needs to be loved, comforted (absent from symptom 8) and cared for, but he cannot trust ('Suspicious', 3) those who have deserted him in his hour of need, although he feels great compassion for those worse off than himself.

This sensitive and vulnerable individual is fearful of the slightest thing and easily startled (he fears robbers, crowds and storms and jumps at noises) but he has no guilty secrets, hence his absence from symptoms 10 and 11.

Such is the extent of his exhaustion that he feels dizzy if he tries to use his mind ('Dullness', 13 and 'Memory, weakness of, words, for', 14) although he is, unlike Thuja, well able to communicate his thoughts if he chooses (absent from symptoms 14 and 15). Despite his physical weakness, he has a strong fighting spirit that reveals itself through symptoms such as 'Quarrelsome' (13) and 'Hurry' (19). Unlike Thuja, he is free from the consuming and destructive effects of guilt (6, 22, 23, 24, and 30) and, although he may be discontented with his lot and weary of living (27), he is not the type to take his own life (29).

Stramonium

The reader should refer to the chapter on Lachesis, pages 283–5, for a fuller picture of Stramonium, which has six of the seven symptoms of the Minimum Characteristic Syndrome of Thuja. More sinned against than sinning, this member of the *Solanaceae* family is, like Natrum Muriaticum, full of bitterness and resentment. Unwanted and unloved, he mistrusts everyone (3) and envies them their good fortune. He tries to rise above his feelings of worthlessness by doing good work ('Occupation, amel.', 4), and paying great attention to small details (1). He is so unsure of himself that he cannot bear being contradicted (5) and he lets rip in a fit of rage, only to feel guilty later for his lack of self-control ('Anxiety, conscience, of', 6) and worried about his future prospects (7).

His fear of being abandoned is so great that he swallows his feelings of resentment ('Talk, indisposed to', 9) and, unlike Thuja, allows himself to be comforted (8).

Although he has nothing to hide, he is afraid of strangers (11) and of being approached (10) because he is haunted by the fears of evil, darkness and solitude.

117

He has problems with thinking ('Dullness', 13), especially on waking, writing (16) and remembering names, people, what he has just said and what he is about to say.

At times, he gives free reign to his homicidal thoughts ('Thoughts, persistent', 22), unchecked by self-reproach (23), but he lacks symptoms 18, 21, 24 and 26 which are indicative of the disruption and discord that Thuja carelessly creates all around him, insensitive to everything except, perhaps, the sound of music. Stramonium is a victim of the effects, both of sycosis – in his dishonesty, conflicts, loquacity, lasciviousness, clairvoyance, megalomania, arrogance and perfectionism, and also of syphilis – in his explosions of violent rage and homicidal urges. In the final stages of his illness he despairs of his redemption (30), gives up on life (27) and decides to slash his wrist or throw himself to his death (29).

The following ten remedies have five symptoms of the Minimum Characteristic Syndrome of Thuja: Baryta Carbonica, Bryonia, Ferrum Metallicum, Ignatia, Lycopodium, Pulsatilla, Sepia, Silicea, Sulphur and Veratrum Album.

Baryta Carbonica

The missing symptoms here are numbers 5 and 6. Baryta Carbonica is typically seen in the slow-witted child who is painfully shy and easily embarrassed. He is so frightened that people will laugh at him that he hides behind the furniture when visitors call at the house.

The Baryta Carbonica adult is a childish simpleton bordering on the mentally retarded. In an attempt to shield himself from the imagined scorn and derision of other people, he dedicates himself to domestic tasks ('Occupation, amel.', 14) with a faultless attention to detail (1). The effects of the syphilitic miasm have eroded his confidence to such a degree that he is incapable of making even unimportant decisions.

He is convinced ('Suspicious', 3) that he is the subject of much gossip, and he avoids people for this reason ('Company, aversion to', 2 and 'Fear, strangers, of', 11). He feels better in his own company ('Talk, indisposed to', 9), although it takes very little to upset him.

He feels so wretchedly alone in the world that, unlike Thuja, he longs for some sympathetic (8) human contact (10).

The syphilitic miasm affects his brain ('Dullness, sluggishness', 13) and his memory; words escape him (14), and he forgets what he is about to do and what he has done or said.

His childish way of dealing with his lack of confidence is to hurry himself up (19) and to pick quarrels with people ('Quarrelsome', 20 and 'Contrary', 21).

The characteristic delusion of Baryta Carbonica that he walks on his knees ('Delusions, knees, that he walks on': 2) provides us with the perfect image of one of society's outcasts who depends for his survival upon the support and generosity of others and is full of self-pity (24).

Bryonia

Bryonia lacks the symptoms 'Occupation, amel.' (4) and 'Anxiety, conscience of' (6) from the Minimum Characteristic Syndrome of Thuja. The reader may remember from our discussion of this remedy in the chapter on Lycopodium that its characteristics are weakness on a physical level, with strong aggravation from motion and a determined strength of will. Driven by a great fear of poverty, he works at his job from morning until night, dreams of work and, when he falls ill, worries about the time he is wasting.

He is a true perfectionist (1) who feels so disadvantaged physically that he responds to opinions that differ from his own with great irritation ('Contradiction, is intolerant of', 5). To minimise the strain of human contact, and the stress headaches caused by people who try to put him down, he avoids others as much as he can (2). On a mental level, the keynotes are: resentment, vexation and the desire to return home. Consequently he is unaffected by signs of people's support (8) and has no time for idle talk (9).

Psoric weakness and sycotic industriousness create a highly volatile individual who is unpredictable and untrusting (3), who is wary, rather than fearful, of strangers (11) and disturbed if they try to come too close (10). His vulnerability is expressed by the churning stomach (25) and the large number of specific fears: the fear of disease (12), poverty, solitude, evil, insanity and death.

He has the sluggish mind that is typical of the sycotic miasm ('Dullness, sluggishness', 13) but suffers no impairment of memory.

His erratic and impulsive nature accounts for the rubrics 'Hurry', (19) and 'Quarrelsome', (20), but he is not aggressively contrary (21) like the self-centred Thuja.

He is completely free from guilt (6), self-condemnation (23) and circling thoughts (22); but his mind is preoccupied with the disease ('Thinking, complaints, of, agg.', 24) which hinders all normal activity and for which he is desperate to find a cure.

His materialistic greed, fear of poverty and despair of recovery are indications of someone who is too attached to this earth to want to leave it – hence his absence from symptoms 26, 27, 28, 29 and 30.

Ferrum Metallicum (*See also* pages 47–8)

Ferrum Metallicum is dogmatic in his assertions and overbearing in his manner. He is too self-assured to need sympathy (8), or to be concerned with other people's motives (3) or with what the future may hold (7). He sets himself very high standards ('Conscientious about trifles', 1) in his work ('Occupation, amel.', 4) by way of sycotic compensation for his physical problems. His conscience (6) protests at his domineering, excitable ('Excitement, night', 18) and argumentative nature. He is easily distinguished from Thuja by the lack of distrust, the absence of anxiety about the future and the dictatorial aspect.

Ignatia

Ignatia affects the nervous system, causing hysteria, great fluctuations of mood and paradoxical and changeable mental and physical symptoms. She expresses her emotions mainly through physical symptoms that develop after anger ('Anger, ailments after': *3*), suppressed anger ('Anger, ailments after, suppressed, from': *2*), anger with suppressed grief ('Anger, ailments after, with silent grief': *3*), mortification ('Mortification, ailments after': *3*), and fright ('Fright, complaints from': *3*). Her unstable and contradictory emotional states only serve to worsen her feelings of insecurity and uncertainty. She feels so guilty for her lack of consistency ('Anxiety, conscience, of', 6) and so confused by the emotional inner turmoil that her self-confidence is non-existent and she finds fault with every little thing she does ('Conscientious about trifles', 1). She will make erratic attempts to get involved in some work ('Occupation, amel.', 4) if left to her own devices ('Contradiction, is intolerant of', 5).

Although she cannot find the reason for her problems within herself, she would not dream of blaming anyone else. She becomes introspective ('Company, aversion to', 2) and withdrawn ('Talk, indisposed to', 9 and 'Consolation agg.', 8). Unlike Thuja, she is not mistrustful (3), anxious about the future (7) or secretive (11), although she is frightened of being accosted (10) by robbers, especially if she wakes in the night.

The emotional instability is responsible for the dulling of the mental faculties (13), and the difficulties in writing (16), although the memory is unaffected (14 and 15). It also accounts for the hurried actions (19) and the argumentative (20) and contrary disposition (21) in this highly-strung, bewildered ('Confusion, dream, as if in', 17), impressionable and likeable patient.

Little as she understands herself, she feels that she is to blame for her lack of constancy ('Reproaches himself', 23 and 'Thoughts, persistent', 22). She does not have symptoms 18, 24 and 25. Her profound religious beliefs intensify her tendency to self-condemnation (30)

In contrast to Thuja, Ignatia does not take her problems so much to heart and would not want to take her own life (27 and 29), except on the very rare occasion when the violence of her suppressed emotions gets the better of her and she kills herself in a fit of hysteria.

Lycopodium

While it is true that Lycopodium has seven of the first nine symptoms in common with Thuja, his essential nature is completely different. The picture of Thuja is a unique mixture of egotism, guilt, irascibility, mental dullness and degeneracy, whereas the sycotic Lycopodium toils ceaselessly to prove that he is neither useless nor ineffectual ('Occupation, amel.', 4). He is one of life's great perfectionists ('Conscientious about trifles', 1) who is justly proud of his intelligence. He hates being contradicted (5) because it offends his pride and shakes his confidence. Unlike Thuja, he has a great fear of being alone, although he will express his need for company in the most roundabout and complex way, because he has a basic distrust ('Suspicious', 3) of people and feels at his most vulnerable in their company ('Company, aversion to', 2). Paradoxically, he is both better and worse when alone, like Ambra Grisea, Bovista and Phosphorus.

He is too arrogant to feel guilty (6) or anxious about the future (7), although he does have anticipatory anxiety, the delusion that he has neglected his duty, a love of power and the fear of being unable to reach the destiny that Fate has reserved for him. Beneath the facade of superiority and reserve (8, 9 and 10), he hides great weakness of character, while Thuja hides a predilection for immoral and self-indulgent acts. Lycopodium's mental sluggishness (13) comes from liver dysfunction and circulatory disturbances that are improved by walking in the open air. He keeps such a tight hold on himself that his body rebels by feeling uncomfortably hot in tight clothing and enclosed spaces. Whereas Thuja feels weighed down by the heavy burden he has to carry, Lycopodium feels much better when he is on the move – his feelings of anxiety, confusion and dullness are all dispelled by walking in the open air.

He is a strict self-disciplinarian who blames himself for failing to reach his unrealistically high standards ('Reproaches himself', 23).

With the affinity for gastric complaints and fluctuations of appetite, which can increase with eating, and be either easily satisfied or insatiable at night, it is not surprising that he suffers from apprehension in the stomach (25). In Thuja, this symptom takes on the entirely different sense of duplication when considered alongside symptoms such as the sensation of being pregnant, of foetal-like movements in the abdomen, and of protusions like fists from the abdomen.

When Lycopodium believes that he has lost the fight, he falls into a state of utter despondency (27) and indifference. In one of his authoritative lectures on materia medica, Kent says: 'The world may come to an end, or the whole family may die or the house may burn up' (*Lectures on Homoeopathic Materia Medica*, p. 646). In despair ('Despair, religious', 30), his thoughts turn to suicide (29), especially when he wakes in the morning. When the sycotic aspect is predominant this remedy may easily be confused with Thuja; but when given appropriately, it will bring love into the patient's life, banishing pride and vanity, and penetrating deep into the psyche to reveal the emotional suffering caused by the deprivation of paternal love. Fear of solitude, compassion for the suffering of others and weeping when thanked are symptoms that complete the picture of Lycopodium.

Pulsatilla (*See also* pages 64–5)

Pulsatilla has six of the first nine symptoms of Thuja. So great is her desire for approval that she always tries to be perfect ('Conscientious about trifles', 7) and when she feels ill or depressed she withdraws into herself ('Company, aversion to', 2 and 'Talk, indisposed to', 9), because she does not wish to drain her friends or push them away ('Suspicious', 3). She feels guilty ('Anxiety, conscience, of', 6) because she is afraid of growing up, and the young Pulsatilla mother weeps for the loss of her innocence. She would like to postpone her maturity indefinitely and is intimidated by all thoughts of the future (7). She lacks symptoms 4, 5, 10 and 11 – far from avoiding people, she will actively seek them out.

Pulsatilla is not such a heavily sycotic remedy as Thuja and lacks symptoms 17 and 20. If she hears that someone is in trouble, she will hurry (19) to finish whatever she is doing and rush to their side. Her capricious nature accounts for the symptom 'Contrary' (21), rather than any real wish to be obstructive. She imagines that she has done wrong, or made a mistake, and reproaches herself (23) constantly ('Thoughts, persistent', 22), especially at night. She feels worse when she thinks (24) or talks about her problems. Like the wind that dispels the gloom, her problems can be blown away by a kind word. Pulsatilla, the windflower, is like a gentle, lonely child who is too afraid to show how she really feels.

Sepia

The cuttlefish is the only mollusc that leaves her eggs once she has laid them. Emotional indifference is the key to this tri-miasmatic remedy. Sepia has seven of the first nine symptoms of Thuja, lacking 6 and 7. She is indifferent to her loved ones, and her husband is the prime target for her envy of the male sex. Just as the cuttlefish makes its escape behind a cloud of ink, so does Sepia try to avoid people (2) by lying down with her eyes closed and her mouth shut ('Talk, indisposed to', 9). She hates fuss and sympathy (8) and feels much better when alone. Devoid of all love for humanity, she is driven by the need to compete with and prove herself against the opposite sex (hence symptoms 1, 3, 4 and 5 and the irritability before menses, 'Irritability, menses, before': 2, which Thuja does not have).

She is too tough to succumb to fear, hence the absence from symptoms 10 and 11; neither is there anything wrong with her memory, except when she gets tired. Her mind slows down (13) at times when her energy is low and her circulation becomes sluggish, such as in the afternoon, after eating and after coition. Such complete emotional detachment means that she never feels the slightest trace of guilt (6 and 23), but she can eventually become drained and deadened by her very indifference, to the extreme where she sees no point at all in carrying on (27) and wants to die (29).

It might be difficult to distinguish between Thuja and Sepia in one-sided sycotic cases, but the secret lies in the presence or absence of guilt; there is almost always some element of guilt in a Thuja case, while the Sepia fear of poverty could be mistaken for anxiety about the future.

The vehemence with which Sepia defends her principles, her immediate willingness to let others take the blame, the total refusal to conform, the single-mindedness of her ambition and the way she dismisses her family, give us some idea of the measure of her indifference. She may say that she is afraid of being alone or that her husband might leave her, or that she hates herself, but if you read between the lines and listen to what she leaves out, you will hear the true voice of Sepia. As a cured Sepia patient once told me: 'Before the remedy, I used to miss my husband when he went away because I was frightened of being alone but, when he came back, I was glad to see him only for the extra help around the house. I begrudged the attention I had to give him. Now that I am cured, I find that I miss him because I love him, I can't wait to see him again and I enjoy doing things for him; I used to think that I had a lot to put up with, but now I realise that I just didn't know how to love.'

Silicea

The Minimum Characteristic Syndrome of Silicea is lack of self-confidence, timidity, perfectionism and obstinacy. Unlike Thuja, he is not addicted to the pursuit of pleasure and is neither averse to company (2) nor anxious for the future (7). He is acutely conscious of his inadequacies, and rather than manipulating circumstances to suit himself, he is always measuring himself against other people and trying to achieve some recognition of his worth through diligent ('Occupation, amel.', 4) and painstaking (1) efforts. The paradox of Silicea is that he wants to stand on his own two feet but also needs a crutch to lean on. When he feels strong, he can be stubborn, irritable and intolerant of contradiction (5); and when he feels weak he needs to be taken in hand and told exactly what to do. Whereas Thuja feels exposed and threatened by consolation, Silicea feels undermined (8). Silicea does not have the Thuja fears of people (10 and 11), although he is very self-conscious about appearing in public.

His physical debility affects and weakens the mind ('Dullness', 13). His feeble attempts at self-assertion account for symptoms 19 and 21 ('Hurry' and 'Contrary'). When life gets too much (27) he may try to drown himself (29).

While Thuja and Silicea may have certain features in common, such as obstinacy, perfectionism, industriousness, and intolerance of contradiction and of consolation, Silicea will gaze at the physician with an expression of great reverence that reveals how much faith he has in the doctor's wisdom and power to relieve him of his suffering.

Sulphur

Here, symptoms 4 and 5 are missing from the Minimum Characteristic Syndrome of Thuja. As discussed in the chapter on Lycopodium, the essential characteristics of Sulphur are egotism, lethargy and congestion – the conceited philosopher who looks at the world through rose-tinted spectacles. Whereas Thuja's life is devoted to the pursuit of pleasure at other people's expense, Sulphur will do anything for a quiet life. Thuja's deceitful and secretive ways of operating contrast sharply with the almost child-like cheerfulness with which Sulphur greets the world; he just cannot take life seriously.

Unlike Thuja, Sulphur is quite aware that his mind is not as good as it should be. When in health, he pays great attention to detail (1), probably to save himself the bother of having to repeat the task. He is too wrapped up in himself to be able to see the good in others ('Suspicious', 3). He worries about the future (7) because he, unlike Thuja, is frightened of failure and poverty.

While Thuja uses people for his own ends, Sulphur remains aloof. He avoids people (2), either because he cannot be bothered to talk (9) or because they drain his energy. Although he is not aggravated by consolation (8), it can disturb him and bring tears to his eyes because, despite his selfish nature, he worries about his friends.

He is too emotionally detached to be afraid of strangers (10 and 11).

As one would expect of this apathetic patient, his mind is slow (13) and his memory poor (the reader should refer to the chapter on Lycopodium for a fuller discussion of this). However, he will talk at length about his optimistic hypotheses and can express himself well enough, unlike Thuja (15).

He gets lost in his own little world ('Confusion, dream, as if in', 17) and will react angrily ('Quarrelsome', 20 and 'Contrary', 21) if his quiet reveries are disturbed. At times he is impulsive ('Hurry', 19) and excitable ('Excitement, night', 18).

Unlike Thuja, Sulphur indulges in no morbid self-analysis, hence the absence of symptoms 23, 24 and 25. He clings to his fantasies ('Thoughts, persistent', 22), such as the delusion that his dirty, old clothes look wonderful ('Delusions, old rags are as fine as silk': 3), whereas Thuja has the fixed idea that his soul is separated from his body.

As he nears the end of his life, he has to face the fact that he has accomplished absolutely nothing, and he is swamped by feelings of guilt ('Anxiety, conscience, of', 6). In his despair (30), he gives up on life (27) and tries to end it all (29) by drowning.

125

Veratrum Album

Here, suspicion (3) and intolerance of contradiction (5) are missing. This remedy is discussed in greater depth in the chapter on Lachesis, so suffice it to say that Veratrum Album is characterised by lack of self-confidence, timidity, and fear of evil, of misfortune and of the future (7). This tri-miasmatic remedy is consumed by an overwhelming ambition that demands fulfilment at any price. On his way up the ladder, he will use people for as long as they have something to offer. He cannot afford to be mistrustful (3) or intolerant ('Contradiction, is intolerant of', 5) if he wants to keep people on his side.

He is hard-working ('Occupation, amel.', 4) and exacting ('Conscientious about trifles', 1). He treats his superiors with great respect, but his inferiors bear the full brunt of his ruthlessness, although he can feel guilty afterwards ('Anxiety, conscience, of', 6). His scheming mind works better when he is on his own ('Company, aversion to', 2 and 'Talk, indisposed to', 9). He remains detached, even when people offer him sympathy (8).

Although Veratrum is generally fearful of the dark side of life, he lacks the specific Thuja fears (10 and 11). His mind is dull (13) and he forgets people and what he has just said.

The perfect diplomat in all his dealings, he makes it his business not to be difficult (21), although he can be impatient (19) and argumentative (20) at times.

Whereas Thuja believes that he is under the control of a superhuman power (22 to 25), Veratrum Album goes one stage further: he states, clearly and categorically – that he is in direct communication with God or that he is Jesus Christ.

Sooner or later he swings to the other extreme, to the conviction that God has deserted him, and a profound depression takes hold of him as he realises that he has been left stranded, cut off from both humans and God ('Despair, religious', 30). At times he sits brooding in silence, and at others he is gripped by a sudden, violent urge to curse and swear and destroy everything within reach; episodes of violent mania, during which he may swallow his own excrement, alternate with periods of taciturnity.

One day he will jump to his death from an open window (29).

5

Medorrhinum

DESCRIPTION

In the preceding chapter on Thuja Occidentalis, we discussed the concepts of individuality and altruism, how the tendency for egotism can start as a compensatory reaction of the small child to the world around him and how the quality of altruism can foster the realisation of what Hahnemann considered to be humanity's highest ideals and greatest potential for maturity and self-development. The sycotic miasm blocks such a beneficial process. In cases where psora and syphilis are involved, despair, fearfulness and feelings of inadequacy combine to create the deep feelings of insecurity that are so characteristic of the tubercular diathesis. In an attempt to counteract the trend towards destruction and certain death, the vital force reacts by creating proliferation and overgrowth.

Hence, it is clear that all feelings of insecurity and attempts at self-affirmation are simply indications of a deeply ingrained constitutional predisposition or miasm.

In Medorrhinum, the elements of sexuality and aggression are tempered by a strongly tubercular influence that is not present in Thuja. A typical example of this is the Medorrhinum baby who, unlike the overweight Thuja child, is small, pale, weak, underweight and anaemic, with chronic catarrh and adenoids, and as slow in his mental and physical development as the Baryta Carbonica child.

Although Thuja and Medorrhinum are both considered to be typical sycotic remedies, the tubercular taint is much more marked in the latter, and their mental and physical pathologies are quite different.

Thuja's symptom picture is of fully developed sycosis, whereas Medorrhinum is a tubercular remedy with the beginnings of sycosis. In Medorrhinum the emphasis is on destructive urges and feelings of insecurity, rather than on the tendency for proliferation, and these form the basis for the mental and physical symptomatology.

A sluggish mind, an aggressive sexuality and a propensity for anti-social behaviour are the sycotic aspects of the remedy. His physical problems make him feel inadequate and vulnerable, and he tries desperately to repress his true nature and behave in more socially acceptable ways that are quite unfamiliar to him.

Both Medorrhinum and Thuja have a guilty conscience for their sins – the former reacts with tubercular insecurity and fearfulness, while the latter hits back with an aggressive egotism. The three main aspects of Medorrhinum are guilt, insecurity, and fear; in Thuja, they are guilt, egotism, and irritability. In Medorrhinum, these aspects are closely interlinked, and form the basis for the whole mental framework. Kent did not attach the same importance to the nosodes as he did to the other remedies. This is demonstrated by the fact that there are many symptoms of Medorrhinum in his materia medica which cannot be found in his *Repertory*. I have turned, therefore, to Allen's *Materia Medica of the Nosodes*, which I believe to be the best study.

The physical symptoms of the Medorrhinum baby are far more impressive, on first sight, than its mental ones. According to the materia medica, the classic picture is one of nasal catarrh, conjunctivitis, a sweaty face with herpetic eruptions, a pale yellowish complexion with yellow at the edges of the scalp, a large head, an excoriating nappy rash, and a tendency to lie in the knee-chest position; in addition to this, there are burning pains, and a sycotic family background, possibly, although not necessarily, with a history of venereal disease. On a mental level, the outstanding characteristic is 'Restlessness': 2). The Medorrhinum child is a veritable *enfant terrible*: hyperactive, moody, rebellious and wild.

When his natural hyperactivity is controlled, his temper becomes worse, especially during the daytime, in accordance with the general time modality of the remedy ('Daytime': 2). Syphilinum, by contrast, is worse from sunset to sunrise. As soon as the sun starts to set, the child becomes happy and playful ('Mood alternating': *1*, 'Cross through day, exhilarated at night, wants to play', H. C. Allen, *Materia Medica of the Nosodes*, p. 299; 'Exhilaration': *1*, with the sub-rubric 'night': 2 – only remedy).

His basic lack of confidence makes him timid ('Timidity': *1*)and fearful. Darkness frightens him ('Fear, dark': 2) and he feels too uneasy to sleep ('Restlessness, night': 2). While others sleep, he wakes up frightened (Waking, as from fright': 3). It will soon become apparent that this symptom is significant when found in the adult.

The main characteristics of the Medorrhinum child are similar to those of Baryta Carbonica: timidity, anxiety and nocturnal fears, with delayed development and slow growth.

Medorrhinum has a very bad memory, a common feature of sycosis. In fact, there are only two rubrics in Kent's *Repertory* where Medorrhinum features in black type: 'Memory, weakness of' and 'Hurry'. Medorrhinum is one of our greatest weakness of memory remedies: he cannot even remember what he has just finished reading ('Memory, weakness of, read, for what has': *2*); he forgets the names of his best friends, and even his own name ('Memory, weakness of, names, for proper': *2*, 'Forgetful, name, his own': *2*); he loses the thread of the conversation ('Forgetful, words, of, while speaking': *2*); he makes mistakes in pronunciation and spelling, and words seem wrongly spelt ('Mistakes, spelling, in': *2*); if he is distracted in mid-sentence, he loses the train of his thoughts ('Memory, weakness of, said, for what has': *2* and 'Memory, weakness of, thought, for what has just': *2*) and cannot recollect them ('Memory, weakness of, say, for what is about to': *2*); in addition to this, he is unable to find the right words to express himself ('Memory, weakness of, words, for': *1*).

His problems are greatly magnified in the consulting room, with the additional stress created by his anticipatory anxiety and fear of disease, aspects of the remedy that will be explored later in greater depth. He finds it very difficult to give his symptoms to the homoeopath ('Great difficulty in stating her symptoms, loses herself and has to be asked over again', Allen, *op. cit.*, p. 296). I consider that two further rubrics should be added to the repertories – 'Memory, weakness of, stating her symptoms, for': *2*, and 'Stating her symptoms, great difficulty in, loses herself and has to be asked over and over again': *2*. If he has not come to the consultation armed with a list of all the symptoms carefully recorded in a notebook, he has to be prompted repeatedly by the physician to explain what he means.

The memory is bad for abstract things such as names, thoughts and words, rather than for the more concrete things that Thuja has trouble remembering, such as events that have happened. Medorrhinum should be added to the rubric 'Memory, weakness of, expressing one's self, for'. The lack of memory is aggravated by the inability to concentrate, especially on abstract subjects ('Concentration, difficult': *2* and 'Difficulty in concentrating his thoughts or mind on abstract subjects', Allen, *op. cit.*, p. 296). 'Concentration, difficult, abstract subjects': *2*).

The difficulty of self-expression, caused by the sudden vanishing of his thoughts ('Thoughts, vanishing of': *1*; 'Thoughts, loss of, caused by sensation of tightness in brain': *2*, Candegabe; 'Momentary loss of thought, caused by sensation of tightness in brain', Allen, *op. cit.* p. 296), is often accompanied by a sensation of constriction around the head, or of a weight on the vertex ('Dullness': *1*; 'Dullness, from weight on vertex: *1*, Candegabe; 'Weight on vertex, which seems to affect mind' Allen, *op. cit.*, p. 296) – a strange, wild feeling ('Wild feeling in head': *2*) that defies explanation.

The typical sensations of sycosis are those of constriction and protrusion, or drawing outwards, and they are present in several head symptoms of Medorrhinum, for example, 'Eye, pain, drawing outward': *1* and 'Head, constriction, band or hoop': *1*.

The remedy's peculiar combination of a sluggish mind, anticipatory anxiety ('Anticipation, complaints from': *1*) and the tendency to rush things ('Hurry': *3*) distinguishes it from all others. The two latter symptoms have far-reaching implications. The deterioration of his mental faculties shatters his self-confidence ('Confidence, want of self': *1*, Candegabe) and brings on the anticipatory anxiety ('Seems to herself to make wrong statements . . .' 'Dread of saying the wrong thing when she has headache' Allen, *op. cit.*, p. 296; 'Mistakes, headache, during': *1*, Candegabe). All intellectual effort places a great stress on his mind and creates tremendous anxiety and tension.

The symptom most frequently associated with this remedy is 'Hurry' and its precise meaning will be discussed at a later stage. For now, suffice it to say that it describes a state of uneasiness that compels him to walk faster than his mind can function; and deadlines put him under so much pressure that he cannot think straight ('Anxiety, time is set, if a': *1*). The anxiety and rushing about tires him out and he loses his ability to think ('Dullness, thinking, unable to, when weary' *1*, Candegabe), talk ('Talk, indisposed to, when weary, or listen, to talk': *1*, Candegabe) and listen. His head starts to ache with the typical sensation of a tight band, and he falls into a state of utter prostration: 'Could not read or use mind at all from pain in head' (*Op. cit.*, p. 296). 'Prostration of mind, headache, during': *1*, Candegabe and 'Head, pain, confusion, mental, with': *1*, Candegabe.

The slightest mental exertion disturbs and irritates him ('Irritability, reading, while': *1*, 'Irritability, writing, while': *1*; 'Irritability, trifles, from':*2*, *Synthetic Repertory*, Vol. I, 'Excitement, reading, while': *1* and 'Excitement, trifles, over': *1*). He tries to avoid headaches by writing down everything that he has to remember, even trivial things; he cannot trust his memory and thinks he is always making mistakes ('Conscientious about trifles': *1*, Barthel, *Synthetic Repertory*, Vol. I).

In a state of perpetual restlessness and mental exhaustion he lets the work pile up ('Undertakes everything, perseveres in nothing': *1*) and sinks into a state of agitated depression that allows him no rest. He promises himself that he will sort it all out tomorrow, but tomorrow never comes ('Dullness of memory and desire to procrastinate, because business seemed so lasting, or as if it never could be accomplished', Allen, *op. cit.*, p. 296; 'Procrastinate, desire to': *3*, Candegabe). The following morning, he wakes up feeling tired and lethargic ('Indolence, morning, waking, on': *1*, Candegabe), and cannot be bothered to do anything, even enjoyable things.

He cannot set his mind to his work ('Work, aversion to mental': *1*), and if he tries to do any ('Work, impossible': *2*) he is driven mad with frustration and despair ('Work, seems to drive him crazy, owing to the impotency of his mind': *1*).

He has no stamina to see things through to completion, due to the combination of restlessness, hurriedness and impatience ('Impatience': *2*), even with small things ('Impatience, trifles, about': *2*). His perception of time becomes distorted, and past events that once seemed to rush through his life are now remembered as if they had happened over a longer time span, and time seems to pass too slowly ('Time, passes too slowly': *2*). It is like a film shot at high speed that, when it is projected on to the screen, gives the illusion that everything is happening slowly. This also explains the delusion that the events of the day happened a long time ago ('Dazed feeling; a far off sensation, as though things done today occurred a week ago', Allen, *op. cit.*, p. 296). Furthermore, his distorted perception of time can confuse the present with the past ('Mistakes, time, in': *1*, with the sub-rubric 'confounds present with past': *1*), unlike Anacardium who confuses the present with the future.

He is too disorientated and confused ('Confusion of mind': *2*) to give a coherent account of his past. Everything has an unreal and dreamlike quality ('Dream, as if in a': *1* and 'Delusion, unreal, everything seems': *2*) and even familiar things seem strange to him ('Delusions, strange, familiar things seem': *1*).

I would like to make one last point about the question of anxiety and hurriedness. At the beginning of this chapter I said that Medorrhinum's guilt was a reaction to his unstable sycotic behaviour and that it was accompanied by tubercular feelings of insecurity and fear. In fact, I would go so far as to say that the determining factors of Medorrhinum are guilt and fear. Hurriedness is significant in that it expresses his wish to escape from the aggressive impulses that are buried deep in his subconscious; impulses that are projected on to the outside world in the guise of fears of external aggressors.

The classic mental picture of the Medorrhinum patient is someone who is speedy, anxious and fidgety, ('Restlessness, anxious': *2*, Candegabe) especially at night ('Restlessness, night': *2*): it is as if he is trying to run away from himself in the belief that he has committed an unforgivable sin ('Anxiety, conscience, of': *2*) for which he will go to Hell, and he prays to God to save his soul ('Anxiety, salvation about': *2* and 'Despair, religious': *1*). His only hope of salvation lies in religion, and he begs for God's mercy with fanatical devotion ('Religious affections': *2*), knowing that the remorse he feels ('Remorse': *2*) in no way atones for his sins.

At times he is dominated by fear and anxiety, and his nerves are perpetually on edge. It is as if he knows the dangers and catastrophes that lie ahead ('Excitement, anticipating events, when': *1*). Medorrhinum has a talent for fortelling the future with astonishing accuracy ('Clairvoyance': *1*, and '. . . news coming to her seems to touch her heart before she hears it' Allen, *op. cit.*, p. 297) and is profoundly upset by bad news that seems to him to be a form of divine punishment ('Bad news, ailments from': *2*). He lives in permanent dread of a sign from above that something bad is about to happen ('Fear, happen, something will': *2*, Candegabe; 'Fear, evil of': *1*, Candegabe).

His fears of the dark ('Fear, dark': *2*) and of divine punishment disturb his sleep, and he wakes up in the middle of the night in distress. He hates not being able to see properly in the darkness, and he has the terrible conviction that some evil has happened, accompanied by strange symptoms of heaviness and heat in the head that make him feel that he is going mad ('Waking, fright, as from': *2*, Barthel, Vol. III, 'Woke at an early hour with a frightened sensation, as if something dreadful had happened', Allen, *op. cit.*, p. 297; 'Delusions, happened, that something terrible had': *1*, Candegabe).

His fear of disease, especially of cancer, is so great that he will exaggerate every tiny symptom and make mountains out of molehills ('Fear, disease, of impending': *2* and 'Fear, cancer of': *2*, *Synthetic Repertory*, Vol. I). It is as if he expects at any moment to see a physical manifestation of his disturbed, inner state.

As his disease progresses, he loses all hope of recovery ('Despair, recovery': *1*, Barthel, Vol. I) and refuses to entertain the idea that he might be getting better: 'Is sure that she is worse, knows she is not going to live, cannot see any improvement, even when it is pointed out' (Allen *op. cit.*, p. 297). He feels that death is near ('Death, presentiment of': *2*), and when people are with him he talks about it calmly enough, but when he finds himself alone he becomes afraid ('Fear, death, of, alone, when': *1*, Candegabe).

Another aspect of Medorrhinum's anticipatory anxiety is the tendency to be startled easily, especially by noise ('Sensitive': 2 with the sub-rubric 'noise, to': 2, 'Starting, startled': 2; with the sub-rubrics 'noise, from': 2 and 'from sleep': 2).

He is touchy and oversensitive to everything that affects him personally and will brood for hours over a harsh word or hurtful comment ('A word or look of seeming harshness puts her in despondency for hours', Allen, *op. cit.*, p. 297; 'Sensitive, rudeness, to': 1, Candegabe and 'Offended, easily': 1, Candegabe).

Tormented by fear and guilt, he turns inward; the miasm that blocks his spiritual development and potential for altruism also nurtures his ego, and he becomes completely self-centred and wrapped up in his own little world ('Selfishness': 1 and 'Egotism': 1).

In accordance with the typical time modalities of the sycotic miasm, his moods alternate between bad temper during the day and exhilaration at night ('Mood, alternating': 1; 'Cross through day, exhilarated at night, wants to play', Allen, *op. cit.*, p. 299). Depressed and fearful in darkness, he cheers up in the evening ('Cheerful, evening': 1), as if released from the chains of his illness, but the joy is tinged with sadness as he knows that he cannot be merry for long ('Cheerful, sadness, with': 1); there is nothing permanent or solid about his feelings of well-being and, as soon as he confronts reality and starts to think about his state of health, he feels bad again ('Thinking, complaints, of, agg.': 2). He feels so bad that he can easily begin to cry ('Weeping, tearful mood': 2), especially when he talks about himself ('Weeping, telling of her sickness, when': 2), and if someone lends a sympathetic ear he cannot control the tears ('Weeping, spoken to, when': 2; 'Cannot speak without crying', Allen, *op. cit.*, p. 297; 'Weeping, cannot speak without crying': 2, Candegabe).

Beneath the cloak of sycosis, there lies a deep and heavy depression. Some tension is released when the long-repressed tears find an outlet ('Weeping, ameliorates symptoms': 2 and 'Spirits in the depths, weighed down with heavy, solid gloom, amel. by torrents of tears.', Allen, *op. cit.*, p. 297).

Weary of life ('Loathing, life': 1, Candegabe) and crushed by the weight of his unresolved conflicts, he sees suicide as the only solution ('Suicidal disposition': 1 with the sub-rubric 'shooting, by': 1), but he is too full of guilt and fear to pick up a gun and he sinks into a state of complete apathy ('Indifference, hell, did not care if he went to heaven or': 1, Candegabe).

Delusions and Sensations

We have already discussed how the suppression of Medorrhinum's subconscious impulses brings about the speediness and the desire to escape. These impulses are projected on to the outside world and become transformed into delusions of persecution in a subconscious attempt to absolve himself of all guilt. The powerful, abstract fear created by his inner world is transformed into specific fears of material things from which he can protect himself. He sees animals ('Delusions, animals, of': *1*), and rats ('Delusions, rats, sees': 1, with the sub-rubric 'running across the room': *1*); he thinks that people are animals and rats ('Delusions, animals of, persons are rats, mice, insects etc.': *2*); he sees people ('Delusions, people, sees': *1*) and faces that peep out from behind the curtains or the bed ('Delusions, faces, sees': *1*); he has the frightening feeling that there is some one behind him ('Delusions, people, behind him, someone is': *1*) and from Allen's *op. cit.*, we have: 'Persons come in, look at her, whisper, and say "come" ' (p. 296). This symptom is made up of four components: 'Delusions, persons, come in, look at her, whisper and say "come" ': *1*, 'Delusions, looking at her, persons are': *1*, 'Delusions, voices, hears': *1*, 'saying "come" ': *1*, 'Delusions, whispers, hears': *1*.

He has the strange sensation that someone is caressing his head ('Delusions, hand, felt a delicate, smoothing her head: *1*). It is hardly surprising that, with all these peculiar sensations, he feels that he is losing his reason ('Delusions, insane, that she will become': *1*). The strong fear of insanity ('Fear, insanity, of': *1*, Barthel, Vol. I) is present in several of Medorrhinum's mental and physical symptoms. For this reason, I would add this remedy to the rubric 'Delusions, persecuted, that he is'.

Dreams

The dream symbolism is similar to that of the delusions and sensations. He has dreams of ghosts and spectres ('Dreams, ghosts, spectres': *2*) that frighten him ('Dreams, frightful': *2*). He has strange dreams of drinking ('Dreams, drinking': *1*). His anxious dreams disturb his sleep ('Sleep, restless': *1*). The Medorrhinum child is so wound up and excited that he wants to stay up all night playing, and the adult lies awake until midnight ('Sleeplessness, midnight, before': *2* and 'Sleeplessness, sleepiness, with': *1*). In the early hours of the morning, he wakes up feeling afraid ('Woke at an early hour with a frightened sensation, as if something dreadful had happened', Allen, *op. cit.*,

p. 297) and cannot get back to sleep again because he feels cold ('Sleeplessness, waking, after, warm, coverings though limbs are cold': 2).

Medorrhinum often sleeps in a particular way, in the knee-chest position with the head bored into the pillow. This keynote is frequently seen in the small child, but is all the more significant when seen in the older child, and the position may bring him relief during an attack of asthma or coughing ('Sleep, position, knees, on the, with face forced into pillow': 1) He may also sleep with his arms over his head ('Sleep, position, arms over head': 1), but never lying with his whole weight on one side.

The General Picture

The main aspects of the remedy are outlined in the following brief summary of the materia medica.

Aggravation

Aggravation of some physical symptoms during the daytime, from sunrise to sunset, in contrast to Syphilinum. However, many sycotic symptoms continue throughout the day and night. Mental symptoms are aggravated at night.

Inflammatory rheumatic pains with oedema that are worse for motion.

Inflammatory rheumatic pains without oedema that are better from motion and worse from cold (Rhus Tox.).

Aggravation from dry cold, touch, thinking of his complaints, heat of the bed.

Amelioration

Amelioration from humid weather (in slightly sycotic cases), lying on the stomach, by the sea, in the open air, when seated or leaning backwards.

Discharges

Profuse, excoriating discharges with itching, and the odour of rotten fish or fish-brine.

Cravings

Craving for stimulants, alcohol, salt, unripe fruit. Ravenous hunger after eating.

Sensations
Trembling throughout the whole body; great nervousness with prostration and restlessness; burning heat in the spinal column and the soles of the feet, feet must be uncovered; of a tight band around the head; of a weight on the vertex and heat, as if he were going mad; that the eyes are protruding.

Generalities
State of collapse, with the desire to be fanned all the time (Carbo Vegetabilis) and desire for fresh air.

Fever
Cold skin, but wants to uncover (Camphor); chill with cold sweat (Veratrum Album).

Eyes
Sensation of sand in the eyes; inflammation of eyelids; discharge.

Nose
Sycotic coryza; post-nasal discharge; nasal catarrh running down throat; snuffles in children and coryza with loss of smell and taste, not relieved by other remedies.

Face
Jaw ache extending to temples; stiffness of jaw and tongue; swelling of submaxillary glands.

Mouth
Small, very sore aphthae; taste of copper.

Abdomen
Recurrent diarrhoea in children with family history of venereal disease; fetid and penetrating odour of stool; fetid oozing from anus with violent itching; sensation of a lump in the rectum; can pass stools only by leaning very far back, with much pain; ascites, with distended abdomen.

Urinary
Intense renal colic with shivering; pain in kidney region ameliorated by profuse urination; bubbling in kidney region; shivering and shaking after urination; dark, ammoniacal urine with a thick, grey film; nocturnal enuresis; diabetes.

Medorrhinum

Female
Sexual desire in single girls, after the menses; ulcers in neck of womb; intense, dragging down menstrual colic with cutting pain, like knives; menses dark, clotted, with stains that are difficult to wash out; profuse menses followed by migraine, with jerking and trembling of the limbs, and neck as stiff as wire; pain in lower abdomen with copious, yellow leucorrhoea; mammae extremely sensitive and cold, with icy nipples; intense, burning pain in left ovary; continuous leucorrhoea, albuminous, like egg-white, acrid, excoriating, with fish-brine odour; itching vagina, worse for scratching, better for bathing with tepid water. Lower abdomen extremely sensitive to touch.

Male
Impotence; persistent, gleety discharge, transparent with streaks of opaque, whitish mucus that leaves yellow stains; frequent erections by day and night; burning in urethra during urination; sensation that a drop of urine remains in urethra after urination; inability to retain urine after 6 p.m.; chronic gonorrhoea; enlarged prostate with frequent and painful urination.

Respiratory
Contraction of throat muscles, better for lying on stomach; cough at night, worse for lying, better for lying on stomach; great oppression of the chest and incessant cough.

Extremities
Gouty and rheumatic pains; arthritic nodosities; Arthritis deformans; sharp, shooting, stitching pains with numbness; stiffness; legs restless, cannot keep them still, worse for rest, better for movement; legs heavy, wooden; weak ankles; balls and soles of feet tender, has to walk on knees; weak knees; burning in feet, has to uncover feet at night.

Generally speaking, Medorrhinum is warm-blooded, better for damp weather, with a tendency to intense, rheumatic pain and a susceptibility to chronic uterine complaints, with associated symptoms.

SYMPTOMS FOUND IN KENT'S *REPERTORY*

	Med.	Thuja	Others
Anticipation, complaints from	*1*	–	2: Arg-n. Gels. *1*: Ars. Lyc. Ph-ac.
Anxiety	*1*	2	large rubric
Anxiety, conscience, of	2	2	large rubric
Anxiety, salvation, about	2	2	3: Ars. Lach. Lil-t. Verat.
Anxiety, time is set, if a	*1*	–	2: Gels. Arg-n.
Bad news, ailments from	2	–	3: Calc. Gels.
Cheerful, evening	*1*	–	large rubric
Cheerful, sadness, with	*1*	–	2: Chin. Nat-m. Phos. Kali-chl. Nux-m.
Clairvoyance	*1*	–	2: Nux-m. Phos.
Concentration, difficult	2	2	large rubric
Confusion of mind	2	2	large rubric
Death, presentiment of	2	–	3: Acon. Apis
Delusions, animals, of	*1*	*1*	3: Op.
Delusions, faces, sees	*1*	–	3: Op. Bell.
Delusions, hand, felt a delicate, smoothing her head	*1*	–	Med. – only remedy
Delusions, insane, that she will become	*1*	–	3: Cimic. 2: Acon. Chel. Manc. *1*: Calc.
Delusions, people, sees	*1*	*1*	2: Stram. Hyos. Bell. Ars. Bry. Puls.
Delusions, people, behind him, some one is	*1*	–	*1*: Anac. Brom. Calc. Casc. Cench. Crot-c. Ruta Staph. Sil.
Delusions, people, beside him, are	–	*1*	
Delusions, persons are rats, mice, insects	2	–	2: Aeth. Cimic.
Delusions, rats, sees	*1*	–	2: Ars. Aeth. *1*: Bell. Calc. Cimic. Stram.
Delusions, rats, sees, running across the room	*1*	–	2: Aeth.
Delusions, strange, familiar things seem	*1*	–	2: Cann-i. Graph. Plat.
Delusions, voices, hears	*1*	–	2: Phos. Coff. Cham. Crot-c. Elaps. Kali-br.

	Med.	Thuja	Others
Despair, religious	1	2	3: Ars. Aur. Lach. Lil-t. Verat.
Dream, as if in a	1	1	3: Nux-m. Op. Stram.
Dreams, dead, of the	2	3	3: Ars. Mag-c.
Dreams, drinking	1	–	1: Dros.
Dreams, frightful	2	1	large rubric
Dreams, ghosts, spectres	2	–	2: Arg-n. Camph. Carb-v. Crot-c. Graph. Kali-c. Sil. Sulph.
Dullness	1	2	large rubric
Dullness, children	2	–	3: Arg-n. Bar-c. Calc-p. Sulph.
Egotism	1	–	3: Plat. 2: Calc. Lach. Pall. Sil. Sulph.
Excitement, reading, while	1	–	2: Coff. 3: Ph-ac.
Excitement, trifles, over	1	–	1: Carl. Chin-a. Cinnb. Lachn. Nit-ac. Phos. Zinc.
Excitement, anticipating events, when	1	–	2: Gels. Arg-nit.
Excitement, writing, while	1	–	Med. – only remedy
Exhilaration	1	1	3: Cann-i. Coff. Lach. Op. Tarent.
Exhilaration, night	2	–	Med. – only remedy
Fear, dark	2	–	3: Cann-i. Stram.
Fear, death	1	–	large rubric
Forgetful, name, his own	2	–	1: Alum. Sulph. Kali-br. Valer.
Forgetful, words of, while speaking	2	–	3: Cann-i. Phos-ac. Arn.
Hurry	3	–	3: Lil-t. Merc. Nat-m. Sulph. Sul-ac. Tarent.
Impatience	2	–	3: Cham. Ign. Nux-v. Sep. Sulph.
Irritability	2	3	large rubric
Irritability, reading, while	1	–	1: Nat-c.
Memory, weakness of	3	2	large rubric
Memory, weakness of, names, for proper	2	–	2: Anac. Crot-h. Guaj. Lyc. Rhus-t. Sulph.
Memory, weakness of, read, for what has	2	–	3: Hell. Lach. Staph.

139

	Med.	Thuja	Others
Memory, weakness of, said, for what has	2	–	3: Hell. Hyos.
Memory, weakness of, done, for what has just	–	1	2: Acon. Bar-c. Calc-p. Hyos. Nux-m. Onos.
Memory, weakness of, persons, for	–	1	–
Memory, weakness of, say, for what is about to	2	1	3: Hell.
Memory, weakness of, thought, for what has just	2	–	2: Cann-i. Cocc. Hyos.
Memory, weakness of, words, for	1	1	3: Bar-c. Plb.
Mistakes, spelling, in	2	–	2: Lach. Lyc.
Mistakes, time, in	1	–	2: Lach.
Mistakes, time, in, confounds present with past	1	–	2: Cic.
Mood, alternating	1	–	large rubric
Religious affections	2	1	3: Hyos. Lach. Lil-t. Sulph. Verat. Zinc.
Remorse	2	–	3: Coff.
Restlessness, night	2	1	large rubric
Sadness	1	3	large rubric
Selfishness	1	–	2: Puls. Sulph.
Sensitive	2	1	large rubric
Sensitive, noise, to	2	–	large rubric
Sleep, position, arms over head	1	1	3: Puls.
Sleep, position, knees, on the, with face forced into pillow	3	–	2: Calc-p. Carc. Lyc. Phos. Tub. (*Synthetic Repertory*, Vol. III)
Sleep, restless	1	2	large rubric
Sleeplessness	2	3	large rubric
Sleeplessness, midnight, before	2	2	large rubric
Sleeplessness, sleepiness, with	1	1	large rubric
Sleeplessness, waking, after, warm, coverings though limbs are cold	2	–	3: Camph. Led. Sec.
Starting, startled	2	–	large rubric
Starting, noise, from	2	–	3: Kali-c. Nat-c. Nat-m. Sil. etc.
Starting, from sleep	2	1	3: Bell. Bor. Hyos. Caust. Spong.
Suicidal disposition	1	1	3: Aur. Nat-s. Aur-m.

	Med.	Thuja	Others
Suicidal disposition, shooting, by	*1*	–	2: Ant-c.
Suicidal disposition, throwing himself, windows, from	–	*1*	3: Aur.
Thinking, complaints, of, agg.	2	*1*	3: Ox-ac.
Thoughts, vanishing of	*1*	–	3: Nux-m.
Time, passes too slowly	2	–	3: Cann-i. Glon.
Time, passes too quickly	–	*1*	3: Cocc.
Unconsciousness, transient	*1*	–	3: Ign. Puls.
Weeping, tearful mood	2	*1*	large rubric
Weeping, spoken to, when	2	*1*	2: Nat-m. Plat. Staph.
Weeping, telling of her sickness, when	2	–	3: Puls. Sep.
Wildness	*1*	–	2: Stram. Verat.
Wild feeling in head	2	–	*1*: Bapt. Lil-t.
Work, aversion to mental	*1*	2	3: Aloe, Bapt. Chel. Chin. Lec. Nux-v. Phos.
Work, impossible	2	–	3: Nat-c.
Work, seems to drive him crazy, owing to the impotency of his mind	*1*	–	2: Kali-p.

SYMPTOMS OF MEDORRHINUM THAT SHOULD BE ADDED TO KENT'S *REPERTORY*

References

Dictionary of Practical Materia Medica, J. H. Clarke
Materia Medica of the Nosodes, H. C. Allen
Lectures on Homoeopathic Materia Medica, J. T. Kent

All quotations are taken from Allen's *Materia Medica of the Nosodes*.

The value which I have given to each symptom is strictly in accordance with the indications given by the above writers. The rubrics in brackets below indicate related rubrics that can be found in Kent's *Repertory*. The 'Comments' provide more information about the rubric when necessary.

('Clairvoyance'.)

Comment: 'Woke at an early hour with a frightened sensation, as if something dreadful had happened.' There are several rubrics that are related to the various aspects of this symptom.

'Concentration, difficult, abstract subjects': *1* (new rubric).

Comment: In contrast to Syphilinum, who forgets concrete facts.

'Confidence, want of self': *1*.

Comment: A result of the dullness of mind. 'Seems to herself to make wrong statements.' 'Dread of saying the wrong thing when she has a headache.'

'Conscientious about trifles': *1*.

Comment: He believes that he gets everything wrong and is afraid of making mistakes, so he writes everything down, even trivial things.

'Delusions, happened, that something dreadful had': *2*.
('Anticipation, complaints from'.)
('Bad news, ailments from'.)
('Death, presentiment of'.)
('Sleep, waking, fright, as from'.)

'Delusions, far off sensation': *1*.

Comment: '. . . as though things done today occurred a week ago.'

'Delusions, looking at her, persons are': *1*.
'Delusions, persons, come in, look at her, whisper and say "come" ': *1*.
'Delusions, voices hears, saying "come" ': *1*.
'Delusions, whisper, hears': *1*.

Comment: Here, one rubric has been subdivided into four and placed on four different pages, so that the prescriber will not miss it.

'Delusions, persecuted, that he is': *1*.
'Delusions, people, beside him, are': *1*.

Comment: Medorrhinum's persecution complex has already been discussed.

'Despair, recovery': *1*.
('Death, presentiment of'.)

Comment: 'Is sure that she is worse, knows she is not going to live, cannot see any improvement, even when it is pointed out.'

'Dullness, head, from weight on vertex': *1* (new rubric).
'Dullness, think long, unable to when weary': *1* (new rubric).
'Dullness, hurried, cannot think at all if hurried': *1* (new rubric).
'Fear, cancer of': *2* (new rubric).
'Fear, death, alone, when': *1*.
'Fear, disease, cancer, of': *2* (new rubric).

Comment: This symptom has been observed in clinical practice.

'Fear, disease, of impending': *1*.
'Fear, evil, of': *2*.
'Fear, happen, something will': *1*.
'Fear, insanity, of': *1*.

Comment: 'Always a feeling of impending danger, but knows not what . . .' 'It is always anticipating, fearing evil will happen, loss of reason or suicide.'

'Indifference, hell, did not care if he went to heaven or': *1* (new rubric). ('Despair, religious')

Comment: The loss of all hope leads to a state of intolerable anguish: '. . . did not care if he went to heaven or hell.'

'Indolence, morning, on waking': *1*.

Comment: 'Always wakens tired in the morning; hates to do anything that must be done, even nice things . . .'

'Irritability, writing': *1* (new rubric).

'Loathing, life': *1*.

'Memory, weakness of, names, for proper, his own name': *1* (new rubric).
'Memory, weakness of, stating her symptoms, great difficulty': *2* (new rubric).

Comment: The patient relies heavily on her notebook.

'Mistakes, headaches, during': *1*.

'Offended, easily': *1*.

Comment: 'A word or look of seeming harshness puts her in despondency for hours.'

'Procrastinate, desire to': *2*.

Comment: 'Dullness of memory and desire to procrastinate, because business seemed so lasting . . .'

'Prostration of mind, headache, during': *1*.

Comment: 'Could not read or use mind at all from pain in head.'

'Sensitive, rudeness, to': *1*.

'Stating her symptoms, great difficulty in': *2* (new rubric).

Comment: 'Great difficulty in stating her symptoms, loses herself and has to be asked over again.'

'Sleep, waking, fright, as from': *2*.

Comment:'. . . as if something dreadful had happened; heavy weight and great heat in head.'

'Suicidal disposition, fear of': *1* (new rubric).
'Suicidal disposition, waking, on': *1*.
'Tendency to suicide, gets up in night and takes his pistol, but his wife prevents him'

Comment: 'It is always anticipating, fearing evil will happen, loss of reason or suicide.'

'Talk, indisposed to, or to listen to talk, when weary': *1* (new rubric).

'Tensive pains in head, with a wild sensation as if she would go crazy.'

'Undertakes, many things, perseveres in nothing': *1*.

'Weeping, speak cannot, without crying': *2* (new rubric).

Comment:
See also 'Weeping, spoken to, when' and 'Weeping, telling of her sickness, when.'

SUMMARY

Medorrhinum is a strongly tubercular remedy with elements of sycotic aggression and sexuality. Due to tubercular feelings of inadequacy, he tends to be more destructive than egocentric. While Thuja provides the picture of sycosis in full bloom, Medorrhinum is the budding sycotic who is still fundamentally tubercular.

Like Thuja, his conscience protests at his unstable and antisocial behaviour – guilt engenders fear in Medorrhinum whereas it provokes an aggressive self-centredness in Thuja. Thuja's three characteristic components are: guilt, irritability and egotism.

Beginning with the two most fundamental aspects of the sycotic miasm, emotional instability and weakness of memory, the mental framework of Medorrhinum can be summarised as follows:

Emotional Instability

This leads to feelings of guilt as his conscience raises its voice in protest.

Related Rubrics
'Anxiety, conscience, of': *2*.
'Anxiety, salvation, about': *2*.
'Religious affections': *2*.
'Remorse': *2*.

Fear

His first reaction to his inner conflicts.

Related Rubrics
'Fear, cancer': *2*.
'Fear, dark': *1*.
'Fear, disease, of impending': *1*.
'Fear, insanity, of': *2*.

Anticipatory Anxiety

This is connected to the fear aspect.

Related Rubrics
'Anticipation, complaints from': *1*.
'Excitement, anticipating events, when': *1*.

Premonitions

This is also connected to the fear aspect. The combination of fatalism and clairvoyance leads him to expect all manner of evils and horrible punishments from above for his imaginary sins.

Related Rubrics
'Bad news, ailments from': *2*.
'Clairvoyance': *1*.
'Delusions, happened, that something dreadful had': *2*.
'Fear, evil, of: *2*.'
'Fear, happen, something will': .

There are three aspects of the fear:

1) Paranoia

Aggressive impulses that are buried deep in the subconscious are projected on to the external world in the form of delusions and dreams; the persistent suppression and projection of subconscious impulses creates a fertile breeding ground for neurosis and obsession.

Related Rubrics
'Delusions, faces, sees': *1*.
'Delusions, people, behind him, some one is': *1*.
'Delusions, people, sees': *1*.
'Delusions, persons, come in, look at her, whisper and say "come" ': *1*.
'Delusions, rats, sees': *1*.
'Dreams, frightful': *2*.
'Dreams, ghosts, spectres': *2*.

2) Desire to Escape

He wants to escape from the influence of his sycotic, aggressive impulses.

Related Rubrics
'Anxiety, time is set, if a': *1*.
'Hurry': *3*.
'Impatience': *2*.
'Restlessness, night': *2*.

3) Extreme Sensitivity
He is hypersensitive to his environment and easily startled.

Related Rubrics
'Sensitive, rudeness, to': *1*.
'Starting, noise, from': *2*.
'Starting, sleep, during': *1*.

Weakness of Memory

Memory weakness for abstract things. He forgets words, proper names, what he has read, what he has said and what he was about to say; he makes mistakes with pronunciation and has great difficulty remembering his symptoms; he has the sensation that his thoughts vanish.

Related Rubrics
'Dullness, children': *2*.
'Forgetful, words of, while speaking': *2*.
'Memory, weakness of': *3*.
'Memory, weakness of, names, for proper': *2*.
'Memory, weakness of, names, for proper, his own name': *1*.
'Memory, weakness of, said for what has': *3*.
'Memory, weakness of, say, for what is about to': *2*.
'Memory, weakness of, for stating her symptoms great difficulty': *2*.
'Memory, weakness of, thought, for what has just': *2*.
'Thoughts, vanishing of': *1*.

Mental Dullness

This is a feeling of heaviness on the vertex that seems to affect the mind. Mental dullness has two aspects:

1) Anticipatory Anxiety
Deterioration of the mental faculties leads to a loss of self-confidence.

Related Rubrics
'Confidence, want of self': *1*.
'Mistakes, headache during': *1*.

2) Hurried Actions
He is in a perpetual state of anxious restlessness that compels him to run faster than his thoughts. Both aspects create a state of mental

exhaustion that is worse when he is short of time or when he is tired. At times like these, he wants neither to talk nor listen when others talk.

Related Rubrics
'Anxiety, time is set, if a': *1*.
'Dullness, think long, unable to, when weary': *1*.
'Prostration of mind, headache during': *1*.
'Talk, indisposed to, or to listen to talk, when weary': *1*.

Mental dullness gives rise to eight more symptoms:

1) Desire to Procrastinate
Depression combines with indifference and aversion to mental work to the point where work seems impossible and the effort of thinking makes him feel as if he is losing his reason.

Related Rubrics
'Indolence, morning, on waking': *2*.
'Procrastinate, desire to': *1*.
'Work, aversion to mental': *1*.
'Work, impossible': *2*.
'Work, seems to drive him crazy, owing to the impotency of his mind': *1*.

2) Irritability
Any mental exertion, whether it be reading or writing, makes him irritable.

Related Rubrics
'Irritability, reading, while': *1*.
'Irritability, writing': *1*.

3) Attention to Detail
He is so frightened of making a mistake that he makes detailed notes of everything, even unimportant things.

Related Rubric
'Conscientious about trifles': *1*.

4) Disorientation in Time
The combination of mental dullness and hurried actions makes him lose all track of time.

Related Rubrics
'Delusions, far off sensation': *1*.
'Mistakes, time, in, confounds present with past': *1*.
'Time, passes too slowly': *2*.

5) Feelings of Unreality

Related Rubrics
'Delusions, unreal, everything seems': *2*.
'Dream, as if in a': *1*.

6) Mood Swings
His state of mind is strongly influenced by his miasmatic inheritance – he is bad-tempered during the day and exhilarated at night. He suffers from bouts of profound depression, interspersed with sparks of cheerfulness in the evening that disappear as soon as he starts to think about his health.

Related Rubrics
'Cheerful, sadness, with': *1*.
'Mood, alternating': *1*.
'Thinking, complaints, of, agg.': *2*.

7) Weeping
He weeps when he speaks or when people ask him how he is.

Related Rubrics
'Weeping, speak, cannot, without crying': *2*.
'Weeping, spoken to, when': *2*.
'Weeping, telling of her sickness, when': *2*.

8) Despair of Recovery
He loses hope of finding a cure and becomes tired of living. His life has lost all meaning and he can see no way forward. He considers suicide as a way out of his problems and does not care if he goes to heaven or hell.

Related Rubrics
'Despair, recovery': *1*.
'Despair, religious': *1*.
'Indifference, hell, did not care if he went to heaven or hell': *1*.
'Loathing, life': *1*.
'Selfishness': *1*.
'Suicidal disposition': *1*.

SCHEMATIC DIAGRAM AND REPERTORISATION

The schematic diagram overleaf illustrates the remedy as summarised in the previous section, with the aspects of emotional instability to the left and deterioration of mental faculties to the right.

Here, we can see how Guilt is connected to Fear, and Fear is connected to Anticipatory Anxiety and Premonitions, with the three related symptoms of Paranoia, Desire to Escape and Extreme Sensitivity.

On the right-hand side, Memory Weakness is connected to Mental Dullness with its related symptoms, Anticipatory Anxiety and Hurried Actions. Mental dullness leads to five symptoms: Desire to Procrastinate, Irritability, Fear of Making Mistakes, Disorientation in Time and Feelings of Unreality.

Four symptoms are connected to the deterioration of the memory: the difficulty in remembering his symptoms, the inability to remember proper names, the vanishing thoughts and dullness from the sensation of a weight on the vertex.

From the two central areas of emotions on the left and memory on the right, both arrows point to the State of Mind – General Reactions. From here, there is an arrow pointing to the bottom left-hand corner where four symptoms illustrate the mood swings, and another arrow pointing to the bottom right-hand corner where three symptoms describe the state of introversion and despair.

COMPARATIVE MATERIA MEDICA

The following six remedies have all the symptoms of the Minimum Characteristic Syndrome of Medorrhinum: Arsenicum, Ignatia, Natrum Muriaticum, Nux Vomica, Phosphorus and Thuja.

Arsenicum

In the words of Paschero: 'Arsenicum suffers from a deep-seated anxiety that emanates from the cells and tissues of an organism whose struggle with the influence of the syphilitic miasm, with its aggressive and destructive impulses, has exhausted him completely.' Arsenicum is characterised by paroxysmal anxiety and mortal anguish that are worse between 2 and 3 a.m., with great restlessness ('Restlessness, night', 2) that drives him out of bed to escape from what he believes to be his imminent death. The influence of syphilis makes him constantly critical of others, neurotic about hygiene and tidiness ('Conscientious about trifles', 22) and apt to blame himself for everything ('Anxiety, conscience, of', 5). The classic symptom 'Fastidious': 2) is a combination of the aspects of meticulousness and fault-finding.

Another major characteristic of Arsenicum is the syphilitic premonition of death. It has been said that the Arsenicum patient has the spectre of death etched on his face. He is convinced that he is going to die, and that his disease will carry him swiftly to his destiny (1). He is tormented by an anxiety that is far worse than the fear of disease; it drives him out of bed at night and has him frantically pacing up and down the room ('Hurry', 4). This nocturnal anxiety and restlessness, with the smell of decay that rises from the depths of his being, is quite different from the Medorrhinum restlessness that brings on the mood swings – day-time bad temper alternating with night-time elation. Arsenicum's premonitions of death are also indicated by the symptoms 'Anticipation, complaints from' (3) and 'Fear, happen, something will' (8).

Mental dullness (6) results from the syphilitic erosion of mental faculties and there are no particular modalities connected to the general weakness of memory.

From the Fear symptoms, Arsenicum has 'Fear, insanity, of' (10) and 'Fear, evil, of' as well as symptom 8. However, we must always bear in mind that the importance of a symptom is only relative to its context in the whole life history of the patient. Medorrhinum's fear of insanity comes from the inner conflict between his emotional

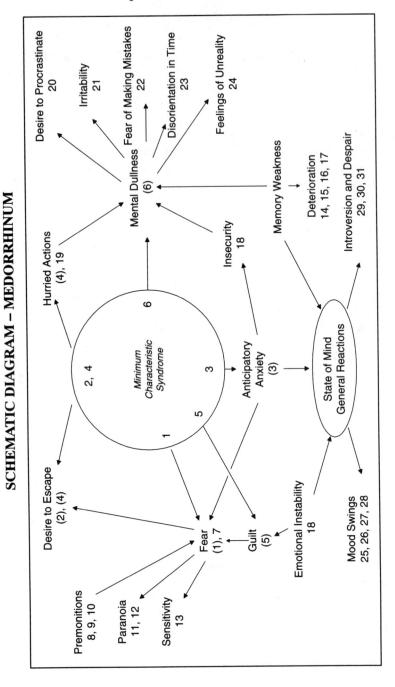

SCHEMATIC DIAGRAM – MEDORRHINUM

Minimum Characteristic Syndrome

1) Fear, disease, of impending
2) Restlessness, night
3) Anticipation, complaints from
4) Hurry
5) Anxiety, conscience, of
6) Dullness

Fear

7) Fear, dark
8) Fear, happen, something will
9) Bad news, ailments from
10) Fear, insanity, of
   *Fear, evil, of

Paranoia

11) Delusions, people, behind him, someone is
12) *Delusions, persons, come in, look at her, whisper and say 'come'

Sensitivity

13) Starting, noise, from

Mental Dullness

14) *Memory, weakness of, stating her symptoms, great difficulty
15) Memory, weakness of, names, for proper
16) Thoughts, vanishing of
17) *Dullness, head, from weight on vertex

Related Symptoms

18) Confidence, want of self
19) Anxiety, time is set, if a

Resulting Symptoms

20) *Procrastinate, desire to
21) Work, impossible
22) Conscientious about trifles
23) Time, passes too slowly
24) Dream, as if in a

State of Mind – General Reactions

Mood Swings

25) Mood, alternating
26) Thinking, complaints, of, agg.
27) Weeping, spoken to, when
28) Weeping, telling of her sickness, when

Introversion and Despair

29) Despair, recovery
30) Despair, religious (of salvation etc.)
31) Suicidal disposition

Note: Asterisked symptoms have not been repertorised. They are included here in order to provide a complete picture of the remedy.

153

REPERTORISATION – MEDORRHINUM

	1	2	3	4	5	6	7	8	9	10	11	13	15	16	18	19	21	22	23	24	25	26	27	28	29	30	31
Med.	1	2	1	3	2	1	2	1	2	1	1	2	2	1	1	1	2	1	2	1	1	2	2	2	1	1	1
Arg-n.	2	2	2	2		3				1					1	2			2							2	1
Ars.	1	3	1	2	3	1		2		1		1						2		1	1	1			3	3	2
Bry.	1	1		2		3				1				2	2			1				1			2		
Calc-c.	2	2		1	2	3	2	2	3	3	1	2		2	1		2			2		1			3	2	2
Ign.	1	2		2		1			2	1					1			3			3		1		1	1	
Kali-c.	3	1		2		3			1			3		1	2						2	2		2	1		2
Lach.	1	1		2		3			1	1	1	2	1	2	1				1	2						3	
Nat-c.	1	1		1		3						3			1		3	2	1		1	1	2				
Nat-m.	1	1		3	2	3		2	2	2		3		2	1					2	1	2			1	1	2
Nux-v.	2	1		2	2	2				2		3			1		1	2	2								
Ph-ac.	2	1	1	2		3		2						1						2		1					1
Phos.	3	2		1	1	3	2	3	1	2			1		1		2			2	2			3			2
Puls.		3		2	1	3	2		1	3			1	2	2			1			2					2	1
Sulph.	1	3		3	2	3			2	1		1	2	1	1			2		2		1				2	1
Thuj.	1	1		2	2	2				1								2		1			1			2	1

Note: Symptoms 12, 14, 17 and 20 are new rubrics and so do not appear in the comparative tables.

Minimum Characteristic Syndrome

1) Fear, disease, of impending
2) Restlessness, night
3) Anticipation, complaints from
4) Hurry
5) Anxiety, conscience, of
6) Dullness

Fear

7) Fear, dark
8) Fear, happen, something will
9) Bad news, ailments from
10) Fear, insanity, of
    *Fear, evil, of

Paranoia

11) Delusions, people, behind him, someone is
12) *Delusions, persons, come in, look at her, whisper and say 'come'

Sensitivity

13) Starting, noise, from

Mental Dullness

14) *Memory, weakness of, stating her symptoms, great difficulty
15) Memory, weakness of, names, for proper
16) Thoughts, vanishing of
17) *Dullness, head, from weight on vertex

Related Symptoms

18) Confidence, want of self
19) Anxiety, time is set, if a

Resulting Symptoms

20) *Procrastinate, desire to
21) Work, impossible
22) Conscientious about trifles
23) Time, passes too slowly
24) Dream, as if in a

State of Mind – General Reactions

Mood Swings

25) Mood, alternating
26) Thinking, complaints, of, agg.
27) Weeping, spoken to, when
28) Weeping, telling of her sickness, when

Introversion and Despair

29) Despair, recovery
30) Despair, religious (of salvation etc.)
31) Suicidal disposition

Note: Asterisked symptoms have not been repertorised. They are included here in order to provide a complete picture of the remedy.

instability and the voice of his conscience. In Arsenicum, guilt is always in the background, and the fears of death and solitude are consequences of his dread of the fate that awaits him.

Arsenicum does not have symptoms 11, 12, and 18 to 24, except for symptom 22 ('Conscientious about trifles'). In Medorrhinum this symptom is an attempt to compensate for his failing memory, while it is one of the keynotes of Arsenicum: the impeccably-dressed gentleman with the gold-headed cane, who is so fastidious, tidy and critical that he cannot tolerate the sight of a badly-hung picture on the wall, (Duprat, *Traité de matière médicale*).

The Arsenicum patient is highly excitable and, like Nitricum Acidum, capable of exploding in a violent fit of anger. He has ailments from anger with great anxiety, with restless anguish that drives him hither and thither; terrible anxiety, especially after midnight, which forces him out of bed; he despairs of ever finding a cure for his illness and believes that he is beyond the help of remedies; he is mean, resentful, selfish, cowardly and full of self-pity.

From the symptoms under the heading State of Mind, he does not have 27 or 28, rubrics that indicate the secretive side of Medorrhinum. His obsessive thoughts drive him to distraction ('Thinking, complaints, of, agg.', 28) and he loses all hope of recovery (29) and salvation (30).

Finally, driven by the destructive urges of the syphilitic miasm, he tries to kill himself by hanging (31).

Ignatia

Ignatia is a completely different personality. It is the picture of psoric anguish with its hysterics, paradoxes, contradictions, changeability and emotional instability. The six symptoms of the Minimum Characteristic Syndrome are linked by Ignatia's hypersensitivity. She is basically someone who is in great need of love and affection and will do her utmost to hold on to the person she loves. She is ashamed of her negative side ('Anxiety, conscience, of', 5) and tries to keep it hidden from view: 'Anger, ailments after, with silent grief': *3*, 'Grief, silent': *3*, 'Mortification, ailments after': *3*, 'Jealousy': *1*, 'Love, ailments, from disappointed': *3*. She gets upset by bad news (9) and is so much at the mercy of her volatile emotions that she fears that they will drive her insane (10). Despite her obsessive nature, she lacks the sycotic paranoia evident in symptoms 11 and 12. The superficial nature of her pathology does not cause deeply ingrained disturbances of the memory, hence her absence from symptoms 14 to 16.

Her emotional instability undermines her self-confidence (18), and she tries to resolve her perpetual doubts, indecisiveness and contradictions with her characteristic obsession for detail ('Conscientious about trifles', 22). Her presence in 'Mood, alternating' (25) needs no explanation; she cries when spoken to (27) because of her paradoxical aggravation from consolation. Although she may lose all hope of recovery (29) and religious salvation (30), the nature of her despair, and indeed of her whole psychological make-up, is too superficial for thoughts of suicide.

Natrum Muriaticum

The Minimum Characteristic Syndrome of Natrum Muriaticum is as follows: unrequited love, suppressed emotions, desire for revenge, dwelling on unpleasant memories.

Fears do not feature prominently in this remedy, whereas in Medorrhinum they are of primary importance. The basis of Natrum Muriaticum is a combination of frustrated emotions and aggression. From this we get the characteristic symptoms of irritability, violence, hatred, rudeness and rage. Guilt ('Anxiety, conscience, of', 5) is an aspect of his general anxiety.

Related to the anxiety and guilt are the three following elements: first, fear, of robbers, storms and that something will happen (8); second, the desire to escape, to avoid people, find solitude and reject all offers of consolation, as it offends him and makes him weepy and full of self-pity; and third, the discharge of emotions, a mixture of mildly hysterical laughter and tears.

He lacks the paranoid and mental deterioration symptoms of Medorrhinum. It is the frustration of his affections, rather than any weakness of memory, that erodes his self-confidence ('Confidence, want of self', 18). He does not appear in any of the memory symptoms and is absent from symptoms 28, 29 and 31. When Natrum Muriaticum is depressed or ill, he cannot weep; neither does he despair of recovery or think of suicide.

There is a fuller discussion of this remedy in the chapter on Natrum Muriaticum.

Nux Vomica

The characteristics of Nux Vomica are as follows: great sensitivity to his surroundings, with irritability, coldness and antiperistaltic contractions of the digestive system. Fearless to the point of recklessness, his fears of disease (1), insanity (10), evil ('Fear, evil, of') and that some-thing will happen (8) are, along with his guilt ('Anxiety, conscience, of', 5), the results of his acute sensitivity and his capacity for destruc-tion and aggression. He is rushed ('Hurry', 4), anxious ('Anticipation, complaints from', 3) and impatient in his attempt to keep up with his stressful life.

He has no paranoid delusions, although his nerves are so on edge that noise can make him jump (13).

The stresses and strains of his life, combined with the abuse of stimulants such as coffee, alcohol and spicy food, bring about the weakness of memory. He has great difficulty expressing himself as his thoughts keep slipping away (16). Eventually his confidence is sapped by exhaustion ('Confidence, want of self', 18) and he, who was once such a hard-working perfectionist (22), begins to hate his work and find it an impossible effort (21). However, his mind is less disturbed and more controllable than Medorrhinum's, and he does not share the same feelings of alienation or try to put things off (20). He finds that time passes slowly (23) because he is so speedy.

He is intolerant of pain ('Thinking, complaints, of, agg.', 26) and impatient with the disease that disables him ('Despair, recovery', 29) but he does not turn to religion for solace (30). In the end, he be-comes exhausted and overwhelmed by a lifetime of toxic abuse of his naturally sensitive constitution; he feels weak, irritable and confused as if intoxicated, and senses that death is near; his thoughts turn to suicide (31) and he may try to end it all by throwing himself from a height although, fortunately, he will usually lack the courage to go through with it.

Phosphorus

The three characteristic features of Phosphorus are as follows: fear, prostration and great sensitivity to all external impressions. Although it possesses all the symptoms of the Minimum Characteristic Syndrome and all the fears, it differs from Medorrhinum in that its picture is not based primarily on sycotic instability, but rather on the state of per-petual anxiety and restlessness that expresses his fear of his tubercular impulses for aggression and destruction.

Phosphorus is a manic depressive ('Mood, alternating', 25) whose moods fluctuate wildly. One minute he can be excited, enthusiastic, compassionate, joyful to the point of euphoria and full of love for all creation; the next minute he can fly into a temper with passionate anger, hatred and violence; and then he may collapse into a state of utter indifference, apathy, depression and exhaustion. Paschero says: 'This is a profoundly weakened organism with a marked tendency for paroxysmal effects prior to the onset of deterioration, senility, atrophy, decay and paralysis.'

The great sensitivity of Phosphorus makes him unable to rest at night (2) but, unlike Medorrhinum, his actions are slow ('Slowness': *3*). Imagination and acute sensitivity combine to exaggerate his perception of reality, and at times he is unable to make clear distinctions between the abstract and the material, or between the intuitive and the rational. He is an artistic, creative and spiritual being. His hurried actions (4) and anticipatory anxiety (3) are results of his hypersensitivity. He is impulsive, bad-tempered and affectionate, a rare combination of irascibility and compassion; he feels guilty ('Anxiety, conscience, of', 5) after an outburst of anger or fit of depression with indifference to his loved ones.

He is generally full of fear and is present in all the Medorrhinum fear rubrics either in black type or italics (1, 7, 8, 10). Unlike Medorrhinum he is afraid of death, solitude and storms, which threaten to devour him like a flame of fire ('Fire, a flame of, seemed passing through him': *1*).

Like Medorrhinum, Phosphorus is clairvoyant and has the feeling that something is lurking in the corner of the room, rather than a suspicion that someone is behind him. Although he can perceive the slightest noise, it does not make him start (13). He does not have the classic Medorrhinum weakness of memory (14, 15, 16) but his mental dullness (6) is brought about by three characteristic features that are worthy of mention: he feels better after eating, cannot concentrate on one thing for very long and understands questions only after they have been repeated. Hence he finds all mental effort impossible (21) but unlike Medorrhinum does not suffer from feelings of alienation as a result. Mental exhaustion and great sensitivity combine to undermine his self-confidence (18).

To summarise, on an intellectual level Phosphorus is intelligent, quick-thinking, perceptive, inquisitive, imaginative, intuitive and creative, but he is also easily distracted and can quickly become drained of energy, weak with exhaustion and in need of bed-rest and food.

He never procrastinates (20) and his sense of order is more concerned with beauty and harmony than with detail (22). His leanings towards the art of meditation and contemplation explain the sensation of being in a dream (24), while in Medorrhinum's case it is an indication of his confused mental state.

From the group of symptoms headed State of Mind he has 'Mood, alternating' (25), for reasons discussed previously, and 'Thinking, complaints, of, agg.' (26) because of his fears. The positive side of Phosphorus is his charismatic charm and affectionate nature, his clairvoyant abilities and his feelings of love for and connectedness with every living thing; with all this on his side, he does not have much cause to weep (27, 28) and he never loses his belief in the powers of medicine (29) and God (30). However, he is capable of contemplating suicide (31) if his depression becomes so bad that it drains all his energy and robs him of his zest for life.

Thuja

The distinction between Thuja and Medorrhinum has already been discussed at the beginning of the chapter – Medorrhinum is characterised by guilt, fear and lack of confidence and Thuja by guilt, egotism and irritability. Although all the symptoms of the Minimum Characteristic Syndrome of Medorrhinum are present in Thuja, their meaning changes in the context of the remedy. Thuja's picture is one of feelings of great aggression and guilt, and while he does not have the specific Medorrhinum fears (7, 8, 10), he is afraid of strangers, being found out and being approached. This is typical of sycosis, with the fears and paranoia being projected on to the world outside.

Thuja does not have Medorrhinum's particular paranoid delusions (11, 12); his delusions include, among others, the sensation of being double or divided into two, of being either fragile or very heavy, and the idea that he has been chosen by God.

He has a weak memory, but with different modalities. He has difficulty with self-expression, but the inability to explain his symptoms is peculiar to Medorrhinum (14). Generally speaking, Thuja has a bad memory for concrete facts, whereas Medorrhinum cannot remember abstract things. Unlike Medorrhinum, Thuja is sure of himself and self-sufficient (18). He is not bothered by time limits (19), and although he is not keen on mental work, he does not find it an insuperable (21) task to be postponed for as long as possible (20). Time seems to pass quickly (23) because of his natural, sycotic slowness. He feels as if he is in a dream (24). From the group of symptoms headed State of Mind, he does not have the symptoms that describe Medorrhinum's changeability, moodiness (25), sensitivity, tearfulness (28), cowardliness and despair of recovery (29).

His fear of exposure makes him cry when spoken to (27). He is so full of doubts that his symptoms increase when he thinks about them ('Thinking, complaints, of, agg.', 26) and he prays fanatically to ward off the encroaching despair (30). Urged on by the impulse to destroy, he may try to kill himself (31).

For a fuller discussion of this remedy, please refer to the chapter on Thuja Occidentalis.

The following seven remedies have five symptoms of the Minimum Characteristic Syndrome of Medorrhinum: Argentum Nitricum, Bryonia, Calcarea Carbonica, Natrum Carbonicum, Phosphoricum Acidum, Pulsatilla and Sulphur.

Argentum Nitricum

This remedy does not have symptom 5, 'Anxiety, conscience, of', which is an essential component of Medorrhinum. Argentum Nitricum lives in a perpetual state of fear, anxiety and agitation that forces him to keep on the move, as if trying to escape from his own impulses. Paschero says of this remedy: 'He is so immature that he is unable to fend for himself and he surrenders himself to anyone who will feed and care for him like a baby.'

Possibly the central symptom of Argentum Nitricum is the feeling of being abandoned, and one can easily imagine the feelings that a baby might experience as it goes through the trauma of the birth process: the feeling of being abandoned as it leaves the mother's womb; the fear of narrow spaces as it tries to pass down the birth canal, with the feeling that walls are closing in on him; and the fear of open spaces and high buildings as it is finally born into the world.

With a background of pseudo-psora, he feels insecure, vulnerable and under attack. Characteristically, he has uncontrollable, destructive impulses that seem to rise up out of nowhere and threaten to overwhelm him. Hence his fear of disease ('Fear, disease, of impending', 1) which represents an imminent danger; he is always on the alert, expecting something to happen that will leave him defenceless. He is afraid of solitude, being attacked and falling from a height. Symptoms 3 and 4, 'Anticipation, complaints from' and 'Hurry', are characteristic of both remedies, but in the context of the syphilitic Argentum Nitricum, the elements of changeability and lack of foresight lend a different meaning to the symptoms.

From the Fear symptoms, he has 'Fear, insanity of' (10) and 'Fear, evil, of'.

The delusions are different: he sees faces and visions that stop him from sleeping (11, 12).

As far as the weakness of memory is concerned (14-16), he is apt to forget word while he is speaking and look to others for help, and he gets blurred vision when he tries to concentrate.

The symptoms 'Confidence, want of self' (18) and 'Anxiety, time is set, if a' (19) have already been discussed. His great anticipatory anxiety is temporarily relieved only when a task is completed, so he always tries to get things done on time (20), despite his fear of failure. He is so speedy that time seems to pass slowly ('Time passes too slowly', 23).

As pathology advances, there is lesional damage to the nervous system, his coordination skills are affected and there is an increasing loss of control and balance.

He feels all alone in the world, afraid of what may happen, fearful of solitude and in a desperate hurry to escape from his own impulses; he looks like a withered, old man who has lost all hope ('Despair, religious', 30), and in his despair he wants to end it all by throwing himself from a high place ('Suicidal disposition', 31), as if attracted by the vacuum created by his own impulses.

To quote Paschero again: 'Argentum Nitricum goes through a process of gradual disintegration, firstly of the mental sphere, with the loss of control and coordination, and later of the digestive system, culminating in the onset of syphilitic locomotor ataxia.'

Bryonia

This remedy does not have 'Anxiety, conscience, of' (5), which shows how ashamed Medorrhinum is of his sycotic, aggressively sexual needs. We have already discussed in preceding chapters how Bryonia devotes himself to his work in an attempt to alleviate his anxiety: he talks and dreams of business, and when he falls ill his most pressing need is to return to his work. Symptoms 3 and 4, 'Anticipation, complaints from' and 'Hurry', are expressions of his anxious determination to complete his work, an anxiety that increases at night ('Restlessness, night', 2) and, as one would expect, when he is ill ('Fear, disease, of impending', 1).

Bryonia does not have the fear of the dark (7) or that something will happen (8) that arise from Medorrhinum's inner conflicts. He has no guilty conscience, but his feelings of vulnerability come out in the fears of poverty, disease (1), evil and insanity (10).

He does not have the paranoid delusions of Medorrhinum (11, 12); rather, in his delirium, he imagines that he is doing business as usual.

His dull mind ('Dullness', 6) cannot retain thoughts ('Thoughts, vanishing of', 16) but there is no specific disturbance of the memory.

He loses confidence in himself (18) because he feels so weakened by psora and so physically incapable of action, with the aggravation from all motion.

However, in the battle against his physical and mental shortcomings, he puts all his energy into his work with conscientious dedication (22) and lets no distracting symptoms (19 – 24) interfere. This is in direct contrast to Medorrhinum, whose essential characteristics are a failing memory and a dull mind.

From the group of symptoms under the heading State of Mind, Bryonia has 'Thinking, complaints of, agg.' (26) and 'Despair, recovery' (29), indicating his frustration at the loss of earnings incurred by his illness.

Calcarea Carbonica

This remedy does not have 'Anxiety, conscience of' (5) from the Minimum Characteristic Syndrome of Medorrhinum. Out of all the symptoms in this group, the fear of disease, 'Fear, disease, of impending' (1), is the most characteristic of Calcarea, who also has all the fear symptoms (7–10). Calcarea Carbonica is slow, deliberate and calculated. He is capable of harbouring deep feelings of hatred and resentment of certain people, even close relatives, and although he cannot bring himself to feel guilty for these feelings, he believes that God will punish him eventually, hence the fear of ghosts, darkness and disease.

Curiously, Calcarea Carbonica has the greatest number of symptoms in common with Medorrhinum. Apart from symptoms 5 and 12, it has all the symptoms of the Minimum Characteristic Syndrome and all the fear and delusion symptoms, but it is a totally different personality. It is not for nothing that Kent tells us that his repertory is only a tool. The materia medica should always have the final word; it is here that we shall discover the true character of the remedy to match the mental and physical symptoms of the patient.

In health, Calcarea Carbonica is slow, secure, successful and self-confident. If he falls ill, he will become apathetic, obstinate, resentful and hateful, with fear arising from the stomach, fear of divine punishment, ghosts, darkness, cruelty and bad news. From the Minimum Characteristic Syndrome, the fear of disease is the most characteristic symptom. It describes a state of apprehension and suspicion that is aroused by the outward expression of his frustration and negativity. He lives in his head, planning everything with great deliberation and forethought, but he has no concept of the wider meaning of life and all metaphysical thought terrifies him. Hence, all his fears are concerned with the unknown, magical underworld. He is afraid of evil ('Fear, evil, of': *3*), insanity (10), thunderstorms, the night-time darkness (7) and that something will happen (8). His clairvoyant abilities disturb his nights ('Restlessness, night', 2) and fill him with fear for the future ('Anticipation, complaints from', 3).

Calcarea does not own his guilt (5), instead he projects it on to the outside world in the form of a sensitivity to noise (13). When he falls ill, his mind goes dull (6) and he cannot think ('Thoughts, vanishing of', 16). Work becomes an impossible effort (21). Unlike Medorrhinum, he remembers all his symptoms and talks about each one with painstaking thoroughness (14) and has no trouble remembering people's names (15). He is unruffled by deadlines (19), unconcerned with detail (22) and unconscious of the passing of time (23), due to his calm and ponderous nature.

From the group of symptoms under the heading State of Mind, his moods fluctuate because he is so sensitive and impressionable ('Mood, alternating', 25), unlike Medorrhinum whose moods change according to the time of day. He is constantly preoccupied with his health ('Thinking, complaints of, agg.', 26) and convinced that he is incurable ('Despair, recovery', 29). The religious inclinations of his childhood are transformed into the religious despair of old age (30) and he is tormented by gnawing doubts about the salvation of his soul. With his avaricious nature and fear of the future, he is destined for a life of spiritual poverty. There is nothing sentimental about Calcarea, so he neither cries when spoken to (27) nor when he talks about his symptoms (28), although the situation can disturb him ('Narrating her symptoms agg.': *3*) and he may cry with rage when reprimanded.

As with all the great destructive remedies, he will eventually become tired of living and turn in on himself, tortured by thoughts of murder, fire and rats; he may then try to put himself out of his misery (31) by slashing his wrists.

Natrum Carbonicum

This remedy is characterised by weakness on both a mental and physical level. He is a misanthropic hypochondriac who shuns company and is profoundly depressed by his physical deterioration. He has no reactive power, with weakness of the digestive system, acid dyspepsia with belching, and weak ankles.

He has a great need for peace and quiet and avoids all distractions. Like all the Natrums he feels both forsaken and resentful and can take a dislike to certain people, including members of his family, for no particular reason, like Calcarea Carbonica.

He can sink quickly into a state of profound dejection where he feels completely overwhelmed by his problems and loses the will to fight. When this happens, he will cut himself off from everyone and find a place where he can lick his wounds in private, although solitude frightens him. The only things that can bring him out of this state are unexpected noises ('Starting, noise from', 13), other people's problems and the sound of gentle, nostalgic music, which can bring tears to his eyes.

From the Minimum Characteristic Syndrome, the most characteristic symptom is 'Dullness' (6); all mental effort wears him out, and reading can bring on headaches and vertigo. The first four symptoms of the Minimum Characteristic Syndrome are easily explained: the first, 'Fear, disease, of impending' (1), by his awareness of his rapid deterioration; the other three arise from the lack of confidence ('Confidence, want of self', 18) that becomes worse as his illness progresses. In health, Natrum Carbonicum can be tough, brave, reliable ('Conscientious about trifles', 22) and positive about his work. He takes his commitments and challenges seriously ('Hurry', 4, and 'Anticipation, complaints from', 3).

Like Calcarea Carbonica, he does not have a guilty conscience (5). His physical weakness makes him vulnerable and fearful of the world, hence the fears of disease, storms, robbers, the future, and evil ('Fear, evil, of': 2). In his delusions and hallucinations he neither sees people (12) nor feels that they are behind him (11), but he believes that he is pursued by enemies, perhaps because he both rejects people and feels deserted by them.

From the group of Memory symptoms, Natrum Carbonicum does not have numbers 15 and 16 – his weak mind causes the loss of memory and a general state of confusion, with vertigo and headaches. He finds it impossible to concentrate on his work (21), but it does not drive him mad because he has already become resigned to a boring life where time seems to stand still (23).

Natrum Carbonicum is a passive victim of fate who has none of the symptoms from the State of Mind section, except 'Mood, alternating'

(25). In the final stages, he becomes so full of ennui and despondency that he cannot even eat a morsel of food without getting ill.

In the early hours of the morning, he may fall prey to suicidal thoughts ('Suicidal disposition, morning': *1*), although he has no serious intentions of ending his life (31).

Phosphoricum Acidum

The characteristics of this remedy are a paralytic weakness of the spine, with great mental and emotional exhaustion, profound apathy and depression. The causation can be emotional trauma, chagrin, grief, disappointed love or overexertion on a mental or physical level; ill effects of grief and mental shock; delirium with stupefaction. The prolonged loss of vital fluids can provoke this symptomatology, with a paradoxical amelioration from stool. Unlike its close relative Phosphorus, it does not weary of life when depressed, and the signs of physical weakness are much slower to manifest following the mental degeneration.

From the Minimum Characteristic Syndrome, symptom 5 is missing. Symptoms 1, 3 and 6 are highly characteristic of Phosphoricum Acidum: 'Anticipation, complaints from' (3), accompanied by the classic diarrhoea, is indicative of the great strain placed on him by an emotional or intellectual challenge; 'Fear, disease, of impending' (1) arises from his condition of great weakness; 'Dullness' (6) describes his typical state of mind, a combination of stupefaction, prostration and total apathy. He shares only two other symptoms with Medorrhinum: 'Thoughts, vanishing of' (16) and 'Dream, as if in a' (24). Like Medorrhinum, he cannot find the right words to express himself.

As far as delusions and hallucinations are concerned, it may be his strong fear of death that makes him hear the ticking of the clock as it marks the passage of time, and see imaginary numbers in the air.

To understand the essential differences between remedies, the symptoms must be considered in the light of the whole dynamic context.

Pulsatilla (*See also* pages 64–5)

From the Minimum Characteristic Syndrome, Pulsatilla has none of Medorrhinum's preoccupation with disease (1). She takes great care with everything she does and worries that she has not done her best ('Anticipation, complaints from', (3), 'Hurry' (4), and 'Conscientious about trifles', 22). Her lack of confidence (18) is exacerbated by the perpetual conviction that she has done wrong. This gives rise to a state of uneasiness ('Restlessness, night', 2) and mental dullness (6) that is aggravated by heat; hot, stuffy rooms bring out her tendency for swelling and inflammation of the veins.

However, the sycotic side of this remedy has much in common with Medorrhinum. Profuse, yellowish-green discharges and leucorrhoea, and a mild but manipulative manner. She is one of the most contrary remedies of our materia medica, with her capriciousness and changeability, and she uses tears and affectionate kisses to get what she wants. Like Medorrhinum, she is warm-blooded and her feet are so warm that she has to uncover them at night, but she does not share the same sleep position (knee-chest) or have inflammation of the perineum.

Her chief concerns are her health and her family, on whom she depends so much that she is terrified of losing them, because she fears solitude and being abandoned. Her immaturity is the stumbling block to her spiritual development, and she feels guilty ('Anxiety, conscience, of', 5) about the selfishness of her fears.

Pulsatilla does not have Medorrhinum's particular delusions (11, 12); rather, her delusions are the product of sexual fantasy, such as the delusions of seeing people, being pursued by enemies and finding a naked man in her bed.

The Memory symptoms, 'Memory, weakness of, names for proper' (15) and 'Thoughts, vanishing of' (16), derive from the lack of confidence (18) and need for order (22) that express her ambivalent need to be both protected and approved of.

The unstable ('Mood, alternating', 25) Pulsatilla is so desperate for love and protection that she will do anything to avoid upsets, and she suppresses her unhappiness with silent resignation. Hence the uncontrollable weeping that can break out suddenly for no apparent reason, or when she talks about her symptoms (28), until she is comforted by some kind words of consolation. She may turn to religion to satisfy her childlike and selfish need for love and affection, and relieve her of the burden of guilt for her wrongdoings and doubts about her salvation. From here it is but one more step to the brink of despair (30) and thoughts of suicide (31) by drowning, a symbolic return to the comfort and safety of her mother's womb.

Pulsatilla does not share Medorrhinum's state of exaggerated expectancy (13, 19), anguish and confusion (21, 23). Medorrhinum's anxiety about his health distresses him deeply, while Pulsatilla is more accepting of her fate, hence her absence from symptoms 26 and 29.

Sulphur

Sulphur is the epitome of the dishevelled and complacent philosopher who is lazy, dirty and warm-blooded. The unpleasant, burning skin eruptions form a barrier between him and the outside world. From the Minimum Characteristic Syndrome, it does not have symptom 3, the anticipatory anxiety which reflects Medorrhinum's anguished approach to life. Sulphur denies that he has any fears, although he is affected by bad news (9) and the threat of evil ('Fear, evil, of': *1*) and insanity (10). Despite his overriding egotism, he has an uneasy conscience ('Anxiety, conscience, of', 5, 'Restlessness, night', 2) about what may happen to his friends. His sluggish circulation makes him lazy and lethargic, and he shouts with rage at anyone who dares to try and shake him out of his idleness; a compensatory reaction to this is 'Hurry' (4).

Because of the lack of any real involvement with the world, he does not have the delusions of Medorrhinum (11, 12). He believes that he is a great, wise man who is dressed in fine silk ('Delusions, old rags are as fine as silk': *3*).

Egotism and guilt explain his fears of robbers, ghosts, high places and failure.

His physical weakness and sluggish circulation dull his mind (6) and affect his memory, but his inability to remember names (15) and keep track of his thoughts (16) is – more than a cause for any real concern – indicative of someone who is engrossed in himself and his fantasies. He locks himself away in his ivory tower so that he does not have to confront his deeply ingrained lack of confidence (18) or bother about people. It should not be difficult to understand, therefore, why he does not figure in symptoms 19, 21 and 23, as he shares none of Medorrhinum's anguished anxiety. In Sulphur, the symptom 'Dream, as if in a' comes (24) from his love of meditation and idle speculation.

Being a completely different remedy from the angst-ridden Medorrhinum, he is absent from symptoms 25 to 29. However, if his guilty conscience gets the better of him and he feels that his life has been a complete failure, he may plunge into the depths of despair (30) and try to commit suicide (31).

6

Natrum Muriaticum

DESCRIPTION

In sickness, the potential for spiritual growth is stifled and the resulting pathology is ruled by a morbid predisposition to disease, which Hahnemann called the 'miasm'. People react in different ways to the frustrations and problems encountered in life, and their reactions are determined, to a large extent, by their individual predisposition to disease. In the same way, a whole range of environmental stress factors, from the natural to the infectious, will affect the individual according to his inherited susceptibilities and genetic make-up.

In Natrum Muriaticum, this predisposition is activated by the disturbance of the salt/water ratio. The remedy's latent susceptibilities to disease are brought out by an imbalance between two of the vital components of all living things: salt and water. The psoric miasm creates in Natrum Muriaticum a feeling of separation from his environment which is expressed, on a physical level, by the salt craving and, on an emotional level, by the need for love to pacify those feelings of insecurity that stem from the cutting of the umbilical cord. In fact, Natrum Muriaticum's emotional needs, and the need to restore the salt/water balance, are felt most keenly during the four phases of life – childhood, adolescence, pregnancy and old age. The equilibrium is disturbed when he has to confront the outside world, with all his inadequacies and problems. The lack of true, nurturing, parental love, which is essential for the development of a secure and confident child, is the fundamental causation of the Natrum Muriaticum picture, with a greater or lesser degree of constitutional mental weakness.

However, the most characteristic and distinguishing symptom of Natrum Muriaticum is the need for affection ('Affectionate': 2). The frustration of his affections in the formative years of life makes an indelible impression upon the young Natrum Mur. It sets the stage for a pattern of behaviour that will repeat itself again and again with every new frustrating experience, as he relives the grief of losing his loved ones. This obsession with the past, the longing to find his lost love, is the second characteristic symptom ('Dwells on past disagreeable occurrences': *3*) from which he refuses to free himself, preferring to grieve for his love ('Love, ailments, from disappointed': *3*), silently and inconsolably ('Love, ailments, from disappointed, with silent grief': *3*.

Love is vital nourishment for Natrum Mur., and the lack of it makes him become angry and aggressive. When his need for love is frustrated, negative feelings rise up against the one who has spurned him, feelings that he tries to suppress for fear of losing the object of his love. Resentment is the third characteristic of this dynamic between love, anger and suppression ('Malicious': *2*) and completes the main outline of the remedy. He bitterly resents the fact that he has to hide his innermost feelings from the eyes of his loved one, through fear of losing her for ever, and he becomes irritable at the least provocation, unable to see the funny side of life and intolerant of the smallest difference of opinion. His fits of temper serve as a valuable escape valve for his inner tension, but he directs them carefully away from the real cause of it all.

This aspect of Natrum Mur. which could be called 'projected anger', reveals the impulsive ('Impetuous': *2*), uncontrollable and irritable ('Irritability': *3*) side of the remedy, whose irritability is typically worse in the morning and at midday ('Irritability, morning': *2* and 'Irritability, noon': *1*) and better in the evening ('Irritability, evening, amel. in': *1*). He detests people who make a fuss and try to comfort him, as they only make him feel more exposed ('Irritability, consolation agg.': *3*). He feels irritable after eating ('Irritability, eating, after': *2*) in the same way as the child who rejects oral substitutes for love. The aggravation before menses ('Irritability, menses, before': *2*) is an expression of the female's competitiveness with men. Natrum Mur. dislikes heat ('Irritability, heat, during': *2*), even the radiance of the sun, a vital manifestation of life and love. The loss of vital fluids adds a physiological dimension to the aggravation after menses ('Irritability, menses, after': *1*).

The more he broods on his problems, the more resentful and bitter he becomes until it begins to colour his whole attitude to life. He becomes so extremely sensitive that he overreacts to everything ('Irritability, takes everything in bad part': *1*), completely loses his sense of humour ('Jesting, averse to': *1*), and takes offence at trivial things, a gesture someone makes or a throwaway line ('Offended, easily': *2*), or the slightest rudeness ('Rudeness, ailments from': *1*); he becomes violent ('Violent': *2*), bad-tempered and quarrelsome

('Quarrelsome': 2), ready to heap the blame on others ('Reproaches, others': 2) in a fit of uncontrollable rage ('Rage, fury': 2). From resentment to hatred ('Hatred': 2) is but one small step, and he will never forgive those who have offended him ('Hatred, persons, of, who had offended': 2).

His outbursts of anger make him ill ('Anger, ailments after': 2) with anxiety ('Anger, ailments after, with anxiety': 1), indignation ('Anger, ailments after, with indignation': 1) and grief that he suffers in silence ('Anger, ailments after, with silent grief': 2).

He looks on the people he loves as sacred mother and father figures on whom he is totally dependent emotionally. If they should ever let him down, the strength and violence of the anger that wells up inside him makes him feel guilty and ashamed of himself ('Anxiety, conscience, of': 2). His anxiety and fear intensify when he tries to relax; as sleep approaches, his subconscious feelings rise to the surface ('Anxiety, evening, bed, in, uneasiness and anxiety, must uncover': 1), and he wakes at 2 a.m. ('Anxiety, midnight, after, 2 a.m.': 1), disturbed by a nightmare ('Anxiety, dreams, on waking from frightful': 2). Like the irritability, the anxiety is worse after eating ('Anxiety, eating, after': 2). He has fearful anxiety ('Anxiety, fear, with': 2), after a fright ('Anxiety, fright, after': 1), about the future ('Anxiety, future, about': 2), about his health ('Anxiety, hypochondriacal': 3), about his salvation ('Anxiety, salvation, about': 1), on going to sleep ('Anxiety, sleep, on going to': 1), while he sleeps ('Anxiety, sleep, during': 2), during a storm ('Anxiety, storm, during a thunder': 1). The female feels anxious before and during the menses ('Anxiety, menses, before': 2, and 'Anxiety, menses, during': 2). He is depressed and dejected, consumed with guilt and despair, with palpitations ('Chest, palpitations, heart, anxiety': 3).

Ashamed and afraid of his uncharitable feelings, his fear symptoms are numerous. He fears that something will happen either to him or to the people he loves and depends upon so much ('Fear, happen, some-thing will': 2), although this fear is secondary to the resentment and murderous anger that can be sparked off by an offensive remark, either real or imagined. The fear that something will happen underlies most of his other fears: the fear of storms ('Fear, thunderstorm, of': 2) is the fear of divine punishment. He is so frightened of his own subconscious that he is afraid of going to sleep ('Fear, sleep, to go to': 1) and his head fills with fantasies and vivid pictures to distract him from sleep ('Fancies, exaltation of, vivid, falling asleep, when': 1). He has a morbid fear of disease ('Fear, disease, of impending': 1) and evil

('Fear, evil, of': 2), and of the world of devils and demons that comes alive at night ('Fear, night': 2). The fear of walking, and of falling while walking, symbolises his fear of asserting himself and is manifested on a physical level by a paralytic weakness ('Extremities, awkwardness, stumbling when walking': 2). He feels that he has been robbed of affection, hence the fear of robbers ('Fear, robbers, of': 2,) and of being robbed. He fears trifles ('Fear, trifles': 2), people ('Fear, people, of': 2) and crowds ('Fear, crowd, in a': 2), and the female Natrum Mur. has fear during the menses ('Fear, menses, during': 2,) that makes her feel that she is going mad ('Fear, insanity, of': 2).

Natrum Mur. is easily frightened ('Frightened easily': 2), shaken by the slightest thing ('Fright, complaints from': 3) and the female is afraid of men ('Men, dread of': 2); she looks for robbers under the bed after having dreamt of them ('Searching on floor, at night for thieves, after having dreamt of them': 1). The patient may, in fact, become totally insane ('Insanity': 2), under the strain of so much nervous tension. He is easily startled ('Starting, startled': 3) by the slightest sound ('Starting, noise, from': 3) and by the slightest thing ('Starting, trifles, at': 2). He starts from fright ('Starting, fright, from': 3), during the heat ('Starting, heat, during': 1), during sleep ('Starting, sleep, during': 2) and on falling asleep ('Starting, sleep, on falling': 2), jerking as if from electric shocks ('Starting, electric shocks through the body, during sleep': 2), that rise up from the feet ('Starting, feet, as if coming from the, wakening her': 2).

This state of nervousness ('Excitement': 3) is intensified at night in bed ('Excitement, evening, bed in': 2), before sleep ('Excitement, sleep, before': 1), on waking ('Excitement, waking, on': 1), and when he is emotionally disturbed ('Excitement, emotional, ailments from': 2) by some bad news ('Excitement, bad news, after': 1).

The stress of so much tension makes him want to run away and hide, even from himself. He is driven by anxious restlessness ('Restlessness, anxious': 2), hurried anxiety ('Hurry': 3), with the fear that time is not on his side, and is intolerant ('Impatience': 2) of the slightest delay ('Impatience, trifles, about': 1), especially with the heat ('Impatience, heat, with': 2). This whole syndrome is a reaction to the feelings of guilt and consequent desire to escape.

A fourth component of the escape dynamic is the desire for solitude. He withdraws from others and shuts himself away. If someone stays with him, he refuses to answer their questions ('Answers, aversion to': 2), and does not wish to be spoken to ('Spoken to, averse to being': 1), because he is irritated and annoyed by idle chatter ('Conversation agg.': *3*), with no desire to speak ('Talk, indisposed to, desire to be silent': *2*) and annoyed by all attempts to bring him out of himself ('Irritability, consolation agg.': *3*), as consolation only makes him more angry ('Anger, consoled, when': *2*), upset ('Consolation agg.': *3*) and sorry for himself ('Weeping, consolation agg.': *3*).

Eventually, even contact with close family annoys the female Natrum Mur. ('Aversion, husband': *1*), and she feels totally alienated, as if she did not belong there ('Estranged, family, from her': *2*). The patient leads a solitary existence, and finds comfort in being alone ('Company, aversion to, amel. when alone': *2*). Separated from the world by a hard rock of resentment, alienated from his family, he misses his childhood home ('Homesickness': *21*), which represents the love and security that have gone from his life. So he avoids people ('Company, aversion to': *3*) and falls prey to a deep sadness that intensifies when he is left alone ('Sadness, alone, when': *2*) to brood on the past ('Thoughts, persistent': *37*), tormented by memories of unpleasant events ('Thoughts, unpleasant subjects, haunted by': *3* and 'Thoughts, tormenting': *3*).

In the silence of the night, he indulges his grief alone ('Sadness, night': *2*), in bed ('Sadness, night, bed, in': *2*), talking to his memories of the dead people that he once loved ('Talks, dead people, with': *1*). He gets more enjoyment from talking to himself than to other people, and feels possibly that his own voice understands him better ('Talking, pleasure in his own': *1*). It is logical, therefore, that the Natrum Mur. baby should be one of the slowest at learning to talk ('Talk, slow learning to': *3*).

He feels so isolated and misunderstood that he wants to cry with grief and anger, although paradoxically he is unable to weep when he wants to ('Sadness, weep, cannot': *3*), while at other times he may weep for no apparent reason ('Weeping, causeless': *2*) and when he does not want to ('Weeping, involuntary': *3*). Natrum Mur. hides his emotions because he is convinced that nobody understands or appreciates him. So he waits until he is alone to cry ('Weeping, alone, when': *2*) and reminisce ('Weeping, past events, thinking of': *2*), and cries in his sleep ('Weeping, sleep, in': *2*). If you try and comfort him he will only cry more ('Weeping, consolation agg.': *3*). He does not want to be spoken to ('Weeping, spoken to, when': *2*) or looked at ('Weeping, looked at, when': *2*) because he believes that you feel sorry for him ('Weeping, pitied, if he believes he is': *2*).

In Natrum Mur., sadness pervades the whole picture of love, anger and suppression. The lifelong obsession with the past, the inability to recover from past hurts, and the feelings of guilt at the damage, real or imagined, that he inflicts on others all depress him deeply ('Sadness': *3*) and rob his life of all pleasure ('Indifference, pleasure, to': *3*). Grief ('Grief': *3*) makes him ill ('Grief, ailments from': *3*). He suppresses his grief and suffers in silence ('Grief, silent': *3*), to the point where he can no longer cry ('Grief, ailments from, cannot cry': *3*), and he worries about what will become of him ('Grief, future, for the': *2*). His worries are justified, as nothing can be done to shake him out of his misery ('Inconsolable': *2*),. and he is impervious to offers of help and consolation.

One of Natrum Mur.'s basic conflicts is between the desire to break away from the family and stand on his own two feet, and the pull of emotional needs which, when frustrated, stir up destructive feelings that fill him with shame and guilt. His guilty conscience undermines his power to be his own person and make his own decisions ('Confidence, want of self': *1*). Impelled by the urge for freedom and ensnared by the chains of guilt, he feels weakened and indifferent to everything, unable to concentrate ('Concentration, difficult': *2*), with a vacant feeling in the head when he tries to apply himself to work ('Concentration, difficult, on attempting to has a vacant feeling': *1*), or on attempting to speak ('Concentration, difficult, talking, while': *2*), and his mind is sluggish ('Dullness': *3*) and confused ('Confusion of mind': *3*), especially after eating ('Confusion, eating, after': *2*), on rising ('Confusion, rising, after': *1*) and when reading ('Confusion, reading, while': *1*). Mental work becomes very difficult ('Exertion, agg. from mental': *3*), he loses his memory ('Forgetful': *2*) for words ('Forgetful, words, of, while speaking': *2*), after eating ('Forgetful, eating, after': *1*) and when he tries to think ('Forgetful, mental exertion, from': *1*).

He lacks ideas ('Ideas, deficiency of': *2*), his thoughts vanish ('Thoughts, vanishing of': *2*) due to his weak memory ('Memory, weakness of': *2*) that makes it difficult for him to express himself ('Memory, weakness of, expressing oneself for': *2*), to work ('Memory, weakness of, labor, for mental': *3*), to remember what has happened ('Memory, weakness of, happened, for what has': *2*), what he has read ('Memory, weakness of, read, for what has': *2*), what he is about to say ('Memory, weakness of, say, for what is about to': *2*) and the right words to use ('Memory, weakness of, words, for': *2*), especially when he is tired ('Memory, weakness of, labor, for mental, fatigue, from': *1*). The result is that he makes mistakes when he speaks ('Mistakes, speaking': *3*) and writes ('Mistakes, writing, in': *2*), saying what he does not mean ('Mistakes, speaking, intend, what he does not': *2*). He gives wrong answers ('Mistakes, speaking, wrong answers, gives': *1*) and misplaces words ('Mistakes, words, misplacing': *2*). In other words, Natrum Mur. does all he can to avoid meaningful and constructive communication with others.

Absorbed in his own little world ('Absent-minded': *3*), brooding on his problems, worrying about what will become of him ('Absorbed, buried in thought, as to what would become of him': *1*), he floats about in a dream ('Dream, as if in a': *2*), paying no attention to what he is doing ('Unconsciousness, conduct automatic': *2*), and dropping things occasionally ('Extremities, awkwardness, hands, drops things': *2*), his lack of coordination being a sign of his desire to separate himself from the world around him.

The aversion to work ('Indolence': *3*), whether on a mental ('Work, aversion to mental': *2*) or physical level, especially in the morning ('Indolence, morning': *2*) expresses his wish to fail.

He is prone to fits of near hysterical laughter that bring some relief to his pent-up emotions ('Hysteria': *3*) and suddenly cheer him up ('Mirth': *1*), especially in the evening ('Mirth, evening': *2*). Fits of hilarity alternate with irritability ('Mirth, alternating with irritability': *1*). However, it is a spurious happiness, tinged with sadness ('Cheerful, sadness, with': *2*), and suffering that makes him laugh too long, too loudly ('Laughing, immoderately': *2*), and incontrollably ('Laughing, involuntarily': *2*). He laughs at serious things ('Laughing, serious matters, over': *2*), and the laughter ends in tears ('Weeping, alternating with laughter': *1*).

This unhappy individual has a curious keynote that is unique to the remedy: 'Cheerful, coition, after': *1*), an activity that represents a degree of maturity and emotional satisfaction rarely achieved by this introverted patient, who is too inhibited to urinate in company ('Company, aversion to, people intolerable to her during urination': *3*).

The fits of hysteria with fainting ('Hysteria, fainting': *2*) provide a release from suppressed obsessive emotions.

Natrum Mur. is a strongly tubercular remedy and the miasm weakens and eventually destroys him. The patient is weak, under-nourished and skinny, too frail to withstand the knocks of life and too thin-skinned to tolerate the slightest injustice ('Mortification, ailments after': *3*). He is easily upset by bad news ('Bad news, ailments from': *2*) that concerns him or other people, as he over-identifies with the hardship of others and tries to appease his guilty conscience by suffering for them ('Sympathetic': *2*). He despairs for himself

('Despair': *2*), without faith or hope of salvation ('Despair, religious, of salvation': *1*) and falls into a state of indifference and ennui ('Weary of life': *2*). He becomes discontented and bored ('Discontented': *3*, with the sub-rubric 'everything, with': *3*), hates his life ('Loathing, life': *3*), and longs for death to put an end to his problems ('Death, desires': *2*). Finally, he is consumed by his tremendous, self-inflicted anger and hatred, and rejects all attempts at reassurance and offers of support with torrents of tears and explosions of rage.

Delusions and Delirium

Both the delusions and the delirium are distorted, dream-like reflections of the patient's subconscious mind. The characteristic time of aggravation for the delirium is the morning ('Delirium, morning, waking, on': *1*) and during a chill ('Delirium, chill, during': *3*), in keeping with the aggravation modalities of most of Natrum Mur.'s symptoms.

The delusions provide more food for thought. Here, the phantom of guilt ('Delusions, images, phantoms, sees': *2*) appears at night ('Delusions, images, night': *1*) in the form of ghosts and spirits ('Delusions, spectres, ghosts, spirits sees': *2*) that he sees as soon as he closes his eyes ('Delusions, spectres, sees, closing eyes, on': *1*). In the longing for his unrequited love, he talks with dead people ('Delusions, talking, fancies herself, as with dead people': *1*) and seems to see them ('Delusions, dead persons, sees': *1*); he hears voices ('Delusions, voices, hears': *1*) in the distance ('Delusions, voices, hears, distant': *1*) and probably imagines that they belong to the dead ('Delusions, voices, hears, dead people': *1*). The aversion to company is expressed by the delusion that the house full of people ('Delusions, house is full of people': *1*), and the feeling of alienation by the delusion that objects appear different ('Delusions, objects, appear different': *1*). The fear of robbers, and of being robbed above all of affection, appears in the delusion of seeing thieves ('Delusions, thieves, sees': *2*) in the house ('Delusions, thieves, sees, house, in': *2*). He is so convinced of their presence that he has the whole house searched ('Delusions, thieves, sees, after a dream, and will not believe the contrary until search is made': *1*).

The delusions are simply the paranoid projection of his subconscious mind and provide a clear illustration of the characteristic syndrome of Natrum Mur. The feeling that he is bereft of all affection is expressed by the delusion that objects appear different; the desire for solitude comes out in the delusion that the house is full; the feelings of guilt are revealed by the nocturnal phantoms; the love disappointment makes him feel as if his affections have been robbed, hence the delusion of thieves in the house: he is so convinced that he is the victim of robbery that he is blind to the fact that he is the perpetrator of the crime. The unrequited love appears in the conversations with dead people; and the final misfortune and misery of his emotional failure is expressed by the delusion that he is wretched when he looks in the mirror ('Delusions, wretched, thinks she looks, when looking in a mirror': *1*), a graphic description of his paranoid projection.

Dreams

The significance of the dreams is very similar. Natrum Mur. is plagued by anxious dreams ('Sleep, dreams, anxious': *3*) as soon as he falls asleep ('Sleep, dreams, anxious, on falling asleep': *2*); he has fantastic ('Sleep, dreams, fantastic': *3*), frightful ('Sleep, dreams, frightful': *3*) premonitions of the future ('Sleep, dreams, visionary': *2*) that appear to be so real ('Sleep, dreams, vivid': *3*) that they continue after he wakes ('Sleep, dreams, continued after waking': *2*), and he cannot believe that he was only dreaming ('Sleep, dreams, true, seem, on waking': *1*). These disturbing dreams ('Sleep, dreams, mind, affecting the': *1*) are typically about crime ('Sleep, dreams, murder': *2*), riots ('Sleep, dreams, riots': *1*) and robbers ('Sleep, dreams, robbers': *3*); they are so vivid that the patient cannot go back to sleep again until the whole house is searched ('Sleep, dreams, robbers, and cannot sleep until the house is searched': *3*). Comments made in the previous section about the delusions can be applied equally to the dreams. The dream that his teeth are falling out ('Sleep, dreams, teeth, pulled out': *1*) is a Natrum Mur. keynote that symbolises his suppressed anger and frustration at the inability to use his teeth to bite and chew, like an infant without teeth.

Insomnia

The characteristic modalities are insomnia from palpitations ('Sleeplessness, palpitation, from': *2*) and shocks ('Sleeplessness, shocks, from': *2*), after waking in distress from a vivid dream ('Sleeplessness, waking, after': *3*) and being unable to go back to sleep in the early hours of the morning, in accordance with the time modalities of the remedy ('Sleeplessness, morning': *1*). To complete the picture, let us add that he wakes early ('Waking, early': *2*), frequently ('Waking, frequent': *2*) and in a state of fear ('Waking, fright, as from': *2*).

Additional sleep symptoms are: sleepiness while reading ('Sleepiness, reading, while': *2*), sitting ('Sleepiness, sitting, while': *2*), after eating ('Sleepiness, eating, after': *2*), during a fever ('Sleepiness, heat, during the': *3*) or a chill ('Sleepiness, chill, during': *2*), as the remedy has a general aggravation from extremes of temperature ('Cold, heat and cold': *2*).

Natrum Mur. has four symptoms related to yawning that are unique to this remedy: 'Yawning, frequent, afternoon, menses, during': *1*, 'Yawning, frequent, evening, riding in a carriage': *1*, 'Yawning, walking in open air, after': *1* and 'Yawning, wine, amel.': *1*.

SUMMARY

Need for Affection

The need for affection is the central issue for Natrum Mur., due to the lack of real parental love in the formative stages of childhood. The fixation on the past and the inconsolable grief for his unrequited love are the clearest expressions of his emotional frustration.

Related Rubrics
'Affectionate': *2*.
'Dwells, on past disagreeable occurrences': *3*.
'Love, ailments, from disappointed': *3*.
'Love, ailments, from disappointed, with silent grief': *3*.

Resentment

Anger with the loved one who has rejected him is quickly suppressed for fear of losing her, creating the dynamic triangle of love, suppressed emotion and resentment.

Related Rubric
'Malicious': *2*.

Irritability

While the true cause of his problems remains blissfully unaware of the strong emotions she has aroused, Natrum Mur. buries his anger, resentment and grief deep in his subconscious, and lets off steam with fits of bad temper and irritability.

Related Rubrics
'Anger, ailments after, with silent grief': *2*.
'Hatred': *2*.
'Impetuous': *2*.
'Irritability': *3*.
'Irritability, consolation agg.': *3*.
'Irritability, menses, before': *2*.
'Irritability, takes everything in bad part': *1*.
'Offended, easily': *2*.
'Quarrelsome': *2*.
'Reproaches, others': *2*.
'Rudeness, ailments from': *1*.
'Violent, vehement': *2*.

Guilt

He feels ashamed of the destructive, negative feelings that have been provoked by the rejection of his love, and resentment leads to guilt.

Related Rubric
'Anxiety, conscience, of': *2*.

Anxiety

Guilt is an expression of anxiety in all its different aspects. His child-like fear of divine punishment and the supernatural accounts for the anxiety he feels about the future, during sleep, on waking from a nightmare and during a thunderstorm, and plunges him into a deep depression with despair, palpitations and indifference to everything.

Related Rubrics
'Anxiety, alternating with indifference': *1*.
'Anxiety, dreams, on waking from frightful': *2*.
'Anxiety, future, about': *2*.
'Anxiety, hypochondriacal': *3*.
'Anxiety, sleep, during': *2*.
'Anxiety, storm, during a thunder'*1*.
'Chest, palpitation, heart, anxiety': *3*.

Fears

Suppressed anger and guilt are related to three different phenomena: fear, the desire to escape and the discharge of emotions. Fear is a direct result of the crippling feelings of resentment and destructive anger brought about by the frustration of his emotions. He is afraid that something will happen to him or to others when he is either awake or asleep. The fears of punishment and robbery are expressed in the fear of storms, crowds and robbers. His fear while walking is an expression of his deep feelings of insecurity. In the female, fear becomes more intense during the menses.

Related Rubrics
'Fancies, vivid, falling asleep, when': *1*.
'Fear, crowd, in a': *2*.
'Fear, falling, of, walking, when': *1*.
'Fear, happen, something will': *2*.
'Fear, menses, during': *2*.
'Fear, robbers, of': *2*.
'Fear, thunderstorm, of': *2*.

Excitability

The projection of fear on to the outside world creates a state of perpetual excitability and hypersensitivity that is worse before he goes to sleep and on waking; the merest thing will terrify him.

Related Rubrics
'Excitement': *3*.
'Excitement, sleep, before': *1*.
'Excitement, waking, on': *1*.
'Fear, trifles': *2*.
'Frightened easily': *2*.

Nervous Reactions

His fearfulness makes him jump up in alarm at the slightest noise, and he is jerked awake at night by the sensation of an electric shock.

Related Rubrics
'Starting, electric shocks through the body during sleep': *2*.
'Starting, feet, as if coming from the, wakening her': *2*.
'Starting, fright, from': *3*.
'Starting, noise from': *3*.
'Starting, trifles, at': *2*.

Desire to Escape

The desire to escape is the second result of resentment and anger. Active expressions of this are the anxious restlessness, hurry (an anxiety about time that he can control) and impatience (an anxiety about time that he cannot control). He wishes to escape from himself.

Related Rubrics
'Hurry': *3*.
'Impatience': *2*.
'Impatience, trifles, about': *1*.
'Restlessness, anxious': *2*.

Desire for Solitude

The first passive expression of his desire to escape is the desire for solitude, a central characteristic of Natrum Mur. that comes from his anxiety. He avoids people and does not want to speak, be spoken to or be forced to reply. He rejects everybody and consolation annoys him, making him feel sorry for himself and reducing him to tears.

Related Rubrics
'Answers, aversion to': *2*.
'Company, aversion to': *2*.
'Consolation agg.': *3*.
'Spoken to, averse to being': *1*.
'Talk, indisposed to': *2*.
'Weeping, consolation agg.': *3*.

Sensation of Isolation

He is eaten up with resentment and cut off from all human contact. He feels alienated from his family and wishes he were with them again. He needs solitude to indulge his grief and brood upon his unpleasant memories. He talks with dead people and discovers that he likes the sound of his own voice.

Related Rubrics
'Company, aversion to, amel. when alone': *2*.
'Estranged, family, from her': *2*.
'Homesickness': *2*.
'Sadness, alone, when': *2*.
'Talking, pleasure in his own': *1*.
'Talks, dead people, with': *1*.
'Thoughts, unpleasant subjects, haunted by': *3*.

Absent-Mindedness

The second passive expression of his desire to escape is the way he distances himself from reality by becoming absent-minded. He is obsessed by thoughts of what will become of him and has the sensation of being in a dream. While he goes about his daily business, his mind is elsewhere, and he becomes clumsy through inattention.

Related Rubrics
'Absent-minded': *3*.
'Absorbed, buried in thought': *2*.
'Extremities, awkwardness, hands, drops things': *2*.
'Unconsciousness, conduct, automatic': *2*.

Emotional Discharge

This is the third reaction to resentment and suppressed anger. He has outbursts of hysterical laughter, moods of mirth and melancholy alternating with irritability. The laughter is involuntary and exaggerated. He laughs at serious matters and ends up crying.

Related Rubrics
'Cheerful, alternating sadness with': *2*.
'Hysteria': *3*.
'Laughing, immoderately': *2*.
'Laughing, involuntarily': *2*.
'Laughing, serious matters, over': *2*.
'Mirth, alternating with irritability': *1*.
'Weeping, alternating with laughter': *1*.

Suppression and Expression of Emotions

His severely repressed emotions break out at inconvenient times. He finds that he is unable to cry when he wants to, but sometimes he weeps for no apparent reason and without wanting to. He weeps on his own and when others look at him or try to comfort him, because he thinks they feel sorry for him. He weeps when thinking of his problems.

Related Rubrics
'Sadness, weep, cannot': *3*.
'Weeping, alone, when': *2*.

'Weeping, causeless': *2*.
'Weeping, consolation agg.': *3*.
'Weeping, involuntary': *3*.
'Weeping, looked at, when': *2*.
'Weeping, past events, thinking of': *2*.
'Weeping, pitied, if he believes he is': *2*.

Inability to Concentrate

His intellectual development is hindered by his emotional immaturity and his negative, destructive impulses. He finds it difficult to concentrate on work, and becomes confused and incoherent when he tries to speak. He feels bewildered, empty and indifferent.

Related Rubrics
'Concentration difficult, on attempting to, has a vacant feeling': *2*.
'Concentration, difficult, talking, while': *2*.
'Confusion, talking, while': *2*.
'Indifference, mental exertion, after': *1*.

Weakness of Memory

Amidst all this confusion, he forgets words while speaking and his weak memory, especially for mental work, makes it difficult for him to express himself. He forgets what has happened, what he has read and what he is about to say. He makes mistakes in speaking, and says what he does not mean. He gives wrong answers. His thoughts vanish when he tries to force himself to concentrate. It would seem that all these symptoms conspire to help Natrum Mur. avoid all contact with others and all possibility of constructive thought.

Related Rubrics
'Forgetful, words, of, while speaking': *2*.
'Memory, weakness of, labor, for mental': *3*.
'Memory, weakness of, expressing oneself, for': *2*.
'Memory, weakness of, happened, for what has': *2*.
'Memory, weakness of, read, for what has': *2*.
'Memory, weakness of, say, for what is about to': *2*.
'Mistakes, speaking, intend, what he does not': *2*.
'Mistakes, speaking, wrong answers, gives': *1*.
'Thoughts, vanishing of, mental exertion, on': *1*.

Grief

Overwhelmed by his seemingly endless problems with love and unexpressed emotions, and severely weakened by the tubercular miasm, he sinks into a profound depression from which nothing can rouse him. He is totally indifferent to the good things in life, suffers his grief in silence and makes himself ill. He is unable to express his unhappiness and spends his time worrying about what will become of him.

Related Rubrics
'Grief, ailments, from': *3*.
'Grief, ailments, from, cannot cry': *3*.
'Grief, future, for the': *2*.
'Grief, silent': *3*.
'Indifference, pleasure, to': *3*.

Despair

With his great hunger for love and need for salt, he looks under-nourished, thin and wasted. He lacks the inner resources to deal with emotional trauma and the injustices of life and over-identifies with the pain and suffering of others. He loses all hope and faith in life, becomes bored and discontented with everything and hates his life. He sees death as the only way out of his problems. Nothing can alleviate the pain of living or relieve him of the heavy burden of resentment that he will carry with him to the bitter end, rejecting all offers of comfort and support with anger and tears.

Related Rubrics
'Bad news, ailments from': *2*.
'Consolation agg.': *3*.
'Death, desires': *2*.
'Despair': *2*.
'Despair, religious': *1*.
'Discontented, everything, with': *3*.
'Inconsolable': *2*.
'Loathing, life': *3*.
'Mortification, ailments from': *3*.
'Sympathetic': *2*.
'Weary of life': *2*.

Delusions

The delusions expose the contents of Natrum Mur.'s subconscious mind to the clear light of day and are simply another expression of the characteristic syndrome. The separation from all affection is expressed in the delusion that objects appear different; the desire for solitude in the delusion that the house is full of people. The feelings of guilt are represented by the nocturnal phantoms. The delusion that thieves are in the house, and the conviction that he has been robbed, are expressions of the love disappointments that make him feel as if his emotions have been robbed. The unrequited love brings about the conversations with dead people. The final misfortune and misery of his emotional failure is represented by the graphic delusion that he thinks he looks wretched when he looks in the mirror, a wonderful keynote of his paranoid state.

Related Rubrics
'Delusions, objects, appear different': *1*.
'Delusions, house is full of people': *1*.
'Delusions, images, phantoms, sees': *2*.
'Delusions, talking, fancies herself, as with dead people': *1*.
'Delusions, thieves, sees': *2*.
'Delusions, thieves, sees, after a dream, and will not believe the contrary until search is made': *1*.
'Delusions, thieves, house, in': *2*.
'Delusions, wretched, thinks she looks, when looking in a mirror': *1*.

Dreams

The dreams have a similar significance to the delusions. Dreams full of anxiety and fear express his feelings of guilt. Dreams that continue after waking reveal his separation from reality. The dream of robbers that he searches for after waking is, like the delusion, connected to his feelings of robbed affection. The dream that his teeth are pulled out, a Natrum Mur. keynote that symbolises the toothless infant who is unable to bite and chew, represents frustrated love and the enforced suppression of emotion.

Related Rubrics
'Dreams, anxious': *3*.
'Dreams, continued after waking': *2*.
'Dreams, frightful': *3*.
'Dreams, robbers': *3*.
'Dreams, robbers, and cannot sleep until the house is searched': *3*.
'Dreams, teeth, pulled out': *1*.

SCHEMATIC DIAGRAM AND REPERTORISATION

The Minimum Characteristic Syndrome of Natrum Muriaticum can be represented by a circle in the centre of the diagram overleaf. In the middle of the circle we have 'Malicious' (1), an essential and characteristic symptom of our remedy. To the left-hand side, we have 'Company, aversion to' (2), 'Consolation agg.' (3) and 'Dwells on past disagreeable occurrences' (4), symptoms that demonstrate his deeply ingrained bitterness. To the right-hand side, we have 'Love, ailments, from disappointed' (6), 'Affectionate' (7) and 'Anger, ailments after, with silent grief' (5). These three symptoms describe the anger he feels at having to suppress his emotions after a love disappointment.

From the centre of the circle – Resentment – two arrows point to the right to indicate the increase of anger and tension that the emotional suppression creates. We have 'Offended easily' (8), 'Reproaches others' (9), 'Violent' (10) and 'Hatred' (11) placed at the top, and 'Anxiety, conscience, of' (12), the guilt aroused by his feelings of negativity and aggression towards his loved one, placed below.

A little way to the right, joined by two small arrows, we have the symptoms that describe the three reactions to his underlying resentment:

Fear – 'Fear, happen, something will' (13), 'Fear, robbers, of' (14), 'Frightened easily' (15) and 'Starting, noise, from' (16).

Desire to escape – 'Hurry' (17), 'Company, aversion to' (2), 'Consolation agg.' (3), 'Dream, as if in a' (18), 'Estranged, family, from her' (19) and 'Homesickness' (20).

Emotional discharge – 'Hysteria' (21), 'Weeping, alternating with laughter' (22) and 'Weeping, involuntary' (23).

From the centre of the circle – Resentment – an arrow points to the left, where we have the symptoms connected with depression: 'Mortification, ailments after' (27), 'Sympathetic' (28), 'Indifference, pleasure, to' (29), 'Grief, ailments from' (30) and 'Loathing, life' (31).

An arrow points downwards from the base of the circle towards the symptoms of the intellect that show how the mind is affected by the general state of conflict: 'Concentration, difficult, on attempting to has a vacant feeling' (24), 'Memory, weakness of, expressing one's self, for' (25) and 'Mistakes, speaking, intend, what he does not' (26). Natrum Muriaticum does his best to avoid all positive thought and contact with others.

COMPARATIVE MATERIA MEDICA

Staphysagria

This is the only remedy with all the symptoms of the Minimum Characteristic Syndrome of Natrum Muriaticum. Kent says in his *Lectures on Homoeopathic Materia Medica*: 'One who is in health can easily put aside a controversy, knowing that he has done what is right, but a Staph. patient when he has to control himself goes all to pieces, trembles from head to foot, loses his voice, his ability to work, cannot sleep and a headache follows' (p. 895). He is depressed, bad-tempered and in need of solitude ('Company, aversion to', 2) to nurse his indignation and hurt at the offences he has received ('Dwells on past disagreeable occurrences', 4). The most characteristic symptom is suppressed anger which he suffers in pain and silence (5). Indignation, suppressed anger and an affectionate nature (7) form the *modus vivendi* of Staphysagria and are more important than resentment ('Malicious', 1).

Despite the fact that he is easily offended (8) and critical of others ('Reproaches others', 9), he lacks the violence (10) and hatred (11) of Natrum Muriaticum. It is easy to see why he does not suffer from guilt (12), the lack of which explains the absence of other related symptoms. He is fearful (15) and dwells constantly on past disagreeable occurrences' (4). He feels distant from his wife ('Estranged, family, from her', 19) and longs for a quiet, loving home life ('Homesickness', 20). On a mental level, his mind is so dull that he feels as if his head were made of wood, especially on the forehead; he forgets what he has read but has no problems with self-expression. Easily mortified (27), apathetic ('Indifference, pleasure, to', 29), ill with grief (30) and tired of life (31), he lacks sympathy and compassion (28) for the problems of others that Natrum Mur. takes on board, along with the emotional suffering caused by his love disappointments.

The guiding symptoms of Staphysagria are: hypersensitivity of all the senses, namely touch, noise, taste and smell; aggravation from touch and sexual excesses; clean-cut wounds; diarrhoea from anger; cystitis and lumbago from sexual frustration; scrofula; painful warts.

Five remedies have six symptoms of the Minimum Characteristic Syndrome of Natrum Muriaticum: Ignatia, Lycopodium, Nux Vomica, Platinum and Sepia.

SCHEMATIC DIAGRAM – NATRUM MURIATICUM

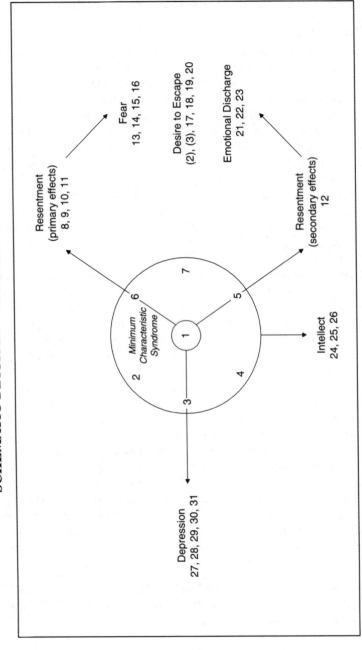

Resentment
(primary effects)
8, 9, 10, 11

Fear
13, 14, 15, 16

Desire to Escape
(2), (3), 17, 18, 19, 20

Emotional Discharge
21, 22, 23

Resentment
(secondary effects)
12

*Minimum
Characteristic
Syndrome*

Intellect
24, 25, 26

Depression
27, 28, 29, 30, 31

Minimum Characteristic Syndrome

1) Malicious
2) Company, aversion to
3) Consolation agg.
4) Dwells on past disagreeable occurrences
5) Anger, ailments after, with silent grief
6) Love, ailments, from disappointed
7) Affectionate

Resentment – Primary Effects of

8) Offended easily
9) Reproaches others
10) Violent
11) Hatred

Resentment – Secondary Effects of

12) Anxiety, conscience, of

Fear

13) Fear, happen, something will
14) Fear, robbers, of
15) Frightened easily
16) Starting, noise, from

Desire to Escape

17 a) Hurry
b) Company, aversion to (passive)
c) Consolation agg. (passive)

Desire to Escape by Distancing Himself from Reality

18) Dream, as if in a
19) Estranged, family, from her
20) Homesickness

Emotional Discharge

21) Hysteria
22) Weeping, alternating with laughter
23) Weeping, involuntary

Intellect

24) Concentration, difficult, on attempting to, has a vacant feeling
25) Memory, weakness of, expressing one's self for
26) Mistakes, speaking, intend, what he does not

Depression

27) Mortification, ailments after
28) Sympathetic
29) Indifference, pleasure, to
30) Grief, ailments from
31) Loathing, life

REPERTORISATION – NATRUM MURIATICUM

	1	2	3	4	5	6	7	8	9	10	11	12	13	14	15	16	17	18	19	20	21	22	23	24	25	26	27	28	29	30	31
Nat-m.	2	3	3	3	2	3	2	2	2	2	2	2	2	2	2	3	3	2	2	2	3	1	3	1	2	2	3	2	3	3	3
Aur.	2	2	—	—	1	2	—	2	1	3	2	3	—	1	1	1	1	—	—	2	3	2	2	—	—	—	2	—	—	3	3
Bell.	2	2	2	—	1	—	—	—	—	3	—	—	—	1	2	—	2	2	—	1	1	1	2	—	1	—	1	1	—	2	2
Chin.	1	2	1	2	—	—	—	1	3	—	—	2	—	—	—	2	—	—	—	—	—	—	—	—	—	—	—	—	—	—	3
Con.	1	2	—	2	1	—	—	—	—	—	—	2	—	2	1	—	1	2	1	1	3	1	—	—	—	—	—	—	1	1	1
Hyos.	2	2	—	2	1	3	—	—	2	3	—	2	—	—	2	—	1	2	—	2	2	2	3	—	—	—	3	2	—	2	2
Ign.	1	3	3	—	3	3	2	—	1	1	2	2	1	2	2	—	2	—	—	—	3	2	3	—	—	—	—	1	—	3	1
Lach.	2	2	—	—	—	2	—	—	2	2	2	—	—	2	2	2	2	2	2	2	3	—	1	—	1	—	3	1	—	3	2
Lyc.	2	2	1	1	3	—	—	2	2	2	—	—	—	1	3	2	1	—	—	1	2	2	—	—	2	—	3	2	1	1	2
Nat-c.	1	—	—	—	1	—	—	—	—	1	1	1	1	—	3	3	1	—	2	—	2	—	—	2	—	—	—	1	1	—	1
Nit-ac.	2	—	1	1	1	1	2	—	—	1	—	2	—	—	2	1	—	—	2	2	3	—	—	—	—	—	1	2	1	1	2
Nux-v.	3	3	1	—	1	1	2	3	2	3	—	1	3	—	2	3	2	—	—	—	3	1	—	—	2	—	1	2	—	2	2
Phosp.	1	1	—	—	—	—	1	1	—	2	—	—	1	2	2	—	1	2	1	—	3	2	2	—	—	—	—	3	—	—	3
Plat.	1	2	2	2	1	—	1	2	—	1	—	1	3	—	1	1	2	—	1	1	3	2	3	—	—	—	2	1	2	2	2
Puls.	—	2	—	—	1	—	2	2	—	2	—	—	—	—	2	—	2	—	—	—	3	2	3	—	—	—	2	—	3	2	2
Sulph.	1	2	—	2	—	—	—	2	1	2	1	—	—	1	2	1	3	2	—	—	2	1	—	—	1	—	2	1	2	2	2
Sep.	—	2	3	2	—	1	—	2	1	2	—	—	—	—	3	—	1	—	2	1	3	1	3	—	—	—	1	—	2	2	2
Staph.	—	—	1	—	3	2	—	2	1	—	—	—	—	—	—	—	—	—	—	2	1	—	—	2	—	—	3	—	1	3	1

Minimum Characteristic Syndrome
1) Malicious
2) Company, aversion to
3) Consolation agg.
4) Dwells on past disagreeable occurrences
5) Anger, ailments after, with silent grief
6) Love, ailments, from disappointed
7) Affectionate

Resentment – Primary Effects of
8) Offended easily
9) Reproaches others
10) Violent
11) Hatred

Resentment – Secondary Effects of
12) Anxiety, conscience, of

Fear
13) Fear, happen, something will
14) Fear, robbers, of
15) Frightened easily
16) Starting, noise, from

Desire to Escape
17 a) Hurry
   b) Company, aversion to (passive)
   c) Consolation agg. (passive)

Desire to Escape by Distancing Himself from Reality
18) Dream, as if in a
19) Estranged, family, from her
20) Homesickness

Emotional Discharge
21) Hysteria
22) Weeping, alternating with laughter
23) Weeping, involuntary

Intellect
24) Concentration, difficult, on attempting to, has a vacant feeling
25) Memory, weakness of, expressing one's self for
26) Mistakes, speaking, intend, what he does not

Depression
27) Mortification, ailments after
28) Sympathetic
29) Indifference, pleasure, to
30) Grief, ailments from
31) Loathing, life

Ignatia

As discussed in previous chapters, Ignatia is a neurotic, hysterical patient who is characterised by rapid changeability and variability of symptoms, a paradoxical nature and extreme emotional sensitivity. The suppression of emotions leads to a wealth of neurological symptoms that are all the physical manifestations of hysteria. Unstable and emotionally disturbed, Ignatia tries to suppress her hysteria – she is one of only three remedies in the rubric 'Grief, silent', along with Natrum Mur. and Pulsatilla; but whereas Ignatia is basically an hysterical patient, Natrum Mur. uses hysteria as a channel for emotional discharge. The psychological framework of Ignatia is predominantly of a superficial nature, whereas in Natrum Mur. it leads to deeper pathology.

Ignatia does not have symptom 4 from the Minimum Characteristic Syndrome which expresses Natrum Mur.'s obsession with the past – the longing for his lost love and the continual dwelling on disagreeable thoughts that have hindered his developing maturity from the early years of his life. The lack of symptom 4, combined with the superficial nature of any malice she might feel (1), are indications of the notorious instability, volatility and paradoxical nature of Ignatia. Furthermore, as she is neither easily offended (8), violent (10) nor full of hatred (11), the accusations she may fling occasionally at other people have no real substance ('Reproaches others', 9). The feelings of guilt ('Anxiety, conscience, of', 12) are aroused by her emotional sensitivity and self-condemnation for her somewhat melodramatic behaviour, rather than any deep-rooted feelings of resentment.

Ignatia does not have the fear that something will happen (13) or the starting from noise (16), examples of the guilt-ridden state of nervous tension that is so typical of Natrum Mur. Ignatia's fear of loss on an emotional level accounts for the fear of robbers (14) and she is easily frightened (15) because of her general hypersensitivity. From the symptoms connected with the desire to escape, she lacks the sensation of isolation (19) that separates the embittered Natrum Mur. from his loved ones. As one would expect, Ignatia has all the symptoms of emotional discharge, and lacks all the symptoms of memory and concentration that encourage Natrum Mur. to withdraw from the outside world. As far as the symptoms of depression are concerned, Ignatia is absent from symptoms 29 and 31, which describe the pseudo-psoric aspect of Natrum Mur.'s depression. Traditionally, Ignatia has always been considered to be a complementary remedy to Natrum Mur. due to its many similarities although, to my mind, its indecisiveness and obsessiveness bring it closer to Silicea, forming a link between these three big polychrests.

Lycopodium

While frustrated affection, suppressed anger, resentment and negativity are essential components of Natrum Mur., a lack of self-confidence is at the heart of Lycopodium's personality. In addition to this central theme, we have an egotistical, dictatorial or servile character with a strongly competitive nature. Whereas the lack of love makes Natrum Mur. withdraw from others and talk only to himself, in the under-confident Lycopodium it makes him sharper, more aggressive and ready to fight. He becomes arrogant, dictatorial and intolerant of contradiction, justly proud of his intelligence, efficiency and perfectionism.

Eventually, Lycopodium begins to lose his grip and, as his insecurities grow, he starts to avoid people ('Company, aversion to', 2), especially those who try to offer him some support ('Consolation agg.', 3), as he refuses to admit his vulnerability to others. The pain of being misunderstood fills him with rage ('Anger, ailments after, with silent grief', 5), and he strongly resents all the unfair treatment he has received, either real or imagined ('Malicious', 1). When he becomes ill, he shuts himself away and broods over the past (4). He has an affectionate nature (7), but his pride protects him from being hurt in love ('Love, ailments, from disappointed', 6). In its tubercular aspect, Lycopodium may be confused with Natrum Mur., as they can both take offence easily (8), blame others (9) and become violent (10), but Lycopodium is quite unlike the embittered Natrum Mur., being devoid of all hatred (11), destructive anger and guilt (12).

Lycopodium has the symptoms related to fear and nervous tension, with the exception of symptom 14, the fear of robbers, which symbolises Natrum Mur.'s fear of being robbed of affection. Lycopodium is too egotistical to feel homesick (20), and too afraid of solitude to withdraw from the family (19). From the symptoms related to the discharge of emotions, he lacks symptom 23, the involuntary weeping. Lycopodium's careful control of his emotions breaks down only when he is either reprimanded or thanked for a noble deed. There is no other remedy who has quite such a monopoly on the memory rubrics. The centre of his pathology is a combination of liver problems and a bad memory, and he finds it nearly impossible to remember people's names. However, he does not hide himself away like Natrum

Mur. – he simply gets embarrassed and tongue-tied ('Memory, weakness of, expressing one's self for', 25). The absence of symptom 29 from the last group of symptoms brings to light an essential difference between the two remedies: a small display of sincere affection and a little help from his friends is all a Lycopodium needs to cheer him up, while Natrum Mur. will feel even more depressed.

Nux Vomica (*See also* page 44)

This remedy has all the symptoms of the Minimum Characteristic Syndrome except symptom 4, the tendency to brood and dwell on the past. Nux Vomica is brave and reckless, living life to the full, with strong feelings of friendship, love and hatred. Although this remedy has the majority of symptoms from 1 to 12, he is quite a different character. Far from being stuck in the past, Nux Vomica is forward-thinking, impatient and hard-working, living more in his head than his body, which he abuses continually with large doses of stimulants such as coffee, alcohol and spices.

He does not have symptoms 13 and 14, symbols of Natrum Mur.'s fear of losing his loved one. However, he has the symptoms of fearfulness ('Frightened easily', 15 and 'Starting, noise, from', 16) that reflect an acute sensitivity to his environment which is comparable only to that of Phosphorus. He is impatient and speedy ('Hurry', 17), and tries to keep people at a distance as he 'desires repose and tranquility': *1*. He may take this to extremes and isolate himself completely from his family ('Estranged, family, from her', 19), but the lack of homesickness (20) shows us that emotional trauma has played no part in this. Nux Vomica's characteristic impulsiveness explains his absence from symptom 23, the involuntary weeping.

He finds life so stressful that he cannot concentrate on his work, and his speech is affected ('Memory, weakness of, expressing one's self for', 25). Like Lycopodium, his absence from symptom 29 gives a different significance to all the other symptoms of depression. Nux Vomica is a mixed miasmatic remedy (tubercular and sycotic) that bears some resemblance to Natrum Mur. However, when sycosis is dominant, with such typically Nux symptoms as perfectionism and industriousness, these similarities become insignificant.

Platinum

This remedy is generally depicted as an arrogant and moody woman who can become wildly excited on both an emotional and a sexual level, and whose mental disturbances can be either simultaneous or alternating with uterine or ovarian complaints. With her wild, arrogant, scornful and hysterical behaviour, this larger-than-life personality is expressed on a physical level by the sensation that the body, or a part of the body, is enlarged while objects and people appear to be small and unimportant.

Platinum is characterised by egotism and a marked superiority complex, which cover up her desperate feelings of abandonment and desertion ('Forsaken feeling': 2). This curious mixture of extremes probably accounts for her changeable mental states and tendency to hysterical outbursts, where brittle cheerfulness can suddenly give way to a bout of morbid depression and introversion. One minute she can be laughing, singing, dancing and whistling, and the next minute she will fly into a sudden rage for no reason at all and try to break everything in sight. Her good moods can change quickly into bad ones, where she wants to be left alone to cry inconsolably and indulge her feelings of abandonment, dredging up those interminable, sad memories of the past. She is haunted by the fear of death, that something will happen, that her husband will leave her and never come back. She has palpitations, tremblings and religious mania alternating with obscene, perverted sexual behaviour.

Such is a broad outline of Platinum, who shares all the symptoms of the Minimum Characteristic Syndrome of Natrum Muriaticum, except the ailments from disappointed love (6) that her pride will not allow. Indeed, she is too arrogant and haughty to permit others to encroach upon her life, so any malicious feelings she may have (1) are very short-lived, and she does not waste her precious time blaming (9) or hating (11) others. Platinum does not consider that she has anything to do with common people. During one of her outbursts of hysteria, she may occasionally take offence (8) and be violent (10). She is frightened (15) of demons, phantoms and people. From the desire to escape symptoms, she feels isolated from her family (19), but not homesick (20), because, as Kent says: 'She imagines that she is of a high-born family and that her friends and relatives are of lowly origin, and looks down upon them' (*Lectures on Homoeopathic Materia Medica*, p. 781). Not surprisingly, she has all the symptoms connected with emotional discharge.

On a mental level she has a weak memory, but the lack of symptoms indicates that she is too self-engrossed to be concerned with anything that happens outside of her own little world. Similarly, we see in the symptoms of depression that she is too proud to feel mortified (27) or feel sympathy for other people's problems (28). The great discrepancy between what she feels to be important and what is important to the rest of society, confirms her feelings of isolation; she becomes ill with grief (30) and tired of living (31).

Sepia

Of all the depressed remedies, Sepia is without a doubt the closest to Natrum Mur., but while the central issue for Natrum Mur. is the need for affection, the essential nature of Sepia is indifference to everything and emotional coldness (7), the clearest expression of this being the aversion to the members of her family. Although the remedy is not in the rubric 'Malicious' (1) in Kent, Sepia does have resentfulness, not because of a love disappointment, but because she feels that life itself has made her emotionally frigid. Emotional indifference is the motivating factor behind her aversion to her husband, who bears the full brunt of her anger and castrating envy. She prefers solitude ('Company, aversion to', 2), grumbles about her wretched life ('Dwells on past disagreeable occurrences', 4) and refuses to be comforted ('Consolation agg.', 3) in her anger, grief and continued frustration ('Anger, ailments after, with silent grief', 5), and finally she becomes totally disillusioned by relationships ('Love, ailments, from disappointed', 6).

She can be easily offended (8), preferring to blame everyone else for her problems ('Reproaches others', 9), and she can at times be violent (10); but she is quite incapable of having feelings and can neither love nor hate (11). With this indifference comes a distinct lack of guilt (12) and fear, with the exception of symptom 15 ('Frightened easily'), although she is, like Natrum Mur., both frightened and fascinated by the sight and sound of thunderstorms. She has all the symptoms related to the desire to escape, except the sensation of being in a dream (18), which is the Natrum Mur. strategy for removing himself from reality by dwelling on the past and brooding over his relationship problems. Sepia has all the symptoms connected with the discharge of emotions and none of the symptoms of the intellect. The symptoms of depression are not sparked off by actual events in her life and she suffers no ailments from grief (30).

The above description has focused on the pseudo-psoric side of Sepia, but when the sycotic aspect predominates there are many more differences between Sepia and Natrum Mur., namely, the compulsive addiction to work, intolerance of contradiction and great attention to detail, as Sepia prepares to engage in a fight to the death with the opposite sex. Whether she is the embittered housewife or the cold, calculating businesswoman, the sycotic aspect of Sepia is much closer to Nux Vomica and Thuja than to Natrum Muriaticum.

Three remedies have five symptoms of the Minimum Characteristic Syndrome of Natrum Muriaticum: Belladonna, Conium and Phosphorus.

Belladonna

It has often been observed that this is the most frequently occurring remedy in Kent: it appears 627 times in the Mind section, to be exact. Belladonna is a plethoric individual – Henri Duprat once said: 'Anges bien portants, démons malades' – jovial and entertaining when well but nervous and irritable when sick. There is a tendency for congestion to the head. He has a hot head and cold feet. The head is sensitive to cold and draughts.

The picture of Belladonna in acutes is easily recognised, and it is not necessary to repeat it here. Instead, let us discuss the chronic picture. When in health, he is calm and composed, but when he falls ill he becomes apathetic and indifferent, crying when reprimanded, afraid of people and noise, wanting to be left alone even though he fears solitude, and irritated by consolation and touch. He becomes quarrelsome, capricious, impulsive and contrary, with an obstinacy similar to Calcarea Carbonica. With much wailing and moaning, and great inner sadness, he can become so hopeless that all he wants to do is drown himself. The variability and alternating nature of his symptoms is a characteristic trait of the psoric aspect of the remedy – he fluctuates between moods of depression and hyperactivity, with anxiety, impatience and hurried movements.

From the Minimum Characteristic Syndrome, he does not have symptoms 4 and 7, which describe how Natrum Mur. dwells on his past love disappointments. His emotions are so intense that he can become violent (10), but not directly at other people, hence the lack of accusations (9), hatred (11) and guilt (12). He does not start at noise (16) or fear that something will happen (13). Unlike Natrum Mur., he is not a victim of frustrated emotion and, while he shares all the symptoms of emotional discharge, he does not feel isolated (19). When he gets depressed, he turns inwards and does not blame others for his problems.

Possibly the central theme of the remedy is the delusion that he is about to receive an injury ('Delusions, injury, is about to receive': *1*,

Synthetic Repertory, Vol. I), as he is unable to discriminate between good and bad. He hates being told off ('Admonition agg.': 2) and reacts with tears and verbal abuse which soon becomes physical, with biting and hitting. Like all the other remedies from the *Solanaceae* family (including Stramonium and Hyoscyamus), this remedy has sudden and violent fits of temper, although the other side of this 'devil' is someone who is caring and compassionate.

Unlike Natrum Muriaticum, who becomes so depressed, worn out and full of bitterness that he loses all zest for life, Belladonna is not indifferent to pleasure (29); it is his uncontrollable aggressive impulses and his inability to tell right from wrong that eventually exhaust him.

Conium

This is a remedy for prematurely old people, celibate men and menopausal women who have been worn down by long, debilitating illnesses. Conium is thin, pale and mentally and physically slow. He is slow to comprehend, and cannot remember dates. His mind becomes lazy and he is incapable of all mental effort, apathetic, indifferent and depressed. He wants no-one to meddle in his affairs so keeps to himself, even though he is afraid of solitude.

With the onset of senility he falls into a profound depression, for no apparent reason, and sits, hunched and motionless, in a corner of the room, letting no-one come near him. He is bad-tempered and touchy, everything annoys or offends him, even the slightest difference of opinion. He has extreme weakness that is worse in the morning, after exertion and after stool. Paresis ascends from the legs, with tremblings, numbness and tingling sensations. He has a weak appetite with heartburn and acrid eructations. There may be impotence, with paresis of the bladder and eyelids. The Conium state can be brought on by the suppression of the sexual appetite, with exhaustion, paresis, apathy and depression.

There are several keynotes that would indicate its use: vertigo on turning over in bed or on the least motion of the head; heavy, drooping eyelids; intense photophobia; painless cancerous tumours; sweat on closing the eyes; cold flatus; sexual desire with sexual fantasies and impotence.

This brief sketch of Conium has been taken from sources such as Clarke, Kent, Nash, Duprat and Voisin, in order to portray the essential differences from Natrum Mur. Conium should be added to the rubric 'Consolation agg.' (3), as Kent clearly includes this symptom in his materia medica. Conium is a profoundly debilitated remedy, with little strength for resentment (1), who suffers from disappointed love (6) but not from anger with silent grief (5). He lives in the past (4) and avoids company (2) because it is painful to be reminded of the time when he was young and healthy. Because of his lack of stamina, he avoids emotional commitment and is undemonstrative (7), even when he feels so sorry for himself that he could cry, like Natrum Muriaticum.

He lacks all the symptoms connected with anger (8 – 11), which confirms Kent's portrait of him as someone whose bad temper and touchiness only serve to make him more depressed and weak. He feels guilty ('Anxiety, conscience, of', 12), vulnerable and full of morbid fears ('Fear, robbers of', 14, 'Frightened easily', 15 and 'Starting, noise, from', 16). However, he does not have the fear that something will happen (13), which stems from the suppressed anger of Natrum Mur. He has the symptoms related to the desire to escape – here again, the lack of homesickness (20) means that he is not bound by the emotional chains of Natrum Mur. The sensations of alienation ('Estranged, family, from her', 19) and of being in a dream (18) are the products of a feeble mind and body. From the symptoms of emotional discharge, he does not have the uncontrollable weeping (23) that bursts out of Natrum Mur. in a pained lament for his lost love.

Phosphorus (*See also* pages 62–4)

Phosphorus lacks symptoms 3 and 4, which describe Natrum Mur.'s obsession with the past and his inconsolable anger. It has a great ability to communicate with the world around him and a sense of belonging to the whole of creation. This sensitive soul is easily exhausted, and when the demands of his artistic and clairvoyant abilities become too much for him, he may withdraw from society, although he is aggravated when alone, with a strong fear of solitude and a desire to be magnetised by others. In one of his more reclusive moods, he may appear to have certain similarities to Natrum Mur., as indicated by his presence in most of the remaining symptoms of the Minimum Characteristic Syndrome; however, he does not have symptom 6, as he tends to become indifferent to his loved ones, rather than disappointed in love.

Unlike Natrum Mur., Phosphorus blames no-one for his own shortcomings (9); and, while he may be one of the most fearful remedies, he does not start from noise (16), possibly because he is not at war with the world but very much part of it. He is so bound up with art and mysticism that he feels at times as if he were on another planet ('Estranged, family, from her', 19), or in a dream-world (18); the lack of homesickness (20) is further confirmation of the indifference to his loved ones, a symptom not shared by Natrum Mur. Being the great extrovert that he is, he has no trouble expressing his emotions (symptoms 21 to 23).

Mental exhaustion can weaken his memory; he may forget what he has read, and make mistakes with writing. However, the lack of the intellect symptoms 24 to 26 suggests that his problems with memory are not emotionally based.

He fluctuates wildly between states of great, clairvoyant ecstasy and listless depression with indifference to everything. He is subject to bouts of depression and despondency, with dramatic outbursts of weeping and the occasional fit of uncontrollable laughter. He has episodes of gibbering delirium, with stupor, drowsiness and lethargy. He can be listless and slow, with no desire to talk. He feels extremely anxious when alone. He feels that life holds nothing for him and wants to die. He is impulsive and subject to sudden fits of anger.

Phosphorus can be distinguished easily from Natrum Mur. by the great fear of solitude and the symptoms of depression. With his love of people and his ability to identify with their problems, he cannot take offence at the things they say (27), as his understanding and capacity for compassion are so great ('Sympathetic': *3*). His exquisite aesthetic sense ensures that he can never become indifferent to pleasure (29).

Six remedies have four symptoms from the Minimum Characteristic Syndrome of Natrum Muriaticum: Aurum, China, Hyoscyamus, Lachesis, Nitricum Acidum and Pulsatilla.

Aurum

Aurum has resentment ('Malicious', 1), aversion to company (2), anger with silent grief (5) and ailments from disappointed love (6) but lacks the need for affection (7) and the tendency to brood on the past (4) that characterise Natrum Mur. Aurum is not aggravated by consolation (3), because the central issues for this remedy are his feelings of abandonment and gnawing guilt ('Anxiety, conscience, of', 12). Natrum Mur., on the other hand, hates fuss and consolation as he feels that it is only an attempt to compensate for the love that was denied him in the past.

The anxiety of conscience, an essential component of Aurum's personality, is so great that he feels as if he had committed a crime. He is self-destructive, angry with himself and so unhappy that he wants to kill himself. He is easily offended (8), violent (10), full of hatred (11) and apt to blame others (9) with syphilitic rage and indignation. However, these symptoms are secondary to the feelings of guilt that they provoke. Nobody can feel quite as worthless as Aurum, when he berates himself for making mistakes, neglecting his duty and losing the affection and estimation of his family and friends – and nobody can feel quite as suicidal as a result. In Natrum Mur. the symptoms of hurt, blame and anger are more prominent, and he is not suicidal.

Aurum is afraid of robbers (14), easily frightened (15) and easily startled ('Starting, noise, from', 16). His negativity comes out in self-destructive anger rather than in the fear that something is about to happen (13).

He does not have the sensation of living in a dream (18), possibly because he feels things all too directly on both a mental and physical level. He does not feel estranged from his family (19) but suffers from homesickness (20), which represents his wish to feel secure and comfortable with people who value him. For this reason, he weeps when he meets his friends ('Weeping, meeting people, when': 2). Natrum Mur., by contrast, avoids his loved ones and weeps when they look at him. Consequently, the meaning of symptoms 22 and 23 ('Weeping, alternating with laughter' and 'Weeping, involuntary') is quite different in the context of each remedy.

Aurum lacks the specific symptoms of the intellect (24–26), as his mind is affected by syphilis in a more general way.

As one would expect from the symptoms missing from the Minimum Characteristic Syndrome, he lacks compassion (28) and indifference to pleasure (29); he is neither affectionate nor stuck in the past, and is not bothered one way or the other by consolation. As his body becomes ravaged by the syphilitic miasm, his feelings of mortification (27), grief (30), and disgust with life (31) increase to the point where he wants to kill himself by throwing himself from the balcony.

China (*See also* pages 55–7)

China has the first four symptoms of the Minimum Characteristic Syndrome of Natrum Mur., but the lack of the remaining symptoms suggests that, unlike Natrum Mur., frustrated affection is not the prime, motivating factor behind his inconsolable grief. He feels rejected and abused, and his wounded ego tries to reassert itself by heaping scorn and criticism on others. He complains bitterly (9) and takes offence at the slightest provocation (8), although he harbours no great feelings of resentment, hatred (11) or violence (10). His feelings of guilt ('Anxiety, conscience, of', 12) are brought out by two important China symptoms that are not present in Natrum Mur., namely, the fear of dogs and the delusion of being persecuted.

Hyoscyamus

For a full description of this remedy, the reader should refer to the comparative section of the chapter on Lycopodium (pages 57–8). The chronic picture is one of anger with silent grief (5), disappointed love (6), resentment ('Malicious', 1) and aversion to company (2). There are the characteristic feelings of jealousy and suspicion, with delusions of persecution where he believes that he is being poisoned, all symptoms that are alien to Natrum Mur. He feels lonely and deserted, and talks to himself and the dead, like Natrum Mur. However, he is not aggravated by consolation (3) and does not dwell continually on the past (4). His resentment stems from the feeling that his friends have deserted him, and left him alone to cope with his tremendous fear of solitude.

Like all remedies from the *Solanaceae* family, he is prone to fits of uncontrollable anger, where he can become violent (10) and full of blame (9), but the explosions soon pass and the anger is much less deep-rooted than the rigid rage of Natrum Mur., with no aftermath of hatred (11) or hurt feelings (8). In other words, the anger is more the product of a hyperactive brain than a manifestation of any deeply engrained resentment. For this reason, there is no fear that something will happen (13) or starting from noise (16), both indications of the state of Natrum Mur.'s nerves under the strain of all that suppressed anger. The fear of solitude is so predominant in Hyoscyamus that he cannot afford to feel alienated from the family (19) or aggravated by consolation (3).

He has a general weakness of memory, forgetting what he has read, said, heard and thought, but he has no difficulty with self-expression. When depressed, he falls into a state of ennui ('Loathing, life', 31), weighed down by sorrow ('Grief, ailments from', 30), with the sensation that everyone is against him and has deserted him.

Lachesis (*See also* page 59)

Lachesis has symptoms 1, 2, 6 and 7 from the Minimum Characteristic Syndrome of Natrum Muriaticum. Traumatic events can bring on a picture of frenzied jealousy, vicious resentment, great anger, arrogance, argumentativeness, eroticism, overbearing behaviour and the slanderous accusations of a wicked tongue. She does not dwell on the past (4) or suffer her pain in silence (5) and she allows no-one to comfort her (3). Unlike Natrum Mur., who almost expects to be criticised and treated badly, she is not easily hurt (8). She feels that the gods have singled her out for her supernatural and clairvoyant powers, and has no qualms about using her destructive abilities for their purposes, hence the lack of fear that something will happen (13). She is a sociable person who would not alienate herself from the family (19), and the remaining symptoms confirm the essential differences between the two remedies. She does not suffer from mortification (27), excessive sympathy (28) or indifference to pleasure (29), but her great capacity for hatred and jealousy can cause her considerable grief ('Grief, ailments from', 30) and ennui ('Loathing, life', 31).

Nitricum Acidum (*See also* pages 66–7)

Nitricum Acidum has four symptoms of the Minimum Characteristic Syndrome of Natrum Muriaticum. The bitterness he feels at the way the world has treated him makes him resentful ('Malicious', 1) and unresponsive to consolation (3), as he broods on the past (4) and longs for affection (7). He is not antisocial (2), angry with silent grief (5) nor disappointed in love (6), symptoms that characterise the hidden suffering endured by the elusive Natrum Mur. From the depths of his bitterness and despair, Nitricum Acidum can look only on the black side, entirely devoid of all faith and hope.

With such low expectations of human nature, he cannot be hurt or surprised by anything that people do (8); he expresses his hatred (11) with curses, torrents of tears and explosions of violent, trembling rage (10), pacified neither by apologies nor excuses. In the aftermath of such an explosion, he will feel guilty (12), fearful (15) and jumpy (16), but he lacks the fear symptoms 13 and 14 that represent Natrum Mur.'s neurotic obsession with his emotional problems. While Natrum Mur. has a kind of love/hate relationship with his loved one, Nitricum Acidum is much less passionate, although he can at times be demonstrative and sympathetic (28). Like Natrum Mur., Nitricum Acidum can feel alienated from his family (19) and unable to concentrate ('Concentration, difficult, on attempting to has a vacant feeling', 24), but the absence of mortification (27) from the symptoms of depression is an indication that the main issue for Nitricum Acidum is the miasmatic predisposition that wields its influence over and above all other factors.

Additional characteristic symptoms of this remedy are: aggravation from touch and noise; jerkings and tremblings; splinter-like pains; stubborn suppurations and fetid discharges; cracks and crusts on the skin; pains which come and go rapidly; and the typical smell of horse urine.

Pulsatilla

Pulsatilla does not have the aggravation from consolation (3), obsession with the past (4) or ailments from disappointed love (6) which account for Natrum Mur.'s particular brand of resentment. Many years of trauma and hardship may take their toll, and Pulsatilla's once pleasant, amenable nature can become hardened and bitter (1).

Although the traditional picture of Pulsatilla is easily distinguishable from Natrum Mur., with its mildness, meekness, docility, tearfulness, and the emotional ups and downs that respond easily to consolation, there is another side to the remedy that is met frequently in clinical practice. She is quiet, reserved, introspective, keeping her suffering to herself, withdrawing from her family when depressed, and wanting to be alone. Through fear of abandonment and solitude, she has forced herself to put up with many injustices and hurts in her life, and she has now had enough. The fear of loss makes her silent and withdrawn in her pain.

The accumulated pain of many traumatic events has left her feeling vulnerable and easily offended (8), but she is incapable of violence (10) and blame (9) for, as Kent says, her irritability and capriciousness always end in tears. Although the male Pulsatilla may be something of a woman-hater, with a strong fear of women and an abhorrence of marriage, hatred is not normally seen in this remedy (11). However, it may be detected in a latent homosexual who is immature, timid and mistrustful.

The constant need for approval and estimation means that she feels guilty and bad a lot of the time ('Anxiety, conscience, of', 12), but there is none of Natrum Mur.'s nervous excitability (13, 16). She is afraid ('Frightened easily', 15) of darkness, ghosts and solitude, but not of robbers (14). As one would expect, there is much crying

('Weeping, alternating with laughter', 22 and 'Weeping, involuntary', 23), hysteria (21) and homesickness (20). She is like a sweet, capricious child whose tears are quickly dissipated by a kind word, like the petals of the windflower that sway in the breeze.

Her timidity inhibits her self-expression ('Memory, weakness of, expressing one's self for', 25). She may be confused with Natrum Mur. when the combination of depression (symptoms 27 – 31), pain and desire for solitude are all present; however, she has none of Natrum Mur.'s deep bitterness, brusque manner and determined refusal to accept all gestures of support.

Two remedies have three symptoms of the Minimum Characteristic Syndrome of Natrum Muriaticum: Sulphur and Natrum Carbonicum.

Sulphur

Sulphur has the resentment ('Malicious', 1), aversion to company (2) and obsession with the past (4) from the Minimum Characteristic Syndrome of Natrum Mur. However, the lack of symptoms 3, 5, 6 and 7 indicates that the cause of his difficulties has nothing to do with hurt feelings and unrequited love affairs.

Sulphur is a supreme egotist, sitting on his backside all day while his mind works overtime, conjuring up wonderful fantasies. In the belief that nothing that involves a lot of effort can be worth having, he adopts the 'sour grapes' attitude to life and takes no interest in anything that does not affect him personally.

Although he does not blame others for his misfortunes (9), he can become easily offended (8), violent (10) and hateful 11), but without the rancour and bitterness seen in the aggrieved Natrum Mur. Sulphur is arrogant, egotistical and naturally impulsive. He feels guilty ('Anxiety, conscience, of', 12) that is he so lazy, apathetic and ineffectual, and this also explains the anxiety he feels for others, especially if they are friends.

Sulphur does not have the fear that something will happen (13), and the fear of robbers (14) is more to do with a self-centred fear of material loss than with any emotional issue. He is easily frightened (15), but does not start at noise (16). A compensatory reaction to the apathy is the tendency to be hurried (17) and impetuous; and a result of it is the withdrawal from reality and dream-like sensations (18). However, Sulphur does not go so far as to withdraw from his family (19), or suffer from homesickness (20); he simply uses people to his advantage and at his convenience.

After a life of indolence and self-absorption, he sees himself as the failure that he is, and sinks into a state of anxiety and despair for the salvation of his soul. He feels profoundly mortified (27) and depressed by the injustices of life and indifferent to everything, even pleasant things (29); life is a huge burden (31) to which suicide, by drowning, seems the only solution. Once more, the lack of compassion for others (28) and sensitivity to grief (30) underline Sulphur's innate self-centredness, confirmed optimism and subtle bitterness.

Natrum Carbonicum

Natrum Carbonicum has resentment ('Malicious', 1), aversion to company (2) and suppressed anger (5).

He is too introverted to respond to consolation (3), and is bothered neither by the past (4) nor by relationship problems (6 and 7). He does not have symptoms 8 to 11, and the fears arise from his feelings of vulnerability ('Fear, robbers, of', 14, 'Frightened easily', 15 and 'Starting, noise, from', 16). He lives in constant fear that he will attract evil or harm, with anxiety and tremblings during the pain and during storms. Natrum Muriaticum's fears centre around the future and the threat of insanity, and make him anxious, speedy and restless – Natrum Carbonicum, by contrast, is too exhausted and lazy to rush about. Other people interest him so little that he has neither a guilt complex (12) nor the fear that something will happen (13).

Like all the Natrums, he feels a great divide between him and his family (19), but the significance of this is greatly modified by the symptoms that are missing from the Minimum Characteristic Syndrome. It is not so much hatred (11) or violence (10) that he feels towards his family, as cold dislike, and here the remedy is closer to Sepia, but without the homesickness (20).

Natrum Carbonicum has a weak mind, with mental confusion and vertigo from the slightest mental effort, but the weakness is general and all-pervasive, without any of the specific rubrics of the intellect (24, 25, 26). From the symptoms of depression, his absence from the mortification and grief symptoms (27 and 30) is further confirmation of his emotional coldness, and any compassion he may feel for others ('Sympathetic') says more about his tendency to hook into other people's negativity than about his caring nature.

7

Kali Carbonicum

DESCRIPTION

A common feature of all the Kali remedies, due to the presence of potassium, is a great emotional instability that brings about dramatic mood swings, from depression to euphoria and apathy to excitement, as the organism reacts with exhausting speed to every little change. The Kali remedies are suited to people who are easily exhausted by stress and whose mental and physical reserves are soon depleted.

Kali Carbonicum is adapted to fleshy, soft individuals with lax fibre and oedematous tendencies. The face is bloated and pale, with a characteristic, bag-like swelling between the upper eyelids and eyebrows. Like Sepia, there is a saddle of freckles across the upper parts of the cheeks and nose and the patient is weak, chilly, pale and anaemic-looking. He is sensitive to draughts and subject to waves of pulsating heat that seem to rise from the stomach to the head.

According to Farrington, the three characteristics of the remedy are perspiration, backache and weakness, especially in the small of the back. The pains are sharp, stitching, stabbing and darting, with a general aggravation from cold, and between 2 a.m. and 4 a.m. As always, any prescription should take into account both the characteristic mental symptoms and the general and particular modalities. The essence of the Kali Carbonicum personality is the totally incapacitating weakness that forces him to become dependent upon others and unable to fend for himself.

Paschero, whose authoritative study has provided the foundations for this work, says of the remedy: 'This is an irritable and bad-tempered patient who is intolerant and discontented with everything, mainly himself ('Discontented': 2, with the sub-rubrics 'everything, with': 1, and 'himself, with': 1), in a perpetual state of conflict and flux. The cause of his discontent and ill humour is the overwhelming nature of his mental and physical weakness ('Confidence, want of self': 2), that forces him to depend on others and makes him incapable of fending for himself.'

My analysis of the remedy is based on these core symptoms. Kali Carb.'s progress is severely hampered by an enormous inferiority complex on both a mental and a physical level. His natural human desire for spiritual development – to realise his potential in life, to grow from a self-centred and irresponsible child into a selfless and mature adult – is thwarted at every turn by a weak constitution that forces him to rely completely on those around him. He is angry ('Antagonism, with herself': 2) and frustrated that he cannot do what he wants, and becomes moody and irritable ('Mood, alternating': 2); his emotions range between anxiety and irritability, fear and anger, vulnerability and self-assertion, depression and excitability.

There follows an analysis of each of these four opposing pairs of symptoms, as they form the essence of his personality.

Anxiety and Irritability

Anxiety
His feelings of anxiety and helplessness stem from a deeply ingrained lack of confidence. He has fearful anxiety ('Anxiety, fear, with': 2) that intensifies during sleep ('Anxiety, sleep, during': 2) and on waking ('Anxiety, waking, on': 2). Sleep and bed are symbols of maternal protection. The four characteristic modalities of his anxiety are: anxiety at night from flatulence ('Anxiety, lying, side, on, right, from flatulence': 1), after breakfast ('Anxiety, breakfast, after': 1), after a chill ('Anxiety, chill, after': 1) and when hungry ('Anxiety, hungry, when': 2). Anxiety can also manifest as restlessness and excitability. There is restlessness before and during the menses, to express the female Kali Carb.'s dissatisfaction with her lot ('Restlessness, anxious': 3, with the modalities 'menses, before': 1, and 'menses, during': 1). Menstruation may cease altogether after a fright ('Genitalia, menses, suppressed, fright, from': 2). Excitability is one of the manifestations of nervousness that, as we shall see in the discussion on the rubric 'Starting, startled', stems from his feelings of helplessness and inability to cope with stress. He has excitement on hearing bad news ('Excitement, bad news, after': 1), and especially when he is hungry ('Excitement, hungry, when': 1 – only remedy). The distress felt in the stomach is typical of Kali Carb. and expresses the need for both emotional and physical nurturing.

Irritability
The counterpart of anxiety is irritability ('Irritability': 3). Kent says in this respect: 'The patient is whimsical, irascible, irritable to the very

highest degree, quarrels with his family and with his bread and butter.' (*Lectures on Homoeopathic Materia Medica*). He becomes irritable from the nervous tension he cannot control, and the irritability has similar modalities to the anxiety: it is worse on waking ('Irritability, morning, waking, on': 2), when he is tired in the evening ('Irritability, evening': 2) and after coition ('Irritability, coition, after': 2), heralding, as Kent says, the break-down of the constitution. The female Kali Carb. has irritability before menses ('Irritability, menses, before': 1), an expression of her discontentment with her weak femininity, and there is irritability from consolation ('Irritability, consolation agg.': 1).

Fear and Anger

Fear

Fear is the external manifestation of his internal anxiety. The fundamental fear of solitude ('Fear, alone, of being': 3) interferes with his desire to liberate himself from the chains of dependence that bind him to other people. He is afraid of dying in solitude ('Fear, alone, of being, lest he die': 2), and of death when alone ('Fear, death, of, alone, when': 1), especially at night in bed ('Fear, death, alone, when, evening, in bed': 1) and while lying in bed ('Fear, lying in bed, while': 1 – only remedy). Death threatens him in other guises, such as the fear of evil ('Fear, evil, of': 1), ghosts ('Fear, ghosts, of': 1), and disease ('Fear, disease, of impending': 3). Many symptoms are felt in the stomach – a whole range of emotions and fears are felt like a constricted knot of anxiety that rises from the stomach ('Fear, stomach, arising from': 2). His feelings of fear and helplessness are intensified by his oversensitivity to his surroundings.

Nervous reactions are typical of this remedy – he is easily startled ('Starting, easily': 3) and jumpy from fright ('Starting, fright, from': 3), noise ('Starting, noise, from': 3), on falling asleep ('Starting, sleep, on falling': 23) and during sleep ('Starting, sleep, during': 3). An unexpected touch may startle him so much that he screams and jumps up ('Starting, touched, when': 3). His skin is so sensitive that he has a real fear of being touched ('Fear, touch, of': 1), similar to Arnica; he is frightened from touch ('Frightened, touch, from': 2 – only remedy), and tries to avoid it at all cost ('Touched, aversion to being': 3); he is easily frightened ('Frightened, easily': 2) by the slightest thing ('Frightened, trifles, at': 3).

Anger

His irritable and debilitated state brings on feelings of inferiority, helplessness, anxiety, fear and tension. Fear engenders anger, for the more fearful a person is, the more anger he feels. As always, the picture of Kali Carb. is created in our materia medica from real human beings with certain morbid predispositions to disease and not from some abstract fantasy. Here we have the whole, unique picture of an individual whose mental and physical symptoms are closely inter-related. The pains of Kali Carb. are disconcertingly unpredictable and unexpected – they can be sharp and cutting like knives, needles or splinters, burning, shooting or darting. Similarly, he recoils sharply from the slightest touch, and his anger at himself, with all his fears and weaknesses, is sharp and pointed. His anger ('Anger': *3*) has the following characteristic modalities: it is worse in the morning ('Anger, morning': *2*), on waking ('Anger, morning, waking, on': *2*) – because waking involves leaving the bed, a mother symbol – and also in the evening ('Anger, evening': *2*) when his lethargy increases. His anger can become violent ('Violent': *1*), causing him to shout uncontrollably ('Shrieking': *3*) at the slightest provocation ('Shrieking, trifles, at': *3* – only remedy): he may attack people ('Striking': *2*) or lash out at imaginary objects ('Striking, about him at imaginary objects': *2*), like the delirious Hyoscyamus. He can be argumentative ('Quarrelsome': *2*), cold and rejecting when angry ('Repulsive mood': *1*), and may let his impulses get the better of him ('Impetuous': *2*). His anger provides a necessary escape valve for his emotions, not a means of self-assertion; he never holds on to it, for fear of frightening away his friends. For this reason, he is neither intolerant of contradiction nor subject to feelings of mortification or suppressed anger, and he is not easily offended. In other words, Kali Carb. does not waste valuable energy nursing his wounded pride, or confronting those who try to hurt or offend; his responses are more indirect, an expression of his inner discontentment ('Discontented': *2*).

Vulnerability and Self-Assertion

Vulnerability

The important symptom here is the fear of solitude, as all his symptoms are aggravated by solitude ('Company, desire for, alone, while agg.': *2*). He has a desperate need for company ('Company, desire for': *3*). He begs piteously for people to stay with him, but treats them like dirt when they do ('Company, desire for, yet treats them outrageously': *2* – only remedy). This rather picturesque and unique symptom may appear in a whole range of subtle guises in clinical practice; for example, the patient who feels that he has to live in close proximity to his family, although in reality he cannot stand them, and will never openly admit to his fear of solitude.

Kali Carb. may be the remedy for the sick child who, like Chamomilla, needs to be held in someone's arms ('Carried, desires to be': *2*) and who gets anxious when he is hungry ('Anxiety, hungry, when': *2*), and the adult who moans continually about every little problem ('Moaning': *3*), with feelings of abandonment ('Forsaken feeling': *1*) and rejection ('Love, ailments, from disappointed': *1*). A debilitated body and weak and disordered mind increase his feelings of vulnerability. He feels confused ('Confusion of mind': *2*), drugged ('Confusion, intoxicated, as after being': *1*), incapable of mental effort ('Dullness': *3*) and coherent speech ('Dullness, speaking, while': *1*), with an unusual amelioration from closing the eyes ('Dullness, closing eyes, on, amel.': *1* – only remedy). Due to a state of extreme apathy, he feels worse whenever he tries to use his mind ('Exertion, agg. from mental': *1*). The apathy affects the memory and he becomes forgetful ('Forgetful': *1*), finds it difficult to express himself ('Memory, weakness of, expressing one's self for': *2*), forgets words ('Memory, weakness of, words, for': *2*), makes mistakes when speaking ('Mistakes, speaking': *2*), misplaces words ('Mistakes, words, misplacing': *1*) and uses them wrongly ('Mistakes, wrong words, using': *1*).

Understandably enough, he does not like being drawn into conversation ('Conversation agg.': *1*), and he experiences an occasional dulling of the senses and the reasoning faculty ('Senses, dullness of': 1, 'Senses, vanishing of': *1*). To detract attention away from his pathetic state, he complains and whines with dogged persistence about anything and everything. Another characteristic symptom of Kali Carb. is his habit of talking nonsense while asleep ('Speech, nonsense, springing up while asleep, on': *1*). This symptom is unique to Kali Carb. and indicative of his difficulty with self-expression. Another interesting feature is the dream of calling out for help ('Sleep, dreams, calling out for help': *1* – only remedy). Kali Carb. will never ask outright for help; he will only let his dreams do it for him. During the night, the moaning will start up again at around 3 a.m. ('Moaning, night, 3 a.m.': *3* – only remedy).

The following quartet of symptoms express in a nutshell the conflicts of Kali Carb.: constant moaning, difficulty in speaking, calling for help in dreams and weeping when telling of his sickness ('Weeping, telling of her sickness, when': *2*).

Self-Assertion

This goes hand in hand with his feelings of vulnerability. Unlike Natrum Carb. and Ammonium Carb., he neither withdraws into himself nor gives up the fight. Instead, he engages in a desperate struggle with lethargy, decay and death that threaten to overwhelm him. His debilitated mind and body are easy prey for all kinds of dietary discrepancies and aversions, and his digestive and liver symptoms increase as he becomes increasingly sensitive on a mental level. Let us recall the words of Paschero: 'The cause of his discontent and ill humour is the overwhelming nature of his mental and physical weakness that forces him to depend on others and makes him incapable of fending for himself.' The conflict between the need for support and the desire for self-affirmation, common to all human beings in their quest for self-development, is expressed here in a way that is peculiar to Kali Carb.

As we have already discussed, he is unable to vent his aggression directly on to his loved ones, for fear of losing their much-needed support, so he goes about it in more convoluted ways, becoming contrary and unpredictable in family and social situations ('Contrary': *2*), sometimes to the point of obstinacy ('Obstinate': *2*). The desire to break free from the chains that bind him to those who help him, and the urgent need to succeed in something to counteract the lethargy, are the motivating force behind his fierce and aggressive tenacity. In fact, he has all the makings of an anarchist, like Causticum and Sepia, with his stubborn and flagrant disregard of all authority, rules and laws, as expressed by the symptom 'Unobserving': *1*.

Depression, Despair and Excitability

This is a remedy of great conflicts and antagonisms – an individual who reacts to the stresses and strains of life in two quite contradictory ways.

Depression

He is basically timid ('Timidity': *3*), especially at night in bed ('Timidity, evening, in bed': *1* – only remedy), dissatisfied ('Discontented': *2*) with himself and everything ('Discontented, himself, with': *1*, 'Discontented, everything, with': *1*), bad-tempered ('Morose': *1*,

Barthel), depressed at night in bed ('Sadness, night, in bed': *1*), in the open air ('Sadness, air, in open': *2*) and when alone ('Sadness, alone, when': *1*), in accordance with the general modalities of the remedy. When night falls, his thoughts become obsessed with the past ('Dwells, on past disagreeable ocurrences, night': *1*), especially when he is alone in his bed ('Thoughts, persistent': *1*, with the modalities 'alone, when': *1*, 'night': *1*, and 'lying, while': *1*); he is tormented by unpleasant thoughts ('Thoughts, tormenting, evening': *1*, 'night': *1*).

He cries ('Weeping': *2*) with frustration and annoyance, not from the need to be comforted, as consolation only makes him feel worse ('Weeping, consolation agg.': *1*). When he is told off, he cries tears of anger ('Weeping, remonstrated with, when': *2*, 'Weeping, admonitions, cause': *2*). He is so dissatisfied with his life that he may cry for no reason at all ('Weeping, causeless': *1*) and without knowing why ('Weeping, causeless, without knowing why': *1*). He may cry during the consultation as he recalls all the sad events of his life ('Weeping, telling of her sickness, when': *2*).

He becomes profoundly depressed and apathetic ('Indifference': *2*), taking no interest even in pleasurable things ('Indifference, pleasure, to': *1*); he is indifferent to those around him, whose company he both needs and rejects ('Indifference, society, when in': *2*) and to work ('Indolence, aversion to work': *2*); he finds that he has no energy for anything or anyone ('Loathing, general': *1*). Too weary to speak ('Talk, indisposed to': *1*), he longs for perfect silence; when he does talk, his speech is incoherent ('Speech, incoherent': *1*) and rambling ('Speech, wandering': *1*) and he mutters in his sleep ('Talking, sleep, in': *3*).

Despair

He suspects that he will never manage to achieve any kind of balance in his life, no matter how hard he might try, and the thought that he might never get any better ('Doubtful, recovery, of': *1*, 'Despair, recovery': *1*) depresses him so much that he loses the will to fight ('Discouraged': *1*). His behaviour degenerates into foolishness ('Foolish behaviour': *1*), chaos ('Chaotic': *1*) and hysteria ('Hysteria': *2*).

Excitability

He can at times become very excitable, impatient, anxious and restless as a sort of defence mechanism to the depression. In an unconscious attempt to counteract the draining effects of apathy and debility, he rushes about, trying to finish impossible tasks quicker than anybody ('Hurry': *2*). He becomes both mentally ('Hurry, mental work, in': *2*) and physically ('Hurry, movements, in': *1*) speedy ('Hurry, occupation, in': *2*). This is the irritable and impulsive housewife who is a veritable whirlwind of activity, whose constant grumbling and complaining may remind us of Sepia, Nux Vomica or Lycopodium. The aspects of anxious restlessness and excitability have already been discussed at the beginning of this chapter.

Delusions, Sensations and Dreams

While these may come from a distorted perception of reality, they offer an insight into the whole picture of the remedy and contain many symbols of great significance.

Delusions and Sensations

In accordance with the general modalities of the remedy, his anxious fantasies intensify during a chill ('Delusions, fancy, illusions of, chill, during': *1*). The sensation that the bed is sinking ('Delusions, bed, sinking, were': *1*) connects with the fear of solitude, the bed being a symbol of maternal protection. The delusion that someone is calling him ('Delusions, calls, someone': *1*) expresses his sensation of solitude and abandonment ('Forsaken, feeling': *1*). His suppressed anger is expressed by the visions of phantoms and images ('Delusions, images, phantoms, sees': *1*), wearing masks ('Delusions, masks, sees': *1*) that frighten him ('Delusions, frightful': *1*) at night ('Delusions, images, phantoms, sees, night': *1*), and there is also the fear that he will be murdered ('Delusions, murdered, that he would be': *1*) or robbed ('Delusions, thieves, sees': *1*). The delusion of birds, a symptom that is shared only with Belladonna and Lac Caninum ('Delusions, birds, sees': *1*), expresses his great desire for freedom. A symptom that is unique to the remedy, the sensation that his head is joined to a passive and helpless body by a neck that is too large ('Delusions, neck is too large': *1* – only remedy), is another expression of his feelings of vulnerability and dependence.

Dreams

Dreams are another reflection of Kali Carb.'s inner conflicts. The dreams of ghosts and spectres ('Sleep, dreams, ghosts, spectres': *3*) express both anger and fear; devilish figures ('Sleep, dreams, devils': *1*) frighten him ('Sleep, dreams, frightful': *3*) with fantastic images

('Sleep, dreams, fantastic': *2*) of rioting ('Sleep, dreams, riots': *1*) and death ('Sleep, dreams, dead, of the': *2*) that will soon be upon him ('Sleep, dreams, death, of, approaching': *1*). He dreams of dangerous situations ('Sleep, dreams, danger': *1*) and of the burden, as heavy as stone, that he carries ('Sleep, dreams, stone lying on him': *1* – only remedy). A keynote symptom is the dream of calling out for help ('Sleep, dreams, calling out for help': *1* – only remedy), which is another expression of helplessness and the need for support.

The lack of sexual energy may lead to impotence and frigidity, although the female expresses herself sexually in amorous dreams before the menses ('Sleep, dreams, amorous, menses, before': *2*), a symptom shared only with Calc. Carb.

The dreams of snakes ('Sleep, dreams, snakes': *1*) could be a phallic symbol, and the fear of loss on an emotional level may account for the dreams of robbers ('Sleep, dreams, robbers': *2*). Kali Carb. not only weeps when telling of his sickness but is also one of the few remedies that dream of weeping ('Sleep, dreams, weeping': *1*). The sitting position both ameliorates his symptoms and makes him fall asleep ('Sleep, position, sitting': *2*). Two more interesting features in the sleep section are that he feels sleepy when eating ('Sleep, sleepiness, eating, during': *3*), a symptom shared only by Phosphorus and Agaricus, and has insomnia after midnight, around 1 or 2 a.m. ('Sleep, sleeplessness, midnight, after': *3*, with the modalities 'after 2 a.m.': *3*, and '1 or 2 a.m.': *3* – only remedy). He is unable to sleep for the circling thoughts in his mind ('Sleep, sleeplessness, thoughts, activity of mind, from': *2*) and the twitching of his limbs ('Sleep, sleeplessness, twitching of the limbs': *2*).

SUMMARY

Lack of Self-Confidence

In the words of Paschero: 'This is an irritable and bad-tempered patient who is intolerant and discontented with everything, mainly with himself, in a perpetual state of conflict and flux. The cause of his discontent and ill humour is the overwhelming nature of his mental and physical weakness that forces him to depend on others and makes him incapable of fending for himself.'

Related Rubric
'Confidence, want of self': *2*.

Changeability

The perpetual state of conflict, irritability and weakness leads to great emotional instability. His moods fluctuate constantly between irritability and apprehension, fear and anger, helplessness and self-affirmation, depression and excitability.

Related Rubrics
'Antagonism with herself': *2*.
'Mood, alternating': *2*.
'Mood, changeable, variable': *2*.

Apprehension

He suffers from feelings of great anxiety and helplessness. He has anxiety with fear, on waking, at night from flatulence when lying on the right side, when hungry and after a chill.

Related Rubrics
'Anxiety, fear, with': *2*.
'Anxiety, hungry, when': *2*. 'Anxiety, chill, after': *1*.
'Anxiety, lying, side, on, right, from flatulence': *1* (only remedy).
'Anxiety, waking, on': *2*.

The anxiety is related to the following symptoms:

Anxious restlessness – This typically affects the female Kali Carb. before and during the menses, symbolising her feelings of inferiority and frustration.

Excitability – Kali Carb. reacts with nervous excitement to stresses such as bad news and hunger. A nervous stomach is characteristic of Kali Carb. and expresses the need for both emotional and physical nurturing.

Related Rubrics
'Excitement, bad news, after': *1*.
'Excitment, hungry, when': *1* (only remedy).
'Genitalia, female, menses, suppressed, fright, from': *2*.
'Restlessness, anxious': *3*, with the sub-rubrics 'menses, before': *1*,
    'menses, during': 1 and 'menses, suppressed, during': *1*.

Irritability

He is generally nervous, jumpy and irritable. He is capricious, quarrel-some and bad-tempered, picking fights with his family and at his place of work. The sub-rubrics for the irritability are similar to those for the anxiety, with aggravation on waking, in the evening, after coition (from debility), before menses (the female's expression of dissatis-faction) and from consolation (the wounded ego).

Related Rubrics
'Capriciousness': *3*.
'Irritability': *3*, with the sub-rubrics 'morning, waking, on': *2*, 'evening': *2*, 'coition, after': *2*, 'menses, before': *1*, and 'consolation agg.': *1*.

Fear

Fear is the external manifestation of his inner anxieties and makes him acutely sensitive and responsive to stimuli, as seen in the abundance of fears, startings and sensitivities.

The fear of solitude is the overriding reason for his continued dependence on others. He fears to be left alone in case he should die, and fears death when lying all alone in his bed. He is terrified of disease. He feels fear in the stomach with constrictions and convul-sions. He is frightened by the least thing, and fears ghosts and evil.

Related Rubrics
'Fear, alone, of being': *3*.
'Fear, alone, of being, lest he die': *2*.
'Fear, death, of, alone, when': *1*.
'Fear, death, of, alone, when, evening in bed': *1*.
'Fear, disease, of impending': *3*.
'Fear, ghosts, of': *1*.
'Fear, lying in bed, while': *1* (only remedy).
'Fear, stomach, arising from': *2*.
'Stomach, constriction, convulsive': *1*.

Nervous Reactions

His perpetual state of tension makes him acutely responsive to external stimuli. Many things make him jump and start, such as fright, noise and unexpected touch, and he is jumpy on falling asleep and during sleep.

Related Rubrics
'Starting, easily': *3*.
'Starting, fright, from': *3*.
'Starting, noise, from': *3*.
'Starting, sleep, on falling': *2*.
'Starting, sleep, during': *3*.
'Starting, touched, when': *3*.

Sensitivity

He is sensitive both to noise and touch. He is both frightened of and averse to touch, and will move his leg sharply away from the slightest touch to the foot. He is oversensitive to the sound of voices.

Related Rubrics
'Fear, touch, of': *1*.
'Frightened, touch, from': *2*.
'Sensitive, oversensitive': *2*.
'Sensitive, noise, to': *3*.
'Sensitive, voices': *2*.
'Touched, aversion to being': *3*.

Anger

His severely weakened state makes him feel inferior, helpless, anxious and overstimulated. It arouses strong feelings of anger which he tries to suppress for fear of abandonment, thus creating a vicious circle of anger, fear and suppression. He is crippled by the fear that his friends will desert him, and his anger acts as an escape valve for the stress of suppressing his emotions, not as a means of self-assertion. For this reason, Kali Carb. is neither easily offended nor intolerant of contradiction. He feels anger on waking, distressed at having to leave the warmth and protection of his bed, and in the evening from exhaustion. He is violent and abusive, shouting uncontrollably, at trifles, and hitting imaginary objects and people. He is quarrelsome, impulsive and hostile.

Related Rubrics
'Anger': *3*, with the sub-rubrics 'morning': *2*, 'morning, waking, on': *2*, 'evening': *2*.
'Impetuous': *2*.
'Quarrelsome': *2*.

Kali Carbonicum

'Repulsive mood': *1.*
'Shrieking': *3,* with the sub-rubric 'trifles, at': *3* (only remedy).
'Striking': *2,* with the sub-rubric 'about him at imaginary objects': *2.*
'Violent': *1.*

Need for Others

His need for others is so great that all his symptoms get worse when he finds himself alone. He begs for company, yet abuses his companions. He feels lonely and deserted by everyone, especially after an unhappy love affair. The infant Kali Carb. whines and moans and demands to be carried. His whining is an indirect way of attracting attention. The constant moaning reaches its peak at around 3 a.m. Four symptoms provide a perfect description of the tormenting conflicts endured by the remedy: the dreams of calling for help, weeping when telling of his sickness, difficulty in speaking and non-stop moaning. His weak and befuddled mind robs him of all self-confidence. He feels confused, as if drugged or intoxicated. His mind is dull and sluggish when he tries to speak or think, with amelioration from closing the eyes. He is forgetful and unable to express his thoughts. He forgets words and makes mistakes in speaking, using the wrong words and putting them in the wrong place. He has temporary losses of consciousness and talks nonsense in his sleep.

Related Rubrics
'Confusion of mind': *2.*
'Confusion, intoxicated, as after being': *1.*
'Dullness': *3,* with the sub-rubrics 'speaking, while': *1,* 'closing eyes, amel.': *1* (only remedy).
'Forgetful': *1.*
'Memory, weakness of, expressing oneself, for': *2.*
'Memory, weakness of, words, for': *2.*
'Mistakes, speaking': *2.*
'Mistakes, wrong words, using': *1.*
'Mistakes, words, misplacing': *1.*
'Senses, dullness of': *1.*
'Senses, vanishing of': *1.*
'Sleep, dreams, calling out for help': *1* (only remedy).
'Speech, nonsense, springing up while asleep, on': *1* (only remedy).
'Weeping, telling of her sickness, when': *2.*

Self-Assertion

He struggles to achieve some kind of independence. He cannot afford to give vent to his anger, lest it should alienate those who support and care for him, so he lets it show indirectly through his perverse behaviour; it is almost as if he takes delight in doing exactly the opposite of what his family and friends expect. His relationships with people become more and more rigid, and he stubbornly refuses to bow to authority. He rebels against all the rules. He needs company, yet abuses his companions. He complains loudly, but rejects all attempts at consolation.

Related Rubrics
'Consolation agg.': *1*.
'Contrary': *2*.
'Obstinate': *2*.
'Unobserving': *1*.

Depression and Excitability

This pair of symptoms describes his habitual response to the stresses and strains of life.

Depression
He is an introverted patient who is dissatisfied with everything, including himself, and prey to fits of ill humour and depression that are worse in bed, in the open air and when alone. He is tormented by unpleasant memories when he is lying alone in his bed at night.

Related Rubrics
'Discontented': *2*, with the sub-rubric 'himself, with': *1*.
'Sadness, alone, when': *1*.
'Sadness, air, in open': *2*.
'Sadness, night, bed, in': *1*.
'Thoughts, persistent': *1*, with the sub-rubric 'alone, when': *1*.
'Thoughts, tormenting, evening': *1*.
'Thoughts, tormenting, night': *1*.
'Timidity': *3*.

Excitability
Engulfed by depression, he becomes restless, hurried, impatient and excitable. In an attempt to compensate for his apathy and debility, he

hurries to get everything done yesterday. He rushes about frantically at work. He is too weak and exhausted to wait for those who are slower than he is, and he hurries them up impatiently. (For a discussion of the remaining two symptoms, please refer to the beginning of this summary.)

Related Rubrics
'Hurry': 2, with the sub-rubrics 'mental work, in': 2, 'movements, in': 1, 'occupation, in': 2. 'impatience': 2.

Weeping

Tears are a strong expression of his general discontentment, and he will cry if comforted or told off. He may cry with anger at the injustice of it all, or for reasons that neither he nor anybody else understands. He weeps when telling of his sickness.

Related Rubrics
'Weeping': 2, with the sub-rubrics 'admonitions cause': 2, 'consolation agg.': 1, 'causeless': 1, 'causeless, without knowing why': 1, 'telling of her sickness, when': 2, 'remonstrated with, when': 2.

Uncommunicativeness

He is too unhappy to speak and wishes for complete silence around him. He cannot communicate with others, as his speech is incoherent and rambling.

Related Rubrics
'Talk, indisposed to': 1.
'Talk, of others agg.': 2.

Indifference

Eventually, apathy overtakes depression and he loses all interest in life; even things that he once enjoyed now bore him to death. He loses his enthusiasm for everything, including work, although he is unlikely to think of suicide.

Despair

He can see no way out of his problems, and thinks that there is no hope for his recovery. As his depression reaches rock bottom, he becomes thoroughly dejected and hopeless.

Related Rubrics
'Despair, recovery': *1*.
'Discouraged': *1*.
'Doubtful, recovery, of': *1*.

Delusions and Sensations

The delusions and sensations are contorted images of reality. The fears of solitude and abandonment are illustrated by the sensation that the bed is sinking and the delusion that someone is calling. The fear of disease is reflected by the delusion that he is sick. The struggle for independence is graphically portrayed by the sensation that his head, and therefore his mind, is bound to his passive and helpless body by a powerfully large neck. The desire for freedom is seen in the delusion of seeing birds, and his anger in the delusion of masks and phantoms, and the paranoid conviction that someone is trying to murder him.

Related Rubrics
'Delusions, bed, sinking, were': *1*.
'Delusions, birds, sees': *1*.
'Delusions, calls, someone': *1*.
'Delusions, images, phantoms, sees': *1*.
'Delusions, masks, sees': *1*.
'Delusions, murdered, that he would be': *1*.
'Delusions, neck is too large': *1* (only remedy).
'Delusions, sick, imagines himself': *2*.

Dreams

Dreams full of visions of ghosts, demons and rioting are expressions of anger, and the dream that death is approaching is about fear. The dream that a stone is lying on him symbolises the heavy burden of his mental and physical condition, and the dream of calling for help reveals his deep fear of destitution and abandonment. These last two dreams are unique to the remedy.

Related Rubrics
'Dreams, calling out, for help': *1* (only remedy).
'Dreams, death, of, approaching': *1*.
'Dreams, devils': *1*.
'Dreams, ghosts, spectres': *2*.
'Dreams, riots': *1*.
'Dreams, stone lying on him': *1* (only remedy).

SCHEMATIC DIAGRAM AND REPERTORISATION

The Minimum Characteristic Syndrome is represented in the diagram overleaf by a circle. In the centre we have symptom 1, 'Confidence, want of self', which encompasses his lack of mental and physical power and his inability to fend for himself. Inside the circle, and to the left of centre, we have the symptoms that express his feelings of anxiety, fear and helplessness in the face of overwhelming physical handicaps and weaknesses, 'Fear, alone, of being' (2), 'Anxiety, fear, with' (3) and 'Company, desire for' (4). To the right of centre, we have the irritable, angry and rebellious aspects that are compensatory reactions to his feelings of vulnerability, 'Consolation agg.' (5), 'Impetuous' (6) and 'Contrary' (7).

Once the basic nucleus of the remedy picture is established, it is not too difficult to see where the remaining symptoms belong. The symptom 'Restlessness, anxious' (31) is an aspect of the anxiety, while the symptoms 'Fear, disease, of impending' (10), 'Touched, aversion to being' (13), 'Starting, noise, from' (12) and 'Fear, stomach, arising from' (11) are all aspects of the fear. The irritability is worse before menses, 'Irritability, menses, before' (9), and the anger is characterised by 'Capriciousness' (15) and the tendency to be 'Quarrelsome' (14), 'Obstinate' (20) and 'Unobserving' (21).

These behavioural extremes strongly affect his emotional stability, 'Mood, alternating' (8), and his moods swing between manic excitability (symptoms 29–32) and heavy depression (symptoms 22–28).

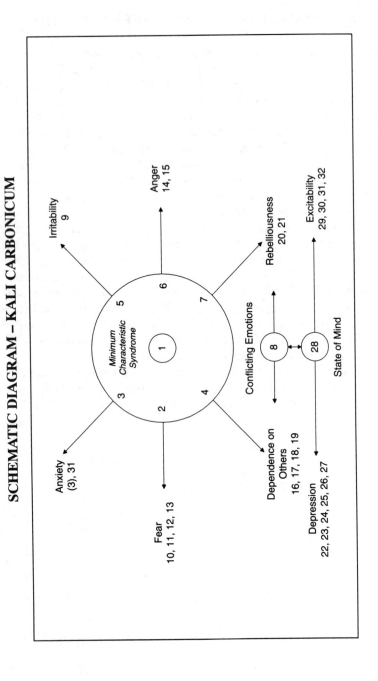

SCHEMATIC DIAGRAM – KALI CARBONICUM

Irritability
9

Anger
14, 15

Rebelliousness
20, 21

Excitability
29, 30, 31, 32

Anxiety
(3), 31

Fear
10, 11, 12, 13

Dependence on Others
16, 17, 18, 19

Depression
22, 23, 24, 25, 26, 27

Minimum Characteristic Syndrome
1

Conflicting Emotions
8

State of Mind
28

3 5 6 7 2 4

Minimum Characteristic Syndrome

1) Confidence, want of self
2) Fear, alone, of being
3) Anxiety, fear, with
4) Company, desire for
5) Consolation agg.
6) Impetuous
7) Contrary

Irritability

8) Mood, alternating
9) Irritability, menses, before

Fear

10) Fear, disease, of impending
11) Fear, stomach, arising from
12) Starting, noise, from
13) Touched, aversion to being

Anger

14) Quarrelsome
15) Capriciousness

Dependence on Others

16) Forsaken feeling
17) Moaning
18) Dullness
19) Memory, weakness of, expressing one's self for

Rebelliousness

20) Obstinate
21) Unobserving

Depression

22) Discontented, himself, with
23) Thoughts, unpleasant subjects, haunted by
24) Weeping, telling of her sickness, when
25) Weeping, remonstrated with, when
26) Indifference, society, when in
27) Loathing, general
28) Despair, recovery

Excitability

29) Hurry
30) Impatience
31) Restlessness, anxious
32) Excitement, bad news, after

REPERTORISATION – KALI CARBONICUM

	1	2	3	4	5	6	7	8	9	10	11	12	13	14	15	16	17	18	19	20	21	22	23	24	25	26	27	28	29	30	31	32
Kali-c.	2	3	2	3	1	2	2	2	1	3	2	3	3	2	3	1	3	3	2	2	1	1	1	2	2	2	1	1	2	2	3	1
Ars.	–	3	3	3	2	–	1	1	–	1	–	1	1	2	2	–	2	1	–	2	–	1	–	2	2	–	–	3	2	2	3	–
Bell.	1	1	1	1	2	–	1	3	–	–	–	–	2	2	2	–	3	3	1	3	–	1	–	–	1	–	1	–	2	1	2	–
Bry.	2	1	1	1	–	2	–	–	–	1	1	–	2	2	3	1	2	3	–	1	–	1	–	–	1	–	1	2	2	2	2	2
Calc.	1	1	2	2	1	–	1	1	1	2	2	2	1	1	1	–	1	3	–	3	2	–	–	–	–	–	2	3	1	2	2	2
Caust.	1	–	3	1	–	1	1	1	2	–	–	–	–	2	–	–	1	2	–	1	2	1	1	–	–	–	–	–	–	–	2	2
Hep.	–	1	2	1	1	3	2	3	–	1	–	–	–	–	1	–	–	2	2	2	–	2	–	–	–	–	–	–	2	2	2	–
Lyc.	2	3	2	3	1	–	1	1	2	1	2	2	1	2	1	–	–	3	–	2	–	1	–	–	–	–	–	–	1	1	–	–
Merc.	1	1	2	1	1	–	2	–	–	1	–	2	1	3	1	–	1	2	2	1	1	1	–	–	–	–	1	1	3	3	1	1
Nux-v.	1	1	1	2	1	3	2	–	2	2	2	3	1	2	1	–	2	3	2	3	–	–	–	–	–	–	–	1	1	3	1	–
Phos.	1	3	2	3	–	1	1	1	–	3	2	–	–	2	2	3	2	3	–	1	–	1	–	3	–	–	2	–	2	–	2	1
Puls.	2	2	2	2	–	–	2	2	–	–	–	–	–	–	–	3	–	3	3	–	–	–	–	–	–	–	–	–	1	2	2	1
Sep.	–	2	2	2	3	3	–	1	2	2	–	–	–	2	–	–	–	3	–	–	1	–	–	3	–	–	–	2	1	3	1	–

Minimum Characteristic Syndrome

1) Confidence, want of self
2) Fear, alone, of being
3) Anxiety, fear, with
4) Company, desire for
5) Consolation agg.
6) Impetuous
7) Contrary

Irritability

8) Mood, alternating
9) Irritability, menses, before

Fear

10) Fear, disease, of impending
11) Fear, stomach, arising from
12) Starting, noise, from
13) Touched, aversion to being

Anger

14) Quarrelsome
15) Capriciousness

Dependence on Others

16) Forsaken feeling
17) Moaning
18) Dullness
19) Memory, weakness of, expressing one's self for

Rebelliousness

20) Obstinate
21) Unobserving

Depression

22) Discontented, himself, with
23) Thoughts, unpleasant subjects, haunted by
24) Weeping, telling of her sickness, when
25) Weeping, remonstrated with, when
26) Indifference, society, when in
27) Loathing, general
28) Despair, recovery

Excitability

29) Hurry
30) Impatience
31) Restlessness, anxious
32) Excitement, bad news, after

COMPARATIVE MATERIA MEDICA

Nux Vomica

This is the only remedy that has all seven symptoms of the Minimum Characteristic Syndrome of Kali Carbonicum. However, it does not have the alternating moods (8) that underlie the fluctuating attitudes of helplessness and rebelliousness. Nux Vomica is characterised by an oversensitivity to everything, with quick, irritable reactions, chilliness and reversed peristalsis. Although he has a need for company, he does not feel worse when alone. He is brave and reckless, a hive of fevered activity, like the typical business executive. This fastidious perfectionist lets nothing stand between him and success.

His lack of confidence (1) results from the combination of a stressful lifestyle and the toxic overload of the digestive system from stimulants such as alcohol, coffee and spices. His fears come not from feelings of vulnerability but from psoric oversensitivity. He does not have the fear arising from the stomach (11). From the group of 'dependence' rubrics, his absence from 'Forsaken feeling' means that his complaining words ('Moaning',17) are not an indirect cry for help. The mental sluggishness ('Dullness', 18 and 'Memory, weakness of, expressing one's self, for', 19) is the result of stress and toxic abuse rather than an indication of any malfunction. Nux Vomica is obstinate in his will to succeed ('Obstinate', 20), while Kali Carb. stubbornly refuses to come to terms with his need for others and to bow to authority (21).

As one would expect of a psoric-sycotic remedy, Nux Vomica does not share the Kali Carb. symptoms of depression (22–27); he gets depressed and irritable after eating and, in the final stages of pathology, becomes tired of living and longs to die, with an impatient despair of recovery ('Despair, recovery', 28) and thoughts of suicide, although he lacks the courage to go through with it. Kali Carb. has neither the wish to die nor suicidal thoughts. Finally, Nux Vom. is impulsive ('Impetuous', 6), perverse ('Contrary', 7), hurried (29), impatient (30) and restless (31), and is not affected by bad news (32).

The following remedies have six symptoms of the Minimum Characteristic Syndrome of Kali Carbonicum: Belladonna, Calcarea Carbonica, Causticum, Lycopodium, Mercurius and Phosphorus.

Belladonna (*See also* pages 197–8)

As already mentioned, this remedy has the largest number of mental symptoms in Kent's *Repertory*. They can be brought on by high fevers, delirium and mania, with violence and excitability. The remedy is sensitive to light, noise, jarring and touch. Symptoms are sudden, intense and violent. The face is fiery red, with dilated pupils; the skin radiates heat. There is violent delirium, with congestion and dilation of the arteries. He sees ghosts, insects and wild animals; he bites and hits those around him, and when the crisis is over he falls into a semi-comatose state, with nightmares and horrible dreams. General characteristics of Belladonna are: the sudden appearance and disappearance of symptoms, congestion of the head, intolerance of sun, cold and touch.

Its affinity for acute inflammatory processes means that it is less often used as a constitutional remedy; however, if all the Belladonna symptoms were extracted from the *Repertory*, the resulting picture would be of great use in chronic states. It is a great remedy for hyperactivity and excitability, with all the symptoms of the Minimum Characteristic Syndrome except 'Impetuous' (6). Duprat says that Belladonna is 'an angel when well and a devil when sick'. The absence of symptoms 9, 11 and 12 is explicable in terms of his psoric excitability, and he is neither competitive (9) nor jumpy (12). He does not have the feeling of abandonment (16) or the disregard for authority (21). Furthermore, symptoms 23, 24, 26 and 28, which describe Kali Carb.'s apathy, despair and tears, are missing and there are no ill effects from bad news (32).

This superficial view of Belladonna may provide the basis for a fuller chronic picture. When he is well, he is calm and easy-going, but when he gets sick he becomes irritable ('Contrary', 7), afraid to be left alone (2), anxious and fearful (3). He prefers company, although consolation and touch annoy him ('Consolation agg.', 5 and 'Touched, aversion to being', 13). He can be argumentative ('Quarrelsome', 14) and difficult ('Capriciousness', 15), and as stubborn ('Obstinate', 20) as Calc. Carb.

He is dissatisfied ('Discontented, himself, with', 22) and, when reprimanded, cries at the injustice of it all; he can get so unhappy that, unlike Kali Carb., he may try to drown himself. His alternating moods and symptoms (8) are psoric in nature; he can be depressed or overexcited, impatient (30), hurried (29) and restless (31).

Calcarea Carbonica (*See also* pages 163–4)

In this remedy, potassium is replaced by calcium. According to Bernard, Calc. Carb. is mentally and physically stable and may stay so for the whole of his life. When he falls ill, stability turns to stubbornness ('Obstinate', 20), resentment and fear ('Fear, stomach, arising from', 11), and he develops an absolute terror of disease, as if it were the clutches of the devil ('Fear, disease, of impending', 10).

Although the remedy is very close to Kali Carb., there are some fundamental differences. All his actions are premeditated, he does not get carried away by spontaneous impulses (6) and has no difficulty with self-expression (19). Symptoms 22, 23, 24 and 26, which express Kali Carb.'s profound self-dissatisfaction, his tendency to dwell on the negative, to avoid people and cry when talking about his problems, are not present in Calc. Carb. Apathy and obstinacy are the essential characteristics of Calc. Carb., while in Kali Carb. they are irritable weakness and the fear of solitude. The former is slow, the latter is hurried. Calcarea can be full of rage and hatred, while Kali does not dare, for fear of solitude. Calcarea is slow and sure, planning everything down to the smallest detail and rationalising everything; the spiritual side of life is too much for his brain to cope with and he has a great fear of the unknown; hence, the fear of the supernatural, evil, storms, darkness, that something will happen, and the night. He is worried and restless (31), and his inner conflicts and guilt are projected on to fears of external things. He has the gift of clairvoyance, and his sensitivity to horrible stories and cruelty account for his fear of the future and poverty.

Causticum

According to Kent, the characteristics of this remedy are despair, anxiety and fear. It is the neediest remedy of our whole materia medica, like the child who needs to hold his mother's hand at night. It is a mixed miasmatic remedy, with tubercular and sycotic traits, which has been weakened by long illnesses or grief, with an overactive imagination that always fears the worst and a great capacity for depression and pain; in the evening, when his premonitions of evil become more intense, he gets the feeling that he has done something seriously wrong. He is an emotional cripple who cannot express his emotions even when people try to console him (5). His anger is expressed indirectly by the tendency to contradict and argue with everyone (14), and he empathises with the pain and suffering of others, although he also has a callous and dictatorial streak. In a predominantly sycotic case, he can be impetuous (6) and contrary (7); the female Causticum will feel irritable before the menses (9), with an anarchic disregard for all social conventions. Causticum's basic feelings of anger and inferiority find their physical expression in paralysis and muscular spasm.

His fears are different from those of Kali Carb. He is afraid of darkness, dogs, and that something bad is about to happen. He hides his weakness behind a dictatorial front, and his ability to identify with the pain of others prevents him from feeling lonely (16). Although he can be as restless as Kali Carb. (31), he does not suffer anything like the same degree of torment and conflict, hence the absence of all of the other symptoms concerned with excitability and depression.

Lycopodium

This remedy is a mixture of self-worship, smug servility and an over-bearing need to dominate others. He does not have symptom 6 from the Minimum Characteristic Syndrome as he is shrewd enough to control his emotions, hide his true feelings and not be indebted to anyone. He is too proud to complain without just cause (17), feel abandoned (16), be afraid of disease (10) or be averse to touch (13); these last two are symptoms that reveal the degree of nervous anxiety that affects Kali Carb. Lycopodium complains only during sleep. He is clever enough to realise that it is wiser not to flout authority (21) or give way to impulses (6). He has none of the symptoms of depression, although he is secretly discontented with himself, and will not openly admit that he is affected by nightmares, bad news, feelings of exhaustion and despair, anxiety and restlessness, or that he weeps when talking about his problems. He covers up his insecurities with a veneer of arrogance, perfectionism and attention to detail that Kali Carb. does not have.

Lycopodium needs to have company around him, but not too near, while Kali Carb. is afraid of solitude but treats those around him very badly. Lycopodium has a dull mind (18) and a weak memory (19), and often tends to forget names. He is difficult ('Contrary', 7), argumentative ('Quarrelsome', 14) and capricious (15), with a stubborn need to defend his dominant position with eloquent speeches and an intolerance of contradiction. When he feels that his strength is failing him, he cries when reprimanded or thanked, because he is basically a shy and vulnerable person who needs a lot of tender care.

Mercurius

Although Mercurius is so intolerant of contradiction that he may even kill the one who dares to contradict (6), it may surprise the reader to know that he does not appear in the rubric 'Impetuous'. The Mercurius picture is typically syphilitic, with marked deficiency of the intellect, mental dullness, slowness to answer and a tendency to regress to childish behaviour. He is prone to bouts of explosive anger and anxious restlessness that impel him to run away from home, as if guilty of a terrible crime. Paschero says: 'His inner feelings of hostility are projected on to the external world in the conviction that the whole world is his enemy; he is suspicious of everyone's motives, including his own, and is afraid of solitude and insanity, with impulses to kill the person who dares to contradict him'.

His desire to escape is not a response to impulsive ideas but an attempt to protect others from his aggression; he is afraid of solitude (2) and seeks company (4) for the same reason. He is full of anxieties and fears (3), and his mental and physical problems make it difficult for him to adjust to the world around him ('Contrary', 7). Apart from the fear of disease that he shares with Kali Carb. (10), he is afraid of insanity and robbers. When something takes his fancy, he can become argumentative ('Quarrelsome', 14), capricious (15), obstinate (20) and thoughtless ('Unobserving', 21).

Mercurius has enough anger in him to make a good anarchist, revolutionary or dictator, if it were not for the fearful guilt that wells up at the sight of a knife. As his depression and discontentment grow (22), his thoughts may turn to suicide if he sees an open window or a sharp instrument, and he sinks deeper into despair (28) and disgust (27). His inability to keep still ('Restlessness, anxious', 31) is a symbol of his quest for perfection and the frantic ('Hurry', 29) and impatient (30) longing for the good life that eludes him in his chaos and confusion.

Phosphorus (*See also* pages 62–4)

According to the French school of homoeopathy, the three characteristics of Phosphorus are fear, prostration and haemorrhagic tendencies. Phosphorus does not have the aggravation from consolation (5) that expresses Kali Carb.'s frustration with his condition of enforced dependence on others.

Phosphorus is heavily influenced by the tubercular miasm, with his outbursts of destructive anger, fearful anxiety (3), restlessness (31), fear of solitude (2) and need for company (4). He suffers from states of intense fear and anger, and is exquisitely sensitive not only to his immediate surroundings but to the whole of creation. The creativity of Phosphorus can be seen in artists and musicians such as Van

Gogh, Chopin and Liszt. Although he is the most affectionate and compassionate remedy of our materia medica, his excitable nature can make him impetuous (6), contrary (7), averse to touch (13), argumentative ('Quarrelsome', 14), capricious (15) and stubborn ('Obstinate', 20). However, the remedy is absent from the rubrics 'Unobserving', 21 and 'Irritability, menses, before', 9.

In a syphilitic case, a love disappointment may push Phosphorus to extremes of chaotic and abusive behaviour, expressing deep hatred and bitterness, although he is unlikely to feel totally abandoned by others (16). Unlike Kali Carb., whose moods fluctuate between the need for protection and the desire to rebel, Phosphorus's emotions ('Mood, alternating', 8) swing between passion and indifference, joy and pain, rage and kindness, and enthusiasm and apathy. He has none of Kali Carb.'s dissatisfaction with life; rather, he has the slow patience (30) of an artistic and creative mind.

The following remedies have five symptoms of the Minimum Characteristic Syndrome of Kali Carbonicum: Arsenicum, Bryonia, Hepar Sulphuris, Pulsatilla and Sepia.

Arsenicum

While Kali Carb.'s anxiety comes from his feelings of inadequacy and his inability to cope, Arsenicum's anxiety lives in the very depths of his subconscious being, as he fights for his life with syphilitic forces of disruption and decay. While Phosphorus may burn to a cinder and Natrum Muriaticum may become dry and withered, Arsenicum rots away. In fact, gangrene is the pathological end result of a process that begins with the inability to control impulses of primitive anger. The Arsenicum patient is painfully aware of the self-destructive urges that will lead him, slowly but surely, to his death and he lives his whole life on the defensive. Arsenicum is characterised by bouts of anxiety and mortal anguish that reach a peak between 2 and 3 a.m. when he jumps out of bed to try and escape his imminent death.

With syphilitic anger and guilt, he constantly blames others and is obsessed by hygiene and order, as revealed by the classic symptom 'Fastidious': 2). He is a miserly old man, thin and chilly, with skin as dry as parchment and breath that smells like the rotting corpse that he will soon become; with a gold-headed cane in his hand, he frowns sternly as he adjusts his jewelled tie-clip and puts the finishing touches to his immaculate clothes.

From the symptoms of the Minimum Characteristic Syndrome, he suffers neither from the insecurity (1) nor the impulsiveness (6) that plague the weak and irritable Kali Carb. Arsenicum is too self-assured to feel irritable before menses (9) or abandoned by others (16), and lacks the inner conflicts that bring about Kali Carb.'s disregard for authority (21). He can, however, become dissatisfied with his lot ('Discontented, himself, with', 22) and hopeless ('Despair, recovery', 28), to the point where he longs for death, and tries to hang himself one night. The elements of impatience (30), restlessness (31) and hurriedness (29) are much stronger in Arsenicum than in Kali Carb., as he tries to escape from the power of his fatal, self-destructive impulses; in Kali Carb. these symptoms are a reaction to his insecurities, fears and feelings of vulnerability.

Bryonia

Bryonia has a strong, forceful personality, a plethoric constitution and a large appetite; he is aggravated by dry cold and by heat. We are all familiar with the main characteristics of Bryonia: irritability, aggravation from the slightest motion, amelioration from pressure and thirst for large quantities at long intervals. However, it is worth taking a closer look as it has most of the symptoms of the Minimum Characteristic Syndrome of Kali Carb., except symptoms 5 and 7. Like the climbing White Bryony plant, Bryonia is a social climber and a capitalist at heart. His great fear of poverty makes him feel unsure of himself ('Confidence, want of self', 1) and he puts all his energy and stubborn determination ('Obstinate', 20) into carving a secure future.

Although he is afraid of solitude (2) and needs company (4), the desire to be alone is far more important, as he is aggravated by the least motion, and does not want to be forced to speak or even think. With intense irritability and anger, he tells everyone to go away and mind their own business; when delirious, he believes that he is busy, has the delusion that he is doing business, and thinks that he is away from home as he tries to escape through the window. He feels imprisoned by his illness and wants to break free to resume his work; his anxiety is so great that it propels him out of bed, in spite of the aggravation from motion.

Like Kali Carb., fear and anger seem to rise from the stomach (11); he is afraid of illness (10) and death. To protect his social position, he complies with others (7) and conforms with the rules of society (21), unlike the rebellious Kali Carb., Causticum and Sepia. He can be capricious (15), argumentative ('Quarrelsome', 14) and intolerant of contradiction. He does not suffer in silence ('Moaning', 17), and his mind is dull and sluggish, with difficulty of self-expression (19). He can be dissatisfied (22), hopeless ('Despair, recovery', 28), hurried (29), impatient (30) and restless (31). He does not have the remaining psoric-tubercular symptoms of Kali Carb.'s depression (23 to 27). The sycotic Bryonia has all the symptoms of the Minimum Characteristic Syndrome, with the exceptions of symptoms 5 and 7 which, like symptoms 9 and 21, express the anger that Kali Carb. feels with the world. Bryonia does not have the tubercular changeability (8) or feeling of abandonment (16) of Kali Carb., and is not affected by bad news (32).

Hopefully, the reader will now have a better understanding of this workaholic in decline, as he lies imprisoned in his bed, unable to move for the pain of his swollen joints and obsessed by worries about work.

Hepar Sulphuris

Paschero says of this remedy: 'Violent anger with urges to kill anyone who dares provoke or offend. Fierce and uncontrollable rage can be unleashed at the slightest provocation. Hateful, serious children who try to destroy everything they can lay their hands on, and malicious adults who take pleasure in doing harm.'

Unlike Mercurius, Hepar Sulph. has no sense of right or wrong. He is violent, impulsive, quick to act, extremely sensitive to pain, touch and cold, and destructive, with sudden urges to kill without remorse. He does not have symptoms 1 and 5 from the Minimum Characteristic Syndrome, the lack of confidence and rejection of support. He is perverse and full of anger.

So it should come as no surprise to learn that Hepar Sulph. has none of Kali Carb.'s fear, weakness or depression; although touch can hurt, he has no aversion to it. The syphilitic taint of the remedy accounts for the dullness of mind (18) and the fear of disease (10), an expression of his fear of divine punishment. He will suddenly give way to his violent, aggressive impulses, like the barber who spontaneously slashes his customer's throat with a knife. He is the most argumentative and fast-talking remedy in our materia medica. With syphilitic impatience (30), restlessness (31) and hurried actions (29), he attempts vainly to escape from himself. Clearly, although the remedy has certain symptoms in common with Kali Carb., it has quite a different basic character.

Pulsatilla (*See also* pages 64–5)

Pulsatilla does not have symptoms 5 and 6 from the Minimum Characteristic Syndrome, which are Kali Carb.'s sycotic reactions to his physical problems. Her changeable nature is indicated by symptoms 7 ('Contrary'), 8 ('Mood, alternating') and 15 ('Capriciousness'), and she is incapable of sustaining an argument (14), of obstinacy (20) or of disregarding others (21). Far from being aggravated by consolation, she positively revels in it (5). She is not irritable before menses (9), but sad and weepy. The only fear she has in common with Kali Carb. is the fear of solitude (2), with the accompanying need for company (4), although she does have other fears such as the fear of ghosts, animals and darkness. As one would expect, she has all the Kali Carb. symptoms of dependence on others (16 to 19). Her insecurities may lead to a deep self-hatred (22), a general state of weariness and disgust (27) and a tendency to weep when talking about her problems. She weeps mild, unprotesting tears that beg for an affectionate hand to wipe them away, quite unlike the abrupt treatment that well-wishers receive from Kali Carb., who complains loudly until people respond, and then treats them badly. Pulsatilla is too changeable and capricious to sink into despair of recovery (28).

When Kali Carb. is depressed, he lets everybody know about it loudly and angrily, and cares little about other people's feelings. The sycotic Pulsatilla, however, is anxious to please everyone and can, as a result, be hurried (29), impatient (30) and restless (31).

Sepia (*See also* pages 60–1 and 123–4)

Here, the minimum syndrome of maximum value is emotional indifference, as seen in the aversion to the members of her family and especially to her husband. She does not have symptoms 1 and 7 from the Minimum Characteristic Syndrome, and the fear of solitude (2) is a combination of self-dislike and morbid fantasy (as seen in the fears of disease, ghosts, thunderstorms and evil). She cannot bear being with her family, and will attack them with sharp, cutting words; but, at the same time, she needs to have people around her (4) to assuage the guilt she feels for rejecting her nearest and dearest. Unlike Kali Carb., she feels better when alone. Kali Carb. rejects consolation because it undermines his self-esteem; Sepia is merely indifferent to it. Kali Carb. is irritable before the menses, while Sepia is both irritable and tearful. Sepia's fears are of a different nature: her fear of disease (10) is the result of her indulgence in morbid self-preoccupation, which also engenders the fear of poverty and the future. In her struggle to assert herself with the opposite sex, she can be extremely argumentative ('Quarrelsome', 14).

Sycosis and syphilis bring their characteristic traits of secretiveness and apathy to her dullness of mind (18); she may rebel against society ('Unobserving', 21) because of her utter indifference to her surroundings, and she is too apathetic to be obstinate (20). Selfishly incapable of giving love, she feels sorry only for herself, and may weep when talking about her problems (24); she may despair of her recovery ('Despair, recovery', 28) and deep down feels guilty for the error of her ways. 'Hurry' (29), 'Impatience' (30) and 'Restlessness, anxious' (31) are sycotic reactions to her general state of stasis and stagnation; at her worst, she can become extremely irritable and bossy.

While there are many similarities between Sepia and Kali Carb., on both a mental and physical level, a careful analysis of each symptom reveals the clear differences between them.

8

Lachesis

DESCRIPTION

Dr Paschero's article on Lachesis, published in the October 1955 edition of *Homeopatía*, is a comprehensive analysis of the mental picture of the remedy. It is a tribute both to his vast experience and his extraordinary, intuitive ability to capture the essence of the remedy – a demonstration of his mastery of what Kent called the skilful art of medicine. The following analysis of Lachesis has been based on Paschero's study and Kent's *Repertory*.

I found Barthel's *Synthetic Repertory*, Volume I particularly helpful when writing this chapter and have included numerous symptoms from this work, as I believe them to be of undoubted value in the study of Lachesis. As the reader will already be aware, these symptoms are indicated as 'Barthel' in my text.

I have analysed a total of 314 rubrics from Kent and a further 290 from Barthel, and have selected approximately 30 of these to represent what I consider to be the essential components of the remedy.

Paschero maintains that Lachesis exemplifies, more than any other remedy, the basic human conflict between the needs of the higher and lower self, the moral dilemma between the dictates of the conscience and the needs of the physical body – in other words, the discrepancy between what is desired and what is attainable in this world.

In Paragraph 20 of Hahnemann's *Chronic Diseases* we learn that oversensitivity and extremes of emotions and reactions are all attributable to the psoric miasm, although the causes of this are not discussed. Presumably, psora is intimately related to the concepts expounded by Keyserling, of existential anguish and basic hunger and thirst, and to Erich Fromm's idea that, when man realises he is set apart from the rest of the natural world by his capacity for wisdom and knowledge, he becomes afraid of the potential for freedom which that implies. However, all theological and metaphysical arguments aside, we should accept the undoubted truth of Kent's affirmation that the effects of psora are deeply engrained upon the human organism; it is not for us to reason why, any more than we should concern ourselves with speculations about the the origins of life itself.

According to Paschero, Lachesis is a remedy of high sexual energy, passion and fear. The mental picture is one of great malice ('Malicious': 2), arrogance ('Haughty': 2), contempt ('Mocking': 2), mistrust ('Suspicious': 3) and criticism ('Censorious': 2). She has a fear of the unknown and of dying suddenly in the night ('Fear, die, he will, if he goes to sleep (after nightmare)': 2, Barthel). Fear becomes the delusion of being chased by enemies ('Delusions, pursued, thought he was, enemies, by': 2), and the need for self-protection brings about the delusion that she is under superhuman control ('Delusions, superhuman, control, under, is': 2).

Paschero considers that her inner feelings of hostility towards the world are outwardly manifested by a marked persecution complex that makes her withdraw completely from others, to nurse her suspicions and depression in total isolation. She rejects everyone's attempts to bring her out of herself and sinks deeper and deeper into a state of total apathy, boredom and despair. When she wakes in the morning, she feels utterly alone and bereft of love, companionship and the will to live.

The more persecuted she feels, the more defensive she becomes, creating an impenetrable vicious circle: she is convinced that she alone is the target for all the evil in the world, and defends herself with all the verbal weapons at her disposal, attacking others with words of angry condemnation, scathing abuse and wounding sarcasm, and flinging absurd accusations around with extraordinary eloquence.

Paschero's description of the mental picture of Lachesis is as follows: 'Feverish mental activity with uncontrollable loquacity that forms an impenetrable barrier between her and the outside world; she disowns all her passionate, sexual feelings and accuses others of having them.'

With this in mind, we will now take a closer look at the character of Lachesis through the repertories.

Basic Anxiety

Every symptom has a meaning, an intention and a result. The meaning or relationship between the rational and the irrational has a unique significance in every patient, and we must look at each case individually to discover the significance of a given symptom in the particular vital attitude or idiosyncrasies of the person. The meaning of the symptom is the 'why' and the intention is the 'what for' and they both assume that there is a result. Therefore, it is difficult, if not impossible, to classify a symptom as psoric, sycotic or syphilitic, when taken in isolation from the whole context of the case. It is especially true of homoeopathy that all analysis must be conducted in the light of the whole picture or life experience of the patient.

Anxiety may well be primarily a psoric symptom, but we must also be aware of the sycotic and syphilitic components. The anxiety of Lachesis is worse in the morning on waking ('Anxiety, morning': *3*, 'Anxiety, morning, waking, on': *3*), in accordance with the general time modalities of the remedy. Other characteristic variations of anxiety are: 'Anxiety, future, about': *2*, 'Anxiety, health, about': *1* and 'Anxiety, salvation, about': *3*. These will be discussed in more detail at a later stage.

Lachesis has the psoric characteristic of uncontrollable anxiety which is intensified at times of general aggravation, indicating the presence of certain disturbances of circulation and imbalances of the nervous system: the anxiety is worse on waking, in the morning, on falling asleep, in the heat, in confined spaces, from touch and after eating. Lachesis has little self-esteem ('Confidence, want of self': *1*) and low mental and physical stamina ('Exertion, agg. from mental': *3* and 'Exertion, physical, agg.': *2*); she feels confused in the morning, on waking, after eating and after sleep ('Confusion of mind': *3*, with the modalities 'morning': *3*, 'morning, waking, on': *3*, 'eating, after': 1 and 'sleeping, after': *1*). Once her mind starts to soar above the clouds ('Absent-minded': *3*), she finds it hard to come down to earth and concentrate ('Concentration, difficult': *3*). She has problems with thinking and comprehending ('Dullness': *3*), especially on waking ('Dullness, waking, on': *3*) and when she tries to read ('Dullness, reading, while': *2*). Her general state is aggravated by any mental exertion ('Exertion, agg. from mental': *3*) and Lachesis is the only remedy to have prostration after eating ('Prostration of mind, eating, after': *1*).

If we take a closer look at the memory rubrics, we find that the memory is extremely good in the evening ('Memory active, evening': *3*) until midnight, like Coffea, but she has a weak memory ('Memory, weakness of': *3*) for past events ('Memory, weakness of, happened, for what has': *2*) and for what she has read ('Memory, weakness of, read, for what has': *3*). She forgets words ('Memory, weakness of, words, for': *2*), proper names ('Memory, weakness of, names, for proper': *1*), the things she has said ('Memory, weakness of, said, for what has': *1*) and done ('Memory, weakness of, done, for what has just': *1*), and has difficulty with expressing herself ('Memory, weakness of, expressing one's self for': *1*). She makes mistakes in speaking ('Mistakes, speaking': *1*), spelling ('Mistakes, spelling, in': *2*) and writing ('Mistakes, writing, in': *3*), and puts words in the wrong places ('Mistakes, words, misplacing': *2*). She feels so disorientated that she does not even know what time it is ('Mistakes, time, in': *2*, 'afternoon, always imagines it is': *2*).

The delusion that time passes too slowly ('Time, passes too slowly': *1*), the mental confusion and prostration after eating combine to create a general sense of disorientation.

At times she feels so confused and disconnected that she does not even recognise her relatives ('Recognize, does not, his relatives': *2*) or surroundings ('Recognize, does not, well known streets': *1*), and her confusion is intensified by walking ('Confusion, walking, while': *2*). She may even lose touch completely with who she is ('Confusion, identity, as to his': *1*) and feel that she is two people ('Confusion, identity, as to his, duality, sense of': *1*, Barthel). Her mind goes blank when she tries to read, speak or write ('Thoughts, vanishing of': *2*, with the sub-rubrics 'reading, on': *2*, 'speaking, while': *2* and 'writing, while': *2*). These are all very small rubrics and there is only one other remedy that is present in all three, the temperamental Cannabis Indica.

Lachesis is quite unable to control the train of her thoughts ('Thoughts, wandering': *1*). Her speech can become badly affected: it is confused ('Speech, confused': *2*), hurried ('Speech, hasty': *3*), incoherent ('Speech, incoherent': *3*), slow ('Speech, slow': *3*), rambling ('Speech, wandering': *3*) and in a different language ('Speech, foreign tongue, in a': *1*).

She is aggressively outspoken, self-centred ('Egotism': *2* and 'Selfishness': *1*, Barthel), malicious, arrogant, contemptuous, critical and mistrustful. Syphilitic destructive tendencies ('Destructiveness': *1*) run throughout the remedy picture and there is a general amelioration from the free flowing of discharges. She is angry ('Anger': *1*), argumentative ('Quarrelsome': *2*), especially when her jealousy is aroused ('Quarrelsome, jealousy, from': *2*), envious ('Envy': *1*) and subject to episodes of violence ('Violent': *1*), with biting ('Biting': *2*) and punching ('Violent, deeds, rage, leading to': *1*). She gets furious at the slightest provocation ('Anger, ailments after anger': *2*) and irritable, especially in the morning and on waking ('Irritability': *2* with the sub-rubrics 'morning': *2* and 'waking, on': *2*). Unique to Lachesis is the extent to which she is plagued by persistent, evil thoughts

('Thoughts, persistent, evil, of': *2*) and surrounded by malice and hatred ('Mischievous': *2* and 'Hatred': *2*).

As the ravages of the syphilitic miasm threaten to overwhelm and destroy her, she employs various means of defence that are peculiar to the remedy and indicative of what really needs to be cured.

Sycotic Defence Mechanism

In health, most people try to alleviate their basic feelings of psoric fearfulness by dedicating their lives to the loving and humble service of others: as they learn to feel more at one with themselves and society, they gain a different perspective on life and eventually lose their fear of death.

In the case of Lachesis, however, there is a compulsion to do everything as quickly as possible ('Hurry': *2*); she bolts her food down ('Hurry, eating, while': *2*) and rushes about like a mad thing ('Quick to act': *2*), working her fingers to the bone ('Industrious': *2*). She feels confused, heavy and depressed in the morning, but her mind wakes up and comes alive as soon as evening falls ('Ideas, abundant': *3*, with the modality 'evening': *3*); she becomes vivacious ('Vivacious': *3*) and highly imaginative, with pleasant, vivid and lively fantasies ('Fancies, exaltation of': *3*, with the sub-rubrics 'pleasant': *1*, 'vivid': *2* and 'lively': *3*). She feels as light as air, a symptom that recurs frequently in the delusions section and is highly representative of the remedy. She loses herself in abstract meditation ('Theorizing': *1*), and either loses her initiative completely ('Initiative, lack of': *1*, Barthel) or takes on several projects at once, only to leave them all half-finished ('Undertakes, many things, perseveres in nothing': *2*), because she is basically chaotic ('Orderly manner, cannot perform anything in': *1*, Barthel), unpredictable ('Mood, changeable': *1*), impatient ('Impatience': *2*) and indecisive ('Irresolution': *3*). She may say that her life is a mess, and her work gives her no satisfaction (Lachesis is not in the rubric 'Occupation, amel.' for this reason).

She will not stop talking, especially in the evening ('Loquacity': *3*, with the sub-rubric 'evening': *3*), jumping from one topic of conversation to another ('Loquacity, changing quickly from one subject to another': *3*) and making eloquent speeches ('Loquacity, makes speeches': *2*). She is even more talkative during the menses ('Loquacity, menses, during': *2*) and in the heat ('Loquacity, heat, during': *2*). Loquacity is a strong characteristic of the remedy and there are very few other remedies in the rubrics I have quoted. One exception to this is Cimicifuga, who also jumps quickly from one subject to another; Voisin says that the difference between the two is that, while Lachesis changes topics but keeps the thread of the conversation, Cimicifuga jumps about wildly in verbal chaos and confusion.

Lachesis can be excessively meticulous ('Conscientious about trifles': *1*, Barthel) but, unlike Lycopodium, finds no satisfaction in work that challenges her intelligence and powers of intellectual reasoning. She ties herself in knots, babbling non-stop ('Answers, hastily': *1*) and contradicting everything that anyone says ('Contradiction, disposition to': *1*), in her need to be the centre of attention all the time. Rather than openly fight for what she wants, Lachesis prefers to go about things in a more convoluted, snake-like way, cheating and lying, like the coils of the *Crotalus Mutus*. She shows with her words and actions that she has a total disregard for what is socially acceptable and advisable ('Contrary': *3*, Barthel) and cannot tolerate the slightest contradiction ('Contradiction, is intolerant of': *1*, Barthel). At the same time, she will set out to destroy her opponents with malicious gossip ('Intriguer': *1*, Barthel), deceit ('Deceitful': *3*), slander ('Slander, disposition to': *1*, Barthel), lies ('Dishonest': *1*, Barthel) and derision ('Contemptuous': *1*). With her hateful, angry words she shows her complete lack of respect for other people's feelings ('Irony, satire, desire for': *2*, Barthel). She is a cruel manipulator ('Cruelty': *2*, Barthel), with no moral sense of duty ('Duty, no sense of duty': *1*, Barthel) or honour ('Honor, sense of h., no': *1*, Barthel); she treats her inferiors with contempt and her superiors with servile respect ('Hard for inferiors and kind for superiors': *1*, Barthel).

The Lachesis husband will be extremely callous towards his family, never buying a single present for his wife and children ('Gifts to his wife or son, husband making no': *3*, Barthel), yet offering great hospitality to every passing stranger. He is a bully ('Dictatorial': *1*) with a passionately jealous, highly sexed, arrogant, cruel and boastful nature ('Boaster': *1*, Barthel).

It may seem to the reader that too much emphasis has been placed on the bad points of Lachesis and that this description is far from objective. However, we must always bear in mind that the remedy picture is not the same thing as the human being who bears those symptoms. Our reasoning spirit allows us all a certain tolerance of our share of miasmatic inheritance, and it is our striving for perfection, to achieve the higher purposes of our existence, as Hahnemann wrote in Paragraph 9 of the *Organon*, that should be given more of our attention than the ravages of inherited disease. The task of the Lachesis patient, and of every other patient for that matter, is to overcome their morbid predisposition to disease.

Love

Feelings of disillusionment and disappointment come easily to the untrusting Lachesis ('Ailments, from disappointment': 2, Barthel) and she is easily frightened ('Ailments, from fright': 2, Barthel), emotionally charged ('Ailments, from excitement, emotional': 1, Barthel), often unhappy ('Grief': 3, Barthel), frequently deceived in love ('Love, ailments, from disappointed': 2) and made to feel jealous ('Ailments, from jealousy': 2, Barthel). If there is an argument happening, you will often find Lachesis in the middle of it ('Ailments, from discords between chief and subordinates': 1 and 'Ailments, from discords between parents, friends': 1, Barthel). She is sensitive to violence ('Horrible things, sad stories, affect her profoundly': 2) and bad news ('Bad news, ailments from': 1) and has been included in the rubric 'Sympathy, compassion': 1 in Barthel's repertory. However, the most important black type symptoms are 'Grief, ailments from': 3, and 'Love, ailments from disappointed': 2. Lachesis is characterised by her sensitivity to 'horrible things' and her lovesick grief; only Ignatia shares this pair of symptoms, but Ignatia's grief is silent while Lachesis lets everyone know about it with her furious rantings and ravings. These two symptoms, possessive love and extreme hatred, are at the heart of what needs to be cured in this remedy.

If she suffers a love disappointment, she tries to run away and hide ('Company, aversion to': 2) in a quiet place where she can feel free to indulge her fantasies ('Company, aversion to, desires solitude to indulge her fancy': 2), and lose herself in nostalgic memories ('Homesickness': 1) of the good times she had with the object of her affection ('Affectionate': 1, Barthel) and sexual desire ('Amativeness': 2 and 'Amorous': 2, Barthel). Her wish to return home ('Home, desires to go': 2) is another expression of the longing to recapture her lost love; however, she may also have the paradoxical wish to travel far and wide ('Travel, desire to': 1), in search of her dreams. With time, she becomes increasingly less outgoing ('Sociability': 1, Barthel) and more withdrawn inside herself. She develops a real dread of marriage ('Marriage, the idea of seemed unendurable': 2), and a misanthropic ('Misanthropy': 1) aversion both to women ('Women, aversion to': 2) and men ('Men, dread of': 1). She refuses to talk to others ('Talk, indisposed to': *1*) and sits muttering to herself ('Muttering': *3*); she wants to be left alone ('Touched, aversion to being': *2*) in peace ('Tranquility': *1*). She loses all will to live ('Weary of life': *1*), especially when she wakes in the morning ('Loathing life': *2*, with the sub-rubric 'morning': *2*).

Fear

Fear is a primary, subconscious response to anger, and Lachesis has great fear of the unknown and of dying in her sleep ('Fear, death, die, fear he will, if he goes to sleep': *2*, Barthel). The fear is exacerbated by the respiratory difficulties and feelings of suffocation that come upon her during sleep, after sleeping or on falling asleep, three modalities that are peculiar to the remedy: the rubrics 'Anxiety, sleep, on going to': *2*, 'Fear, sleep, to go to': *2* and 'Fear, bed, of the': *2* are all variations of the same theme. Her fears of insanity ('Fear, insanity, of': *1*), misfortune ('Fear, misfortune, of': *1*), disease ('Fear, disease, of impending': *1*), thunderstorms ('Fear, thunderstorm, of': *1*), travelling by car ('Fear, riding, when in a carriage': *2*), water ('Fear, water, of': *2*) and evil ('Fear, evil, of': *2*) are all different aspects of the basic fear of divine punishment and death ('Fear, death, of': *2*). The fears of men ('Fear, men of': *1*), people ('Fear, people, of': *1*), contagious, epidemic diseases ('Fear, contagious, epidemic diseases, of': *1*, Barthel), of being poisoned ('Fear, poisoned, of being': *2*) and of robbers ('Fear, robbers, of': *2*) are external manifestations of an inner emotional disturbance.

External Manifestations

To defend herself against the source of her fears, Lachesis convinces herself that she is under the control of a higher being, a superhuman force for evil ('Delusions, influence, is under a powerful': *2* and 'Delusions, superhuman control, under, is': *2*). It is interesting to compare this with the delusions of other remedies: Thuja, for example, believes himself to be under a higher being, but not controlled by it; Platinum and Cannabis Indica have delusions of superiority. Lachesis is the only one who both feels herself to be under superhuman control and influenced by it. This also accounts for her desire to be magnetised ('Magnetized, desires to be': *2*). She believes that she is pursued by enemies ('Delusions, pursued, thought he was, enemies, by': *2*) who are conspiring ('Delusions, conspiracies against him, there are': *1*, Barthel) to harm her ('Delusions, injury, is about to receive': *1*), or that she is already being injured ('Delusions, injury, is being injured': *1*) by those around her ('Delusions, injury, is being injured, by his surroundings': *2*); she believes that she is about to be poisoned ('Delusions, poisoned, he is about to be': *1*, Barthel), or that she has already been ('Delusions, poisoned, he has been': *2*, Barthel), by the medicine she has just taken ('Delusions, poisoned, medicine being': *1*), that there are thieves in the house ('Delusions, thieves, sees, house, in': *2*) and that her time is up ('Delusions, die, time has come to': *1*) and preparations are being made for her funeral.

She sees dead people ('Delusions, dead, persons, sees': *2*), devils ('Delusions, devils, sees': *1*), images and phantoms ('Delusions, images, phantoms, sees': *3*) when she is alone ('Delusions, images, sees, alone, when': *1*), that may be either frightening ('Delusions, images, frightful': *2*) or pleasant ('Delusions, images, pleasant': *2*). She feels that someone is behind her ('Delusions, people, behind him, some one is': *1*) and hears voices that she must follow ('Delusions, voices hears, that he must follow': *1*, Barthel), voices that confess things that she never did ('Delusions, voices, hears, confess things she never did': *1*, Barthel), voices that tell her to steal and kill ('Delusions, voices, hears, steal and kill, that she must': *1*, Barthel). She believes that she is being watched ('Delusions, spied, being': *1*, Barthel), that she has stolen things ('Delusions, stolen something, she has': *1*, Barthel), or that somebody thinks so ('Delusions, stolen, something, or somebody thinks it': *1*, Barthel), and that she is doomed ('Delusions, doomed, being': *2*, Barthel) and lost forever ('Delusions, lost, she is, predestination, from': *2*, Barthel).

With her leanings towards the supernatural and the superhuman, she has the delusion of being double ('Delusions, double, of being': *1*) or that she is someone else ('Delusions, person, thinks she is some other': *2*), floating above the ground ('Delusions, floating in air': *2*) or above the bed ('Delusions, floating in air, bed, is not resting in': *2*) and that she has been lifted into space ('Delusions, space, fancied he was carried into, while lying': *2*) and is lighter than air ('Delusions, body, lighter than air': *1*). She has beautiful visions ('Delusions, visions, beautiful': *1*) when her eyes are closed ('Delusions, visions, closing the eyes, on': *2*), fantastic visions ('Delusions, visions, fantastic': *1*) with clouds of colour ('Delusions, visions, clouds of colors': *1*). She imagines that she hears wonderful, heavenly music ('Delusions, music, fancies he hears': *2*) with the sweetest and most sublime melody ('Delusions, music, fancies he hears, sweetest and sublimest melody': *2*) that comforts her in her world of spectres ('Delusions, spectres, sees': *1* with the sub-rubric 'closing eyes, on': *2*) and snakes that are in and around her ('Delusions, snakes in and around her': *1*). If she reaches a state of complete mental breakdown, she may even start to crawl on the floor ('Insanity, crawls on the floor': *1*).

Other Forms of Fear

The primary subconscious response to anger is, as stated previously, fear of the unknown. This is expressed in Lachesis by her extreme sensitivity to external circumstances ('Sensitive': *2*) such as noise ('Sensitive, noise, to': *2*), reading material ('Sensitive, reading, to': *1*), touch ('Sensitive, touch, to': *2*, Barthel), after using her mind ('Sensitive, mental exertion, after': *2*, Barthel), thunderstorms ('Storm, during': *23*) and shining objects ('Shining objects agg.': *1*). Then we have the startings and jumping from noises ('Starting, noise, from': *2*), on falling asleep ('Starting, sleep, on falling': *2*), on waking ('Starting, waking, on': *2*) as if suffocating ('Starting, waking, on, as if suffocated': *2*). Next, we have the excitement from hearing horrible things ('Excitement, horrible things, after hearing': *2*) and bad news ('Excitement, bad news, after': *1*) that affects her in the morning ('Excitement, morning': *1*), evening ('Excitement, evening': *2*, p. 40) and in bed ('Excitement, bed, in': *1*) at night ('Excitement, night': *2*). She is unable to come to terms with the past and spends a lot of time crying over hurts she has suffered ('Weeping, offence, former, about': *1*, Barthel) and old arguments ('Weeping, vexation, from, old': *1*, Barthel). Her symptoms are always ameliorated by the free-flowing of discharges, and she feels better for a good cry ('Weeping, am.': *1*, Barthel); she cries when telling a story ('Weeping, anecdotes from': *2*, Barthel) and may cry hysterical, spasmodic tears ('Weeping, spasmodic': *1*, Barthel) with convulsions ('weeping, convulsions, during': *1*, Barthel) and epileptic fits ('Weeping, convulsions, from, epileptic': *2*, Barthel). She cries at night ('Weeping, night': *2*) in her sleep ('Weeping, sleep, in': *1*), and from noise ('Weeping, noise, at': *2*). She becomes hysterical ('Hysteria': *3*) after sex ('Hysteria, sexual excesses, after': *1*) and from the suppression of discharges ('Hysteria, suppression of discharges, after': *2*). She has frequent vanishing of the senses ('Senses, vanishing of': *2*). She loses consciousness ('Unconsciousness': *3*) after an outburst of emotion ('Unconsciousness, emotion, after': *3*) and during the menses ('Unconsciousness, menses, during': *3*) and her behaviour becomes automatic ('Unconsciousness, conduct, automatic': *1*) and trance-like ('Unconsciousness, trance, as in a': *3*).

This is a wonderful example of how a collection of symptoms can all fit together to describe the unconscious trance-like state of Lachesis, who is gifted with the power of clairvoyance, controlled by evil superhuman powers and believes herself to be someone else that she can talk to. In a mediumistic trance, she gazes into her crystal ball with her face flushed, her eyebrows raised, her throat hot, swollen and uncovered, warning her clients of the evils that may befall them. A couple of final details to complete the picture are that the fits of unconsciousness are worse during a fever ('Unconsciousness, fever, during': *2*) and in a warm room ('Unconsciousness, warm room': *2*).

Other Characteristics

In Barthel's repertory we find evidence of her affectionate disposition ('Affectionate': *1*, and sensitivity to hurt ('Ailments from mortification': *2*, fear ('Ailments from: fright': *2*), grief ('Ailments from: grief': *3*) and jealousy ('Ailments from: jealousy': *2*); we find that she is ambitious ('Ambition': *2*), hard-working ('Business, desire for': *1*), mortified when things go wrong ('Ailments from: reverses of fortune': *1*), compassionate ('Sympathy': *1*), concerned about her relatives ('Cares, relatives, about': *1*) and other people ('Cares, others, about': *1*) and, if she should be so unfortunate as to lose a child, she will probably never recover ('Ailments from: death of a child': *1*). From Barthel we learn that her syphilitic tendency for indifference and apathy ('Indifference': *2*) can apply not only to the welfare of others ('Indifference, welfare of others, to': *1*) but also to her duties ('Indifference, duties, to': *1*) and work ('Indifference, work, with aversion to': *1*). The human psyche has the potential to produce a whole range of paradoxical emotions and any remedy picture, which is after all modelled on real life, is capable of a number of conflicting and contradictory mental symptoms; I would even go so far as to say that all negative ideas contain within them a seed of the positive.

Paschero says that Lachesis's strong persecution complex is responsible for the state of profound grief ('Grief': *2*) in which she finds herself eventually, sighing deeply ('Sighing': *1*) and withdrawing from all contact ('Company, aversion to': *2*); she becomes afraid of people ('Fear, people, of': *1*) and keeps herself to herself ('Reserved': *1*), silent ('Talk, indisposed to': *1*) and suspicious of everybody ('Suspicious': *3*), especially in the afternoon ('Suspicious, afternoon': *2*), a unique keynote for Lachesis. Suspicion lies at the very heart of this remedy – the complete lack of trust in the world and God is the prime motivating force behind all the anger, hatred, maliciousness, jealousy and envy. She becomes apathetic, bored with life ('Loathing, life': 2), in the morning ('Loathing, life, morning': 2) and on waking ('Loathing, life, waking, on': 2); sadness overwhelms her ('Sadness': 3), especially in the morning ('Sadness, morning': 3) and on waking ('Sadness, waking, on: 2) when she bemoans her fate ('Moaning': 1) and laments ('Lamenting': 2). At these times, she feels quite alone, without a friend in the world ('Forsaken feeling': 2), especially in the morning ('Forsaken feeling, morning': 2) on waking ('Forsaken feeling, waking, on': 2), and her thoughts turn to suicide ('Death, desires': 2).

Paschero continues: 'The essential characteristic of the remedy is the way she projects all her inner feelings of hostility and passionate sexuality onto other people.' She takes offence at the slightest remark ('Offended, easily': 2, Barthel) and believes herself to be the target for all the evil in the world. She feels condemned to damnation and is obsessed by thoughts of evil ('Thoughts, persistent, evil, of': 2). She twists her secret desire for an illicit affair into accusations of her husband's infidelity. She has high sexual energy ('Lasciviousness': 3), even in her dreams ('Sleep, dreams, amorous': 3), and her jealous nature ('Jealousy': 3) can easily get out of hand ('Jealousy, irresistible, as foolish as it is': 2, Barthel). She tends to blame everyone but herself ('Reproaches, others': 2), with abusive language ('Abusive': 1, Barthel) and satirical remarks ('Jesting': 1) that poke fun at people ('Mocking': 2) and have a laugh at their expense ('Laughing, silly': 2). She talks non-stop, full of interminable ridiculous ideas ('Ideas, ridiculous': 3) and gestures ('Gestures, ridiculous or foolish': 2).

Her furious ranting reaches its peak as night falls, and she may become delirious ('Delirium, wild': 1), with violent behaviour ('Delirium, violent': 2) and constant mutterings ('Delirium, muttering': 2). Delirium can be brought on by the loss of vital fluids ('Delirium, loss of fluids, from': 2) or fatigue ('Delirium, fatigue, study, etc., from': 1) and, as night progresses, this state intensifies ('Delirium, night': 3) and her loquacity ('Delirium, loquacious': 3) knows no bounds ('Delirium, changing subjects, rapidly': 3). A Lachesis in the throws of raging jealousy is an impressive sight: her face is red and puffy, her eyes wild and bulging, as she tears at her clothing, gasping for breath and heaping torrents of abuse upon her victim, until she is eventually overcome by the intensity of her emotions and, clutching her chest, falls unconscious to the floor. The ensuing unconsciousness may be a defensive strategy to discourage the most extreme manifestation of her jealousy, the desire to kill ('Kill, desire to': *1* and 'Jealousy, kill, driving to': *1* – P. Schmidt's *Additions to Kent's Repertory*).

The Spiritual Level

As I have said before, a person bears the burden, or carries the cross, of his symptoms rather taking on the actual remedy picture. To take this analogy a little further, the horizontal arm of the cross could be seen to represent the growth of the child into adulthood, as it travels from the left-hand side – symbolising the dependence and need for security of childhood – to the right, a symbol of maturity, responsibility and the service of others. The vertical part could be seen to symbolise the path of the person's spiritual development, with the base representing the earth, materialism, property, and earthly pleasures, and the top representing the transcendence of matter into spirit and the rewards of the soul. Throughout his life, every human being struggles with the conflicts created between these opposing poles.

Lachesis is a wonderfully clear example of these polarities. Her personality split centres around the feelings of strong, inner hostility that become transmuted into the belief that she alone has been singled out for persecution. She is confused by her feelings of duality; in the morning she wakes feeling down and depressed, while in the evening she comes alive ('Exhilaration': *3*) and feels happy ('Cheerful': *3*) and full of fun ('Mirth, evening': *3*). She feels as if she has two wills ('Will, two, feels as if he had two wills': *2*), and has the sensation of being under an evil, superior power. She believes that she is beyond help ('Doubtful, recovery, of': *1*) and despairs for the salvation of her soul ('Doubtful, soul's welfare, of': *3*), a symptom she shares with the notoriously guilty remedies such as Arsenicum, Aurum and Pulsatilla. She may discover religion in a big way ('Religious affections': *3*), and the Lachesis child talks to saints, angels and dead people ('Religious affections, children, in': *2*). Lachesis can be insolent ('Impertinence': *1*, Barthel), pretentious ('Conceited': *1*, P. Schmidt), full of complaints ('Complaining': *2*, Barthel), and protests ('Protesting': *1*, P. Schmidt), with much sighing and lamenting ('Lamenting': *2*); discontented with her lot ('Discontented': *1*), discouraged ('Discouraged': *2*), cynical ('Scepticism': *2*, Schmidt's Additions) and pessimistic ('Pessimist': *1*, Barthel). She looks for solace in meditation ('Meditation': *2*), and mutters to herself when she is alone ('Talks, to himself when alone': *1*, Barthel). Then, like the Phoenix rising from the ashes, she is brought back to life by her own imagination, which creates wonderful fantasies in her mind ('Fancies, lively': *3*) and transports her to another world ('Ecstasy': *2*).

As she reaches the end of her days, bored and exhausted, her thoughts turn to suicide as the only solution to her problems, and she may try to drown herself in a final gesture of defiance at the snake that has been suffocating her all her life ('Suicidal disposition': *2*, with the means 'drowning, by': *2*).

SUMMARY

The mental characteristics of Lachesis are high sexual energy, passion and fear. The subconscious response to anger is fear, which she externalises in many forms. The result is, as Paschero writes: 'feverish mental activity with uncontrollable loquacity that forms an impenetrable barrier between her and the outside world; she disowns all her passionate, sexual feelings and accuses others of having them'.

This forms the basic nucleus of symptoms that go to make up the mental picture of Lachesis from the repertories.

Anxiety

This is primal, psoric anxiety that is worse when she wakes up in the morning and has to come back to the real world. Her fear of divine punishment is expressed by the anxiety for the future and for her salvation.

Anxiety is accompanied by psoric feelings of helplessness and restlessness.

Related Rubrics
'Anxiety, future, about': *2*.
'Anxiety, morning': *3*.
'Anxiety, morning, waking, on': *3*.
'Anxiety, salvation, about': *3*.

Difficulties of Concentration

Lachesis lacks self-confidence and feels confused in the morning, on waking and when she tries to concentrate. The mind is dull and sluggish on waking, on mental exertion, when she tries to read and after eating.

Related Rubrics
'Concentration, difficult': *3.*
'Confidence, want of self': *1.*
'Confusion, morning': *3*, and 'waking, on': *3.*
'Dullness, waking, on': *3.*
'Dullness, reading, while': *2.*
'Exertion, agg. from mental': *3.*
'Prostration of mind, eating, after': *1.*

Memory

Lachesis is one of only two remedies whose memories function better in the evening. However, she forgets words, proper names, what she has read, said and done, and what has happened. She has difficulty with self-expression.

Related Rubrics
'Memory, active, evening': *3.*
'Memory, weakness of': *3.*
'Memory, weakness of, happened, for what has': *2.*
'Memory, weakness of, read, for what has': *3.*
'Memory, weakness of, words, for': *2.*
'Memory, weakness of, names, for proper': *1.*
'Memory, weakness of, said, for what has': *1.*
'Memory, weakness of, done, for what has just': *1.*
'Memory, weakness of, expressing oneself, for': *1.*

Mistakes

Lachesis makes mistakes in speaking, spelling and writing, and misplaces words. She is disorientated and imagines that it is always afternoon. This keynote symptom is connected to the mental confusion, mental prostration after eating and the sensation that time passes too slowly.

Related Rubrics
'Mistakes, speaking': *1.*
'Mistakes, spelling, in': *2.*
'Mistakes, time, in, afternoon, always imagines it is': *2.*
'Mistakes, writing, in': *3.*
'Mistakes, words, misplacing': *2.*
'Time passes too slowly': *1.*

Confusion and Vanishing of Thoughts

At times she may not recognise her relatives, and her confusion while walking may cause her to lose her way. She may lose all sense of her own identity, and have a sensation of duality. Her thoughts vanish when she tries to read, speak and write. These three last symptoms are a keynote for Lachesis, indicating the problems she has trying to control her wandering thoughts.

Related Rubrics
'Confusion, identity, as to his': *1*.
'Confusion, identity, duality, sense of': *1*, Barthel.
'Confusion, walking, while': *2*.
'Recognize, does not, his relatives': *2*.
'Recognize, does not, well-known streets': *1*.
'Thoughts, vanishing of': *2*.
'Thoughts, vanishing of, reading, on': *2*.
'Thoughts, vanishing of, speaking, while': *2*.
'Thoughts, vanishing of, writing, while': *2*.
'Thoughts, wandering': *1*.

Speech Problems

The speech can be confused, incoherent, slow, wandering and in a foreign language. These are all indications of the sense of duality, confusion and chaos that afflict her.

Related Rubrics
'Speech, confused': *2*.
'Speech, foreign tongue, in a': *1*.
'Speech, hasty': *3*.
'Speech, incoherent': *3*.
'Speech, slow': *3*.
'Speech, wandering': *3*.

Anger

The following symptoms are the most characteristic of the remedy: malicious, arrogant, suspicious, a sharp, critical tongue, selfish, egotistical and jealous. The syphilitic aspect comes out in the anger, envy, argumentativeness and jealousy, and the predilection for acts of violence and destruction. She is obsessed by thoughts of evil, hatred and mischief.

Related Rubrics
'Anger, ailments after anger': *2.*
'Censorious': *2.*
'Egotism': *2.*
'Envy': *1.*
'Haughty': *2.*
'Hatred': *2.*
'Jealousy': *3.*
'Malicious': *2.*
'Mischievous': *2.*
'Mocking': *2.*
'Quarrelsome': *2.*
'Quarrelsome, jealousy, from': *2.*
'Selfishness': *1*, Barthel.
'Suspicious': *3.*
'Thoughts, persistent, evil, of': *2.*
'Violent': *1.*
'Violent, deeds, rage, leading to': *1.*

Productivity

Lachesis is a compulsive workaholic who thinks, acts and eats with lightning speed. In the morning, she is confused and depressed; in the evening, she comes alive and her mind fills with ideas and fantasies. Basically, she is all theory and no practice, with many plans and no perseverance to see them through. She is indecisive and intolerant of her messiness and her inability to finish things.

She talks non-stop, uncontrollably, tying herself up in knots and jumping from one topic of conversation to another in a way that only she and Cimicifuga can. The loquacity intensifies in the evening, during heat and during menses.

Related Rubrics
'Fancies, exaltation of': *3.*
'Hurry': *2.*
'Hurry, eating, while': *2.*
'Ideas, abundant, evening': *3.*
'Impatience': *2.*
'Industrious': *2.*
'Industrious, evening': *2.*
'Initiative, lack of': *1*, Barthel.

'Irresolution': *3*.
'Loquacity': *3*.
'Loquacity, changing quickly from one subject to another': *3*.
'Loquacity, evening': *3*.
'Loquacity, heat, during': *2*.
'Loquacity, makes speeches': *2*.
'Loquacity, menses, during': *2*.
'Orderly manner, cannot perform anything in': *1*, Barthel.
'Quick to act': *2*.
'Theorizing': *1*.
'Thoughts, rapid': *2*.
'Undertakes, many things, perseveres in nothing': *2*.
'Vivacious': *3*.

Aspects of Sycotic Aggression

She wants to be the absolute centre of attention, enmeshing others in her own chaos and confusion, and manipulating them to do what she wants with any means at her disposal. In conversation, she will outstrip anybody with her persistent contradictions and her intolerance of other people's points of view.

She will also win any verbal battle of wits with deceit, slander and cruel gossip. She is entirely unscrupulous in her dealings, treating her superiors with servile respect and her inferiors with contempt. She is jealous, arrogant, cruel and tyrannical.

Related Rubrics
'Answers, hastily': *1*.
'Boaster': *1*, Barthel.
'Contemptuous': *1*.
'Contradiction, disposition to': *3*.
'Contradiction, is intolerant of': *1*, Barthel.
'Contrary': *3*, Barthel.
'Cruelty': *2*, Barthel.
'Deceitful': *3*, Barthel.
'Dictatorial': *1*.
'Duty, no sense of': *1*, Barthel.
'Hard, for inferiors and kind for superiors': *1*, Barthel.
'Honor, sense of h., no': *1*, Barthel.
'Intriguer': *1*, Barthel.
'Slander, disposition to': *1*, Barthel.

Emotional Relationships

Lachesis has ailments from grief, disappointed love and bad news. She hates to witness any kind of disagreement or discord among family, colleagues or friends. She is very sensitive to tragic events and unhappy love affairs, a pair of symptoms shared only with Ignatia, although the two remedies are easily distinguished by the silent grief of Ignatia and the infuriated jealousy of Lachesis. The essence of what is to be cured in this remedy is the combination of possessive love and extreme hatred.

Related Rubrics
'Ailments from: discords between parents, friends': *1*, Barthel.
'Bad news, ailments from': *1*.
'Grief, ailments from': *3*.
'Hatred': *2*.
'Horrible things, sad stories, affect her profoundly': *2*.
'Jealousy, as foolish as it is irresistible': *2*.
'Love, ailments from disappointed': *2*.

Unhappiness in Love

If she suffers a love disappointment, her first impulse is to run away and hide in a quiet place where she can indulge her amorous fantasies and revive happy memories of her lost love; she wants to return home, to where the heart is. She also has the desire to travel far and wide, always on the lookout for something better than what she has. She rejects women, men and all idea of marriage. She becomes misanthropic and silent, wanting to be left quite alone to sit and mutter to herself. She becomes tired of living, especially in the morning, on waking, and wants to die.

Related Rubrics
'Affectionate': *1*, Barthel.
'Amorous': *2*, Barthel.
'Company, aversion to': *2*.
'Company, aversion to, desires solitude to indulge her fancy': *2*.
'Fear, men, of': *1*.
'Home, desires to go': *2*.
'Homesickness': *1*.
'Loathing, life': *2*.
'Loathing, life, morning': *2*.

'Marriage, the idea seemed unendurable': *2*.
'Misanthropy': *1*.
'Muttering': *3*.
'Touched, aversion to being': *2*.
'Travel, desire to': *1*.
'Women, aversion to': *2*.

Fear

Fear and anger are closely related. Lachesis is afraid of the unknown and of dying in her sleep, especially when feelings of suffocation or constriction are present before, during and after sleep. She has anxiety on going to sleep, fear of going to sleep, fear at night and fear of the bed. The fears of divine punishment and death are represented by the fears of insanity, misfortune, disease, thunderstorms, water, evil and travelling by car. She is also afraid of men, people, being poisoned and robbers.

Related Rubrics
'Anxiety, sleep, on going to': *2*.
'Fear, bed, of the': *2*.
'Fear, death, of': *2*.
'Fear, death, die, fear he will, if he goes to sleep': *2*, Barthel.
'Fear, disease, of impending': *1*.
'Fear, evil of': *2*.
'Fear, to go to sleep': *2*.
'Fear, insanity, of': *1*.
'Fear, men, of': *1*.
'Fear, misfortune, of': *1*.
'Fear, night': *2*.
'Fear, people, of': *1*.
'Fear, poisoned, of being': *2*.
'Fear, robbers, of': *2*.
'Fear, riding, when in a carriage': *2*.
'Fear, thunderstorm, of': *1*.
'Fear, water, of': *2*.

Delusions

Her delusions serve to protect her from any real danger. She believes that she is controlled by a powerful, evil, superhuman being, that she is pursued by enemies, that she is surrounded by people conspiring against her, wishing her harm; she believes that she is about to be or has been poisoned, that there are robbers in the house, that her time is up and her relatives are preparing her funeral.

She imagines herself dead, sees dead people, devils and visions that are either frightening or pleasant. She feels that someone is behind her. She hears voices that she must follow, confessing things that she has not done; voices command her to steal and kill; she believes that she is being spied upon, that she has stolen something, that she is doomed, a lost soul.

Related Rubrics

'Delusions, conspiracies, against him, there are': *1*, Barthel.

'Delusions, dead, persons, sees': *2*, with the sub-rubric 'corpse, that he himself was dead': *2*.

'Delusions, devils, sees': *1*.

'Delusions, doomed, being': *2*, Barthel.

'Delusions, images, phantoms sees': *3*, with the sub-rubrics 'frightful': *2*, and 'pleasant': *2*.

'Delusions, influence, is under a powerful': *2*.

'Delusions, injury, is about to receive': *1*.

'Delusions, injury, is being injured': *1*, with the sub-rubric 'by his surroundings': *2*.

'Delusions, lost, she is, predestination, from': *2*, Barthel.

'Delusions, people, sees, behind him, someone is': *1*.

'Delusions, poisoned, he has been': *2*, Barthel.

'Delusions, poisoned, he is about to be': *1*, Barthel.

'Delusions, poisoned, medicine being': *1*.

'Delusions, pursued, thought he was, enemies, by': *2*.

'Delusions, spied, being': *1*, Barthel.

'Delusions, stolen something, she has': *1*, Barthel.

'Delusions, superhuman control, under, is': *2*.

'Delusions, thieves, sees, house, in': *2*.

'Delusions, voices hears, confess things she never did': *1*, Barthel.

'Delusions, voices, hears, that he must follow': *1*, Barthel.

'Delusions, voices hears, steal and kill, that she must': *1*, Barthel.

Sense of Control by Superhuman Forces

The feeling of being under the control of an alien influence makes her feel as if she is another person, a duplicate of herself who has been carried off into space and remains suspended in the air, floating above the bed and lighter than air. Fantastic visions of clouds of colour fill her eyes and sublime music fills her ears, while she is haunted by fantasies of phantoms and snakes that invade and surround her.

Related Rubrics
'Delusions, beautiful': *2*, with the sub-rubric 'landscape': *2*.
'Delusions, body, lighter than air': *1*.
'Delusions, charmed and cannot break the spell': *2*, Barthel.
'Delusions, double, of being': *1*.
'Delusions, floating in air': *2*, with the sub-rubric 'bed, is not resting in': *2*.
'Delusions, music, fancies he hears': *2*, with the sub-rubric 'sweetest and sublimest melody': *2*.
'Delusions, person, other, she is some': *2*, Barthel.
'Delusions, snakes in and around her': *1*.
'Delusions, space, fancied he was carried into, while lying': *2*.
'Delusions, spectres, sees': *1*, with the sub-rubric 'closing eyes, on': *2*.
'Delusions, visions': *2*, with the sub-rubrics 'closing the eyes on': *2*, 'fantastic': *1* and 'clouds of colors': *1*.

Sensitivity to Surroundings

She is extremely sensitive to noise, touch, thunderstorms, shining objects, reading material and after mental exertion. She starts nervously from noise, on falling asleep and on waking, with a feeling of suffocation or constriction. She gets easily wound up by horrible stories and news of tragic events, especially in the evening, in bed and at night. She cries when she remembers old hurts and vexations. She feels better for a good cry and cries at night, during sleep and when she hears a noise. She can become hysterical after sex and after the suppression of discharges. She loses consciousness after strong emotions, during menses, during a fever and in a warm room, and falls into a mediumistic trance, where she believes that she is gifted with clairvoyant powers, possessed by an evil, superior force, and that she has become someone else to whom she can talk. She is the stereotypical witch-like fortune-teller with the crystal ball.

Related Rubrics
'Clairvoyance': *1*.
'Excitement, bad news, after': *1*.
'Excitement, bed, in': *1*.

'Excitement, evening': *2*.
'Excitement, horrible things, after hearing': *2*.
'Excitement, night': *2*.
'Hysteria': *3*, with the sub-rubrics 'sexual excesses, after': *1* and 'suppression of discharges, after': *2*.
'Magnetized, desires to be': *2*.
'Senses, vanishing, of': *2*.
'Sensitive, mental exertion, after': *2*, Barthel.
'Sensitive, noise, to': *2*.
'Sensitive, reading, to': *1*.
'Sensitive, touch, to': *2*, Barthel.
'Shining objects agg.': *1*.
'Starting, noise, from': *2*.
'Starting, sleep, on falling': *2*.
'Starting, waking, on': *2*.
'Starting, waking, on, as if suffocated': *2*.
'Thunderstorm, during': *1*.
'Unconsciousness': *3*, with the sub-rubrics 'emotion, after': *3*, 'conduct, automatic': *1*, 'fever, during': *2*, 'trance, as in a': *3* and 'warm room': *2*.
'Weeping, ameliorates': *1*, Barthel.
'Weeping, anecdotes, from': *2*, Barthel.
'Weeping, night': *2*, with the sub-rubric 'sleep, in': *1*.
'Weeping, noise, at': *2*.
'Weeping, offence, from, former or about': *1*, Barthel.

Emotional Vulnerability

In Barthel, we find several references to the emotional vulnerability of Lachesis. She is affectionate, easily hurt, full of grief, jealousy and fear; she worries about her friends and family and, if she suffers the loss of a child, she may never recover from the shock. She has great ambitions and finds it hard to come to terms with failure. In its syphilitic aspect, Lachesis can become indifferent to the welfare of others, to her duties and her work. This is a remedy of great emotional extremes, illustrating the huge range of emotions inherent in the human psyche.

Related Rubrics from Barthel
'Affectionate': *1*.
'Ailments from: death of a child': *1*.

'Ailments from: fright': *2*.
'Ailments from: grief': *3*.
'Ailments from: jealousy': *2*.
'Ailments from: mortification': *3*.
'Ailments from: reverses of fortune': *1*.
'Ambition': *2*.
'Business, desire for': *1*.
'Cares, full of, others, about': *1*.
'Cares, full of, relatives, about': *1*.
'Indifference': *2*.
'Indifference, duties, to': *1*.
'Indifference, welfare of others, to': *1*.
'Indifference, work, with aversion to': *1*.
'Sympathy': *1*.

Effects of Anger

She feels angry and resentful that life has destroyed her faith and envies those who still have some. She becomes depressed, withdrawn, suspicious and silent except for the occasional sigh of boredom. Every morning, she wakes feeling extremely depressed and lonely; moaning and lamenting that all her friends have deserted her in her hour of need, she feels that there is nothing left for her but to die.

Related Rubrics
'Company, aversion to': *2*.
'Death, desires': *2*.
'Fear, people, of': *1*.
'Forsaken feeling': *2*, with the sub-rubrics 'morning': *2*, 'waking, on': *2*
'Lamenting': *2*.
'Loathing, life': *2*, with the sub-rubrics 'morning': *2*, 'waking': *2*.
'Moaning': *1*.
'Reserved': *1*.
'Sadness': *3*, with the sub-rubrics 'morning': *3*, 'waking, on': *3*.
'Sighing': *1*.
'Suspicious': *3*, with the sub-rubrics 'afternoon': *2*, 'evening': *2*.
'Talk, indisposed to': *1*.

Persecution Complex

She is offended easily and feels persecuted by the whole world, lost and doomed for ever. Thoughts of evil dominate her mind and her desire for some extramarital excitement becomes converted into the paranoid conviction that her husband is being unfaithful to her. She is given to violent scenes of sexual jealousy and erotic dreams that fuel her jealousy to the point of insanity; she heaps wild accusations on her victim, her cutting words dripping with contempt and irony as she unleashes the full flood of her ridiculous ideas and gesticulations.

Related Rubrics
'Gestures, ridiculous or foolish': *2*.
'Ideas, ridiculous': *3*.
'Jealousy': *3*.
'Jealousy, brutal from, gentle husband becoming': *1*, Barthel.
'Jealousy, irresistible, as foolish as it is': *2*, Barthel.
'Jesting': *1*.
'Lasciviousness': *3*.
'Laughing, silly': *2*.
'Mocking': *2*.
'Offended, easily': *2*, Barthel.
'Reproaches, others': *2*.
'Sleep, dreams, amorous': *3*.
'Thoughts, persistent, evil, of': *2*.

Delirium

The intensity of her rage reaches a peak at night and she becomes violent and delirious, wild and voluble. To repeat Paschero, 'A Lachesis in the throes of raging jealousy is an impressive sight: her face is red and puffy, her eyes wild and bulging, as she tears at her clothing, gasping for breath and heaping torrents of abuse upon her victim, until she is overcome by the intensity of her emotions and, clutching her chest, falls unconscious to the floor, in a final effort not to succumb to homicidal impulses.'

Related Rubrics
'Abusive, husband insulting wife before children or vice versa': *1*, Barthel.
'Delirium, changing subjects rapidly': *3*.
'Delirium loquacious': *3*.
'Delirium, muttering': *2*.
'Delirium, night': *3*.

'Delirium, violent': *2*.
'Delirium, wild': *1*.
'Kill, desire to': *1*.

Emotional Instability

Lachesis acts and feels as if she were two people; when she wakes up in the morning, she feels lonely and sad but, as soon as evening falls, she comes alive and feels happy to the point of exhilaration. She feels as if she had two wills, one the voice of her conscience and the other the commands of a superior force for evil. She fears she is doomed to feel like this for ever. Lachesis children talk obsessively of saints, angels and death. In the perpetual struggle between right and wrong, she becomes peevish, arrogant, cantankerous, discontented, discouraged, cynical and pessimistic. She seeks solace in quiet meditation and talks to herself when alone. Like the phoenix rising from the ashes, she refuses to give up the fight and her fantastic imagination creates wonderful, ecstatic visions as she is carried away up into the ether. In the final stages, she becomes utterly bored with life, and suicide seems to be the only possible solution; in a final gesture of defiance at the viper who has kept her in its grip throughout her whole life, she tries to drown herself.

Related Rubrics
'Cheerful': *3*.
'Cheerful, evening': *2*.
'Complaining': *2*, Barthel.
'Conceited': *1*, P. Schmidt.
'Discontented': *1*.
'Discouraged': *2*.
'Doubtful, recovery, of': *1*.
'Doubtful, soul's welfare, of': *3*.
'Ectasy': *2*.
'Exhilaration': *3*.
'Fancies, lively': *3*.
'Fancies, pleasant': *1*.
'Impertinence': *1*, Barthel.
'Lamenting': *2*.
'Meditation': *2*.
'Mirth, evening': *3*.
'Pessimist': *2*, P. Schmidt.

'Protesting': *1*, P. Schmidt.
'Religious affections': *3*.
'Religious affections, children, in': *2*.
'Sadness, waking, on': *3*.
'Scepticism': *2*, P. Schmidt.
'Suicidal disposition': *2*.
'Suicidal disposition, drowning, by': *2*.
'Talks, himself, to, only when alone': *2*, Barthel.
'Will, two, feels as if he had two wills': *2*.

SCHEMATIC DIAGRAM AND REPERTORISATION

Passionate anger, high sexual energy and anxiety are the main mental characteristics of this remedy. Anger and fear are intimately related; rather than own to her innermost feelings, she prefers to place the blame on other people.

For this reason, we have placed the symptoms connected to the projection phenomena in the centre of the diagram overleaf. To the left, we have the symptoms that describe the basic anxiety, lack of confidence and dullness of the intellectual faculties. The various ways in which Lachesis expresses her anger have been grouped together and placed in the upper right-hand corner. The Fear symptoms are in the upper left-hand corner. Lachesis tends to react to stress either with fear or anger, and disowns her feelings as a means of self-defence. Symptoms that try to compensate for the anxiety and lack of confidence have been grouped together under the headings Work and Relationships with Others; those who are healthy have the potential to achieve freedom and maturity through these aspects of life, while those who are sick find nothing but problems and obstacles in these areas. Below the centre, we find the group of symptoms headed 'Emotional instability', as the state of mind is wholly influenced by all preceding symptom complexes.

COMPARATIVE MATERIA MEDICA

Lycopodium

Lycopodium is the only remedy that has eight of the ten symptoms of the Minimum Characteristic Syndrome of Lachesis, but it differs from Lachesis in its very essence, the lack of self-confidence. He is shrewd, intelligent and arrogantly competitive He uses his fastidiousness and industriousness to prove his superiority over others, and covers up his feelings of insecurity and helplessness, symbolised by the fear of not arriving at his destination, with a powerful and domineering nature ('Dictatorial', 9). However, the absence from symptoms 5 and 6 provides evidence of the basic differences between the two remedies.

Lachesis feels rejected and forsaken, and is full of rage, fury, hatred, envy and ridiculous ideas, such as the fear that God will kill her while she sleeps because she is under the influence of a superior, evil force. She is full of resentment and the desire for revenge; Lycopodium becomes resentful ('Malicious', 1) if he suspects (3) that he is not held in high enough esteem by others. Jealousy (7) creates a desire for revenge in Lachesis and an inferiority complex in Lycopodium. Lachesis blames others for the lack of love in her life; Lycopodium ('Reproaches others', 8) complains about the lack of support. Lachesis is an articulate fast-talker who jumps from one topic of conversation to another, and her words are full of envy, suspicion and malice; Lycopodium's eloquence ('Loquacity', 10) is skilful, fluent, persuasive and self-centred, impressing his audience with his emotive and knowledgeable phrases.

Like Lachesis, Lycopodium has trouble remembering what he has read (14), as well as proper names and words; in fact, his appalling memory plays a large part in his lack of confidence. He is more irritable than dull on waking (12). Lachesis's poor memory for past events is convenient, allowing her to reformulate or embellish the past as it suits her. Lycopodium has no confusion of identity (15).

As stated earlier, it is often said that a person can work to attain spiritual freedom through the service and love of others. Lycopodium does not have the work ethic (20) of Lachesis or the tendency to take on more than he can chew (22). He is quick ('Hurry', 21), intelligent and fastidious and gets great satisfaction from doing a job well; hence his presence in the rubric 'Occupation, amel': *1* where Lachesis does not appear. Lycopodium is absent from symptoms 25 to 27, which fuel Lachesis's desire for revenge and destruction. Lycopodium is less afraid of evil (23) and robbers (24) than of the solitude and darkness

SCHEMATIC DIAGRAM – LACHESIS

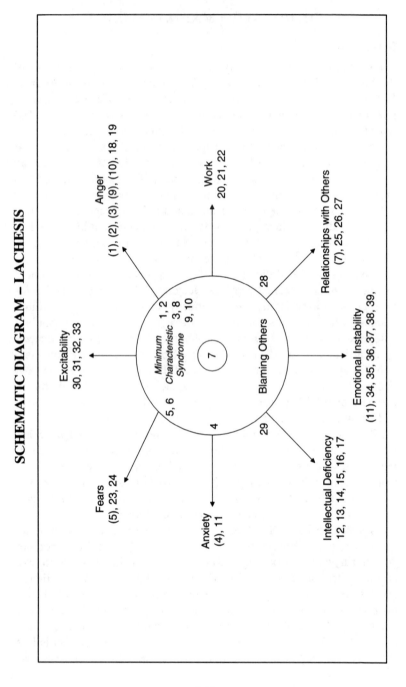

Minimum Characteristic Syndrome

1) Malicious
2) Haughty
3) Suspicious
4) Anxiety, morning, waking, on
5) Fear, sleep, to go to
6) Forsaken feeling
7) Jealousy
8) Reproaches others
9) Dictatorial
10) Loquacity

Anxiety

11) Despair, religious (of salvation etc.)

Intellectual Deficiency

12) Dullness, waking, on
13) Memory, weakness of, happened, for what has
14) Memory, weakness of, read, for what has
15) Confusion, identity, as to his
16) Speech, hasty
17) Speech, wandering

Anger

18) Censorious, critical
19) Contradict, disposition to

Work

20) Industrious

21) Hurry
22) Undertakes, many things, perseveres in nothing

Fear

23) Fear, evil, of
24) Fear, robbers, of

Relationships with Others

25) Love, ailments, from disappointed
26) Hatred
27) Homesickness

Blaming Others

28) Delusion, pursued, thought he was, enemies, by
29) Company, aversion to

Excitability

30) Starting, sleep, on falling
31) Clairvoyance
32) Magnetized, desires to be
33) Excitement, horrible things, after hearing

Emotional Instability

34) Sadness, morning, waking, on
35) Mirth, evening
36) Complaining
37) Meditation
38) Loathing, life
39) Suicidal disposition

REPERTORISATION – LACHESIS

	1	2	3	4	5	6	7	8	9	10	11	12	13	14	15	16	17	18	19	20	21	22	23	24	25	26	27	28	29	30	31	32	33	34	35	36	37	38	39
Lach.	2	2	2	3	2	2	3	2	1	3	3	3	2	3	1	3	3	2	1	2	2	2	2	2	2	2	1	2	2	2	1	2	2	3	3	2	2	2	2
Aur.	2	1	2	2	–	3	1	1	1	2	3	–	–	–	–	1	1	1	2	3	1	–	1	1	2	2	2	2	1	1	–	–	–	2	–	2	1	3	3
Caust.	1	2	3	2	2	–	–	–	1	1	–	–	–	–	–	–	–	2	2	1	1	–	2	2	2	1	2	–	–	2	2	–	–	1	–	1	1	1	1
Chin.	1	1	2	2	1	1	–	3	–	–	–	1	–	–	–	1	1	1	1	1	2	–	1	2	1	–	–	2	2	1	1	–	–	2	2	1	1	3	2
Hyos.	2	2	2	2	–	–	3	2	2	3	2	–	–	2	3	3	3	1	2	2	1	–	–	1	3	–	1	2	2	–	1	–	–	–	1	1	2	1	2
Lyc.	2	3	3	2	–	–	–	2	2	–	–	–	2	2	3	3	3	2	2	–	3	–	1	–	–	–	–	1	1	3	3	–	–	–	2	2	2	2	–
Merc.	1	1	2	–	1	–	–	1	1	–	1	–	–	–	1	1	1	1	1	–	3	–	2	1	–	–	2	–	–	2	2	–	1	1	–	–	–	3	1
Nat-m.	2	1	–	1	1	–	2	2	–	1	–	–	–	–	–	2	2	1	2	1	2	–	2	2	3	2	2	3	3	2	2	3	–	–	2	2	–	3	2
Nux-v.	3	1	1	2	1	–	–	2	1	1	2	3	1	–	2	1	1	2	2	1	2	–	1	1	1	–	1	3	–	2	2	–	–	–	–	1	2	2	1
Phos.	1	1	1	2	–	3	2	–	–	2	2	–	–	–	–	2	2	–	–	–	1	–	2	2	–	1	–	1	–	2	–	–	–	–	1	2	–	3	2
Puls.	–	–	2	3	–	–	–	1	–	–	2	–	–	–	–	2	2	1	1	1	2	–	1	1	–	1	2	2	2	–	1	–	–	–	–	–	1	1	1
Staph.	–	2	3	1	–	2	1	1	–	1	3	1	–	1	2	2	3	–	–	–	3	–	1	1	2	–	2	–	1	–	–	–	–	–	2	1	2	1	2
Stram.	3	2	3	–	–	–	–	–	–	3	–	–	–	1	1	2	2	1	–	1	1	–	1	1	–	–	1	2	–	–	1	–	–	1	–	2	1	1	2
Sulph.	1	3	3	–	–	1	–	1	–	1	–	–	–	–	–	1	1	3	3	1	1	–	1	1	–	–	–	1	–	3	3	–	1	–	2	2	2	2	1
Verat.	1	3	2	–	–	–	–	–	–	2	–	–	–	1	1	–	1	2	2	1	1	–	1	1	2	1	1	1	–	–	–	–	–	1	–	–	–	–	1
Anac.	2	1	2	1	–	–	–	1	–	1	–	1	1	–	2	2	2	–	1	1	–	–	1	1	–	3	–	3	1	1	1	–	–	1	–	–	–	–	2
Arn.	1	1	1	1	–	–	1	1	–	1	–	1	1	–	1	1	1	2	2	1	1	–	1	1	–	–	1	–	–	1	1	–	–	–	1	1	–	–	–
Ign.	1	1	1	1	–	–	–	–	–	–	1	–	–	–	–	2	2	1	1	2	2	–	2	–	3	–	2	3	–	1	–	–	1	–	1	1	1	–	–
Plat.	1	3	–	1	–	2	–	–	–	–	1	1	–	–	–	2	2	2	2	1	1	–	1	1	–	–	–	2	–	–	–	3	–	–	1	–	1	2	1
Calc.	2	1	–	–	–	1	–	–	–	–	2	–	–	–	–	1	1	1	1	1	1	–	–	3	2	–	–	1	–	–	1	3	2	1	1	–	1	2	2

Minimum Characteristic Syndrome

1) Malicious
2) Haughty
3) Suspicious
4) Anxiety, morning, waking, on
5) Fear, sleep, to go to
6) Forsaken feeling
7) Jealousy
8) Reproaches others
9) Dictatorial
10) Loquacity

Anxiety

11) Despair, religious (of salvation etc.)

Intellectual Deficiency

12) Dullness, waking, on
13) Memory, weakness of, happened, for what has
14) Memory, weakness of, read, for what has
15) Confusion, identity, as to his
16) Speech, hasty
17) Speech, wandering

Anger

18) Censorious, critical
19) Contradict, disposition to

Work

20) Industrious

21) Hurry
22) Undertakes, many things, perseveres in nothing

Fear

23) Fear, evil, of
24) Fear, robbers, of

Relationships with Others

25) Love, ailments, from disappointed
26) Hatred
27) Homesickness

Blaming Others

28) Delusion, pursued, thought he was, enemies, by
29) Company, aversion to

Excitability

30) Starting, sleep, on falling
31) Clairvoyance
32) Magnetized, desires to be
33) Excitement, horrible things, after hearing

Emotional Instability

34) Sadness, morning, waking, on
35) Mirth, evening
36) Complaining
37) Meditation
38) Loathing, life
39) Suicidal disposition

that bring him face to face with his dark side, with all its weaknesses and vulnerabilities; he is basically in great need of affection, too proud to indulge in nostalgia (27) and too nice to hate (26), and can be moved to tears by a show of gratitude. Like Lachesis, he feels persecuted by his enemies (28) and tries to hide himself away, ('Company, aversion to', 29), despite his fear of solitude, in the belief that he is about to be supplanted by people who have called his bluff; Lachesis feels persecuted and singled out as a target for all the evil in the world and withdraws from people in order to protect herself.

Lycopodium jumps and starts on falling asleep (30), as well as when the doorbell rings, because of the nervous tension and fear he feels in the stomach; in Lachesis, this symptom is indicative of her fear of suffocating and dying in her sleep. Lycopodium is absent from symptoms 31 and 32, which are related to Lachesis's extrasensory powers of communication with the supernatural; neither does he figure in symptom 33, which illustrates Lachesis's fear of violence.

Lycopodium is absent from symptoms 35, 37 and 39, which express the emotional instability of Lachesis, her penchant for astral travel and her utter boredom with life in the final stages.

The following four remedies have seven symptoms from the Minimum Characteristic Syndrome of Lachesis: Aurum, Natrum Muriaticum, Nux Vomica and Veratrum Album.

Aurum

Aurum does not have the fearful, anxious and jealous outlook on life (symptoms 4, 5 and 7 from the Minimum Characteristic Syndrome) that illustrates Lachesis's deep fear of divine punishment. Aurum's guilt complex stems from a syphilitic desire for destruction coupled with crippling feelings of insecurity. Paschero says of Aurum: 'He is basically an irritable, quick-tempered patient who cannot bear the least contradiction; he is prone to violent explosions of uncontrollable rage that can bring about his own destruction.'

Like Lachesis, Aurum can be resentful ('Malicious', 1), arrogant ('Haughty', 2), critical ('Reproaches, others', 8), domineering (9) and talkative (10); but whereas Lachesis is full of envy and jealousy, Aurum has strong feelings of criminal guilt and angrily tries to inflict violent punishment on herself. Aurum's feelings of mistrust (3) and abandonment (6) come from the firm belief that she is evil, unworthy of people's trust and that she has neglected her duty; in Lachesis, they reflect her feelings of persecution.

270

Aurum has none of the symptoms related to the intellectual deficiencies (12 to 17), but the miasmatic influences of psora and syphilis make her critical ('Censorious', 18) and contradictory (19). Her guilt at neglecting her duty makes her work twice as hard ('Industrious', 20) and twice as fast ('Hurry', 21), although she lacks perseverance ('Undertakes, many things, perseveres in nothing', 22).

Aurum has all the symptoms under the headings of Fear, Relationships with Others and Blaming Others (23 to 29), which provides further proof of the fact that a remedy should never be prescribed on the basis of symptoms taken in isolation from the rest of the case, but on the whole life experience and character of the patient. It is the meaning, intention and result of each symptom that give the remedy its particular, individual character. In Lachesis, the miasms of syphilis and sycosis combine to create a picture of tremendous malice, pride, self-centredness, jealousy and envy. In Aurum, the syphilitic miasm creates a picture of great self-destruction and deep depression. Aurum lacks the sycotic leanings towards the supernatural, and does not have symptoms 30, 31 and 32. In typically syphilitic style, she internalises her guilt and, unlike the sycotic Lachesis who externalises all her feelings, does not suffer from hearing horrible things (33).

Aurum does not have symptoms 34 and 35, which illustrate the sycotic nature of Lachesis's fluctuating emotional state, with sadness in the morning and happiness in the evening. In the final stages of pathology, Aurum becomes totally bowed down under the weight of unremitting self-abuse and self-reproach, and sits lost in deep thought ('Meditation', 37) about all the wrong things she has done in her life; she despairs of religious salvation (11) and eventually turns her back on life (38) and tries to kill herself (39) as a last-ditch attempt to escape the merciless torture of the enemy within.

Natrum Muriaticum

Natrum Muriaticum has 7 of the 10 core symptoms. The determining factor here is the craving for affection ('Affectionate': *2*) that he did not get from his parents in his formative years. He is obsessed with the past ('Dwells on past disagreeable occurrences': *3*) as he searches desperately for love. Frustration turns to anger, anger is suppressed and festers away in the form of resentment. Unlike Lachesis, Natrum Mur. is neither mistrustful (3), domineering (9) nor forsaken (6), symptoms that illustrate how Lachesis converts her need for affection into a need for absolute control; to assuage her feeling that she is hated and hounded by all, she uses all her powers of manipulation to bend people to her will.

Natrum Mur. cannot remember past events (13) or what he has read (14) because he wants to forget his unhappy past. Although he can be critical ('Censorious', 18), he is too emotionally repressed to venture a difference of opinion (19). He suffers his feelings of grief ('Grief, silent': *3*) and hatred (26) in silence as he broods over his unrequited love ('Love, ailments, from disappointed', 25), wallowing in nostalgic memories ('Homesickness', 27) and, like Lachesis, talking to the dead and taking pleasure in the sound of his own voice. He is full of bitter resentment for his fate and withdraws from the world, rejecting all offers of support and consolation. Lachesis, on the other hand, thinks about the past with a mixture of hatred and happiness, and wants to be alone to give free rein to her fantasies. Unlike Natrum Mur., Lachesis uses her powers of clairvoyance (31) and trance (32) to sharpen her extrasensory perception. Natrum Mur. looks in the mirror and thinks he looks wretched ('Delusions, wretched, thinks she looks, when looking in a mirror': *1*), while Lachesis believes that she is under the control of superhuman forces. Both remedies are full of hatred (26), resentment ('Malicious', 1), criticism ('Censorious', 18), blame ('Reproaches others', 8), startings (30) and fears ('Fear, evil, of', 23 and 'Fear, robbers, of', 24), and they are both afraid of thunderstorms ('Thunderstorm, during': *1*). However, Natrum Mur. does not have that tremendously destructive anger, extreme mistrust and raging jealousy that make Lachesis so sensitive to stories of horrible things (33); Natrum Mur. suffers his sibling jealousy in silence, wanting to cry but unable to.

Like Lachesis, Natrum Mur. feels happy in the evening (35), weary of life (38) and suicidal (39); but Lachesis has far greater emotional instability with her swings of mood from depression, loneliness, boredom and sluggishness on waking to cheerfulness to the point of hilarity in the evening, with mental clarity and feverish activity. Natrum Mur. can also be hysterical, with joy alternating with irritability and sadness. He laughs at serious things and the laughter soon turns to tears. He is not demanding enough to complain out loud (36), but keeps his regrets to himself. Eventually, he reaches the point where all he sees is pain and injustice in the world, and he can no longer bear to go on living without faith or hope, full of bitterness, sadness and discontentment. He may reject life altogether and try to shoot himself. Lachesis, on the other hand, ends up feeling overwhelmed by the feelings of suffocation and constriction that have haunted her all her life, and gives into them by throwing herself into the river.

Nux Vomica

This remedy is characterised by an extreme sensitivity to stimuli, irritability, chilliness and antiperistaltic contractions of the digestive system. It does not have symptoms 5, 6 and 9, which describe Lachesis's feelings of abandonment and fear of the unknown. Nux Vomica is totally fearless and exercises his authority without recourse to manipulation. He is extremely sensitive to the slightest offensive remark and, if his pride is hurt, he will not forgive easily ('Malicious', 1). He is proud of his sense of duty ('Haughty', 2), jealous of his affections (7) and a tireless worker who speaks out ('Reproaches others', 8) if he suspects (3) that people are not pulling their weight. He is a fastidious and impatient perfectionist who can be super-critical of others ('Censorious', 18) and self-opinionated ('Contradict, disposition to', 19); he is ambitious and better for occupation. His absence from symptom 22 suggests that he is more effective and efficient at his work than Lachesis. Neurological disturbances and mental exhaustion are the result of years of toxic abuse from drugs, food and alcohol, with consequent difficulties with self-expression and remembering words. He is afraid of evil (23), but not of robbers (24). He suffers from love disappointments (25) and his exaggerated reflexes bring about impulsive and violent behaviour, startings (30) and strong reactions to hearing horrible things (33), rather than feelings of hatred (26) and persecution. He is much more confrontative than Lachesis and acutely perceptive without the need for the trappings of clairvoyant and trance-like powers (31, 32). He lacks the emotional swings described by symptoms 34 and 35, is too impatient to sit still in meditative thought (37), and complains loud and long (36) about his pains and suffering; he may lose all interest in life and think of a way to end it all, but his courage fails him at the last moment.

Veratrum Album

This remedy does not have anxiety on waking (4), fear to go to sleep (5) or jealousy (7), which express Lachesis's desire to escape from reality and the fear of the contents of her subconscious mind, symbolised by the suffocating on waking. The feelings of suffocation and constriction around the neck, the need to keep windows and doors open for fresh air, the intolerance of the slightest touch and the need to loosen her clothing are all indicative of disturbances of circulation, on a physical level, and of a persecution complex, on a mental level. Veratrum Album has none of these symptoms, although its varied and numerous symptoms are worth closer study. However, a true understanding of its character can only be gained in clinical practice, when prescribed to patients with a Veratrum picture.

Veratrum Album is characterised by lack of confidence, timidity and indecisiveness, with a fear of evil (23), misfortune and the future. It is a tri-miasmatic remedy with a burning social ambition. He will use any means at his disposal to achieve his ends, and shamelessly toadies to anyone who can be useful, although when he reaches the top he will arrogantly cast aside all those who have helped him; he is domineering (9) and cruel, with high sexual energy. In his lonely ('Forsaken feeling', 6) climb to the top of the social ladder, he boasts with excessive pride ('Haughty', 2), blames others for his faults (8) and is constantly on the lookout for danger ('Suspicious', 3).

He knows exactly what he wants, hence his absence from symptom 15, and is critical of others ('Censorious', 18), although he is too clever to jeopardise his position by revealing his private thoughts (19). Like Lachesis, he works hard ('Industrious', 20) and fast ('Hurry', 21) and lacks perseverance (22); but, whereas Lachesis can never finish anything before she gets hopelessly tied up in theory and hypothesis, Veratrum Album is restless to the point of hyperactivity and feels better when occupied: 'Busy restlessness, he undertakes several things, but is always soon weary and accomplishes nothing' (Allen, *Encyclopedia of Pure Materia Medica*, p. 75).

Herein lies the essential difference between the two remedies: Veratrum Album accomplishes nothing because he is always looking for the best, most suitable path to success and, in doing so, represses his emotional needs.

He suffers from disappointed love ('Ailments from: love, disappointed', Barthel) but hates no-one (26), believing that he has no enemies. While Lachesis feels persecuted by her enemies (28), Veratrum is persecuted by fear ('Fear, evil, of', 23 and 'Fear, robbers, of', 24), not by those whom he uses and then rejects. He does not fear people, start from noise or on falling asleep (30). He is absent from symptoms 31, 32 and 33 as, far from being a witch-like figure with a crystal ball, under the influence of a superhuman malevolent force, he believes that he is Christ incarnate, or at the very least in direct communication with God. Veratrum Album is similar to Lachesis and Hyoscyamus in the moral tussles between good and evil, obscene and brazen behaviour and the search for salvation in religion ('Despair, religious', 11).

Although Veratrum may feel unhappy when he wakes up (34), the evening is the worst time for his depression, in direct contrast to Lachesis who livens up at this time (35). Veratrum becomes cheerful at night-time. Barthel's repertory includes Veratrum in the rubric 'Complaining' but not in the rubric 'Meditation' (37). He also lacks the aggravation on waking that is so characteristic of Lachesis. When Veratrum reaches the time in his life when he realises that he has strayed a long way from his path, his mind fills with nostalgic memories of the past ('Homesickness', 27) and he feels completely alone, forsaken by God and tired of life (38), with a desperate wish to kill himself by throwing himself from a height (39).

The following seven remedies have six symptoms of the Minimum Characteristic Syndrome of Lachesis: Causticum, China, Hyoscyamus, Mercurius, Phosphorus, Staphysagria and Stramonium.

Causticum

Kent says that the essential features of this remedy are anxiety, despair and fear. Causticum can be domineering (9), like the controversial politician or statesman who hides his basic cowardice by aggressively asserting his opinions above those of others (19). It is a tri-miasmatic remedy with malice (1), pride (2), mistrust (3) and a critical disposition (18).

Causticum suffers from a deep depression that cries out for sympathy; possibly the most outstanding characteristic is the child's fear of solitude at night, as he clings to his mother whimpering and crying 'Don't let them hurt me!' and 'Let me out of here!'

He also has a fear of dogs and that something will happen to him or his loved ones, with feelings of excessive compassion and guilt especially in the evening.

He is anxious on waking ('Anxiety, morning, waking, on': 2) and in the evening when he fearfully wonders what will becomes of him, especially before going to sleep. However, unlike Lachesis, he is not afraid of going to sleep (5) and is too needy of support to let others desert him (6) or make him jealous (7).

Causticum has none of the symptoms of intellectual deficiency (12 to 17) or those related to work (20 to 22). It is a remedy of many fears, such as the fear of evil (23) that arises from his feelings of guilt. He suffers from love disappointments (25) and nostalgia (27). Causticum is more aggressive in speech than in actions and is neither violent nor hateful (26); his views are controversial bordering on anarchic, and he can be domineering with people less powerful than himself.

He does not have Lachesis's persecution complex (28), but is afraid of strangers and, unlike Lachesis, needs to have people around him (29).

The suppression of his anger and the fear that something will happen to him account for the starting on falling asleep (30) but he lacks the clairvoyant sensitivity of Lachesis (31 to 33) and her fascination with violence.

While Lachesis wakes feeling sad (34) and spends the evenings in a cheerful mood, Causticum is overcome with despair, anxiety and fear in the evening; he is full of dark forebodings about the fate of his loved ones and moans ('Complaining', 36) constantly with fear and regret about the suffering he sees all around him; this reinforces his sense of futility ('Loathing, life', 38) and his suicidal tendencies (39).

China

China does not have the powerful personality of the possessive Lachesis and is consequently not present in the rubrics of fear (5), jealousy (7), domination (9) and loquacity (10). As discussed in previous chapters, China is irritably apathetic, indifferent, deeply depressed, insensitive and averse to company. He is a highly frustrated individual, full of stubborn resentment ('Malicious', 1) and arrogance ('Haughty', 2), blaming everybody but himself (8) for his misfortune, trusting no-one (3) and feeling persecuted (28) and lonely (6).

He is beset by anxieties on waking ('Anxiety, morning, waking, on': 2), not only because he feels so apprehensive about what the day will bring, but also because his nocturnal dreams and fantasies have been banished by the harsh reality of daylight. If he feels happy at this time, it is probably because his nocturnal fantasies turn into blissful daydreams. Unlike the jealous, domineering, loquacious and sensual Lachesis, China locks himself away inside his head and blames society for everything.

China dreams all night long and feels sluggish on waking (12); he gets so caught up in his nocturnal world of fantasy that he loses all touch with reality, feels confused as if intoxicated or in a dream and talks nonsense ('Speech, wandering', 17) but, unlike Lachesis, he never loses sight of who he is (15).

He is industrious (20) in theory rather than in practice, all talk and no action, and criticises the work of others to divert attention away from his own laziness.

China is a very fearful remedy; he is afraid of evil (23) and dogs and believes that he is being hounded by his enemies.

He does not have the Relationship with Others symptoms 25, 26 or 27 but, if someone lets him down, he feels that the whole world is against him and becomes inconsolable in his feelings of abandonment, resentment and moral indignation.

Finally, he becomes worn out by the empty promises of his nocturnal dream world ('Meditation', 37) and finds that life holds nothing for him ('Loathing, life', 38). Unlike Lachesis, he does not plummet to the depths of religious despair (11), but looks on suicide as a quick and easy solution to his problems (39), although he lacks the courage to go through with it.

Hyoscyamus

These are highly emotional and impressionable people who suffer from alternating and simultaneous states of manic excitability and depression with nervous spasms. As previously mentioned in the chapter on Lycopodium, this is a member of the *Solanaceae* family, which is characterised by periods of delirium and manic depression.

In both Hyoscyamus children and adults one sees a damaged or underdeveloped nervous system with a tendency for arrogant (2) and suspicious (3) behaviour. If they are disappointed in love (25), they will bear a grudge for years to come ('Malicious', 1); although there is not the same sense of abandonment (6) as in Lachesis, they have the delusion of being deserted ('Delusions, deserted, forsaken': *1*) and can feel intensely jealous (7) of others. Hyoscyamus is loquacious (10) when excited but lacks the remaining core symptoms, 4, 5 and 9, which illustrate Lachesis's connections with other worlds.

In keeping with the remedies of the *Solanaceae* family, his lapses of memory are more general than those of Lachesis, in that he not only forgets what he has read (14) but also what he has said and heard. When excited, he will talk very fast (16) and disjointedly (17); but while Lachesis has the power to malign and wound with her eloquent words, Hyoscyamus stammers and stutters his drunken and incoherent drivel.

As already discussed in the chapter on Lycopodium, Hyoscyamus owes its lack of confidence to the psoric miasm and its suspicious nature to the sycotic miasm. There is a strong persecution complex with the delusion that he is being poisoned or chased by enemies (28) and he withdraws from people (29), trying to hide his compulsive behaviour, confusion and sexual jealousy. To bolster up his low self-esteem, he is quick (21), meticulous and conscientious at his work (20). The syphilitic aspect of the remedy comes out in the feelings of disorientation and the highly critical (18) and argumentative nature (19). His weak and confused mind makes him angry but he has no deeply ingrained feelings of hatred (26). The generally poor memory and the confusing sensation of being in a dream make him homesick (27) and, as familiar things seem strange to him, he is unaware of the fact that he is already at home.

He is not afraid of robbers (24), although he is frightened of solitude, people, being poisoned and other evils (23). He not only has a persecution complex but also the delusions that someone calls him, people harm him and animals devour him; the opposite side of this particular coin are the delusions that he is possessed by the devil, that he is a devil or criminal and that he sees birds and plucks out their feathers.

In the final stages, he loses his memory completely and is tormented by feelings of guilt; he feels guilty of some unpardonable crime, and believes that he is not worthy of divine mercy; frustrated, exhausted and confused, he believes that he has lost the affection of his friends and sits muttering to himself, overwhelmed by grief, afraid of being poisoned and angry with the whole world; he shouts, laughs, attacks people and beats at horrible visions on walls with his fists. In his more tranquil moments, he sits and thinks (37) about the mess he is in and how much he hates life (38); he seriously considers drowning himself ('Suicidal disposition', 39) in a final attempt to find peace and maternal protection.

Lachesis and Hyoscyamus have similarities in the symptoms concerning the way they relate to others: they are both jealous (7), stuck in the past ('Homesickness', 27), emotionally frustrated ('Love, ailments, from disappointed', 25) and lonely (6). Their jealous natures can lead them both to committing a crime of passion ('Jealousy, crime, to a', Barthel); Lachesis suffers from jealousy with frightful images ('Jealousy, images, with frightful', Barthel), Hyoscyamus can be driven to kill for jealousy ('Jealousy, kill, driving to', Barthel). Lachesis can do nothing to control her jealousy ('Jealousy, as foolish as it is irresistible': 2, Barthel), and the male may be driven to wife-beating as a result ('Jealousy, strike his wife, driving to', Barthel). Hyoscyamus has raging jealousy ('Jealousy, rage, with', Barthel) that may drive him to suicide ('Love, disappointed, suicidal disposition from', Barthel). However, while Lachesis will justify her actions with outlandish ideas and accusations, Hyoscyamus becomes tongue-tied, violent or suicidal. He cannot justify himself, is basically weak and pathetic, and is dominated by the fear of solitude.

Mercurius

From the Minimum Characteristic Syndrome, Mercurius does not have anxiety on waking (4), feelings of abandonment (6), jealousy (7) and loquacity (10), which express Lachesis's particular dynamic of possessiveness, mistrust, anxiety and malicious slander. The syphilitic Mercurius has anxiety at night; anxiety and fear are etched upon his face and feelings of restlessness and guilt make him want to run away and hide from his destructive impulses to kill himself and others.

He is full of resentment (1), mistrust (3) and blame (8). The absence of ailments from disappointed love (25), hatred (26), industriousness (20), amelioration from occupation and conscientiousness indicates that his arrogance (2) and bossiness (9) do not conceal a lack of confidence, as in Lycopodium, or a deep need for affection, as in Lachesis; rather, they are syphilitic signs of mental deterioration and confused impulses to kill anyone who dares contradict. Syphilitic remedies are aggravated at night, hence the fear of going to sleep (5)

Like Lachesis, he has a weak memory for what he has read (14), as well as for dates, names, places and people. He may be exceptionally advanced in some areas of development ('Precocity': *1*), but more often than not we see the chaotic and childish side of the remedy. He does not suffer from a confusion of identity (15) so much as a confusion of location, losing himself in well-known streets. Although he is quick both in speech (16) and action 27), his mind works slowly and his answers are slow and rambling 17), unlike the verbal adroitness of Lachesis.

Impulsively destructive and aggressive, he imposes his revolutionary, anarchic ideas with damning indictments ('Censorious', 18) and intolerance ('Contradict, disposition to', 19) of other people's points of view. In the midst of chaos, he longs for his lost paradise ('Homesickness', 27), not from disappointed love as we have seen (25), but from a guilt-ridden wish to recapture the days when life was easier and more simple.

Like Lachesis, he has the delusion that his enemies pursue him (28). Inner feelings of hostility become twisted into the beliefs that everyone is his enemy, that he is surrounded by enemies, that animals are about to attack him, that he is surrounded by criminals and that he is a criminal himself; hence the fears of evil (23), robbers (24) and going to sleep (5) and the nervous starting on falling asleep (30).

Unlike Lachesis, he cannot find comfort in the supernatural dimensions of life; he has neither clairvoyant abilities (31), the desire to be magnetised (32), religious despair (11) nor the need to meditate (37).

Complaining loudly (36) and furiously about his lot, he becomes tired of life (38) and works himself up into a suicidal rage (39) where he becomes afraid of the lethal potential of open windows and knives.

Phosphorus

For a more detailed discussion of this remedy the reader should refer to the chapter on Lycopodium. The following four symptoms from the Minimum Characteristic Syndrome of Lachesis are not found in Phosphorus: feelings of abandonment (6) and jealousy (7), which are aroused in Lachesis when other people let her down, and reproach (8), expressed by the torrents of abuse and accusations that Lachesis gives vent to when she does not get her way. Lachesis is suspicious, resentful, dictatorial and loquacious and her fear of going to sleep (5), the fourth symptom not found in Phosphorus, represents the fear of divine punishment, with anxiety on waking, a generally low time for the remedy.

By contrast, Phosphorus is sensitive to all internal and external impressions. He is afraid of solitude because that means being separated from his environment; he needs to be in perpetual communion with his fellow beings and with God; but he is easily drained by people and subject to violent mood swings from passionate fervour, love, hatred and rage to utter indifference, with the desire for peace and quiet and the need to withdraw completely.

The fearful Phosphorus has a feeling of helplessness ('Helplessness, feeling of': *1*), not to be confused with the forsaken feeling that carries with it an implied criticism of others, a symptom not found in Phosphorus (8). This affectionate and supportive remedy has no jealousy (7), although his extreme sensitivity can lead to feelings of resentment ('Malicious', 1); he can find it hard to trust people ('Suspicious', 3) because he is so wary of being misunderstood. He has a great need to make his presence felt and uses his vivid imagination to pretend that he is somebody important, hiding his vulnerability and fear of solitude with a sycotic disguise of overbearing arrogance.

He feels the presence of God and does not fall prey to religious despair (11).

Both remedies have 'Dullness, waking, on' (12) and 'Confusion, identity, as to his' (15). Phosphorus's lack of stamina leads to frequent bouts of exhaustion and a weak memory for what he has read (14) and difficulty in concentrating. He has a lively and entertaining way of expressing himself and tends to wander off the point (17), led by his inquisitive mind, acute perceptions and general apathy.

Unlike the proud and possessive Lachesis, Phosphorus is not disposed to find fault (18) or contradict others (19). However, he is unable to control his impulsive outbursts of rudeness and, while Lachesis does not care whom she hurts when her jealousy is aroused, Phosphorus is afraid of the strength of his anger and the harm that it can do.

Both remedies are hard-working (20) and hurried (21); Lachesis lacks perseverance (22) while Phosphorus tries to compensate for his lack of stamina with artistic and aesthetic excellence.

In Phosphorus, the fears of evil (23) and robbers (24) are aspects of his general fearfulness, while in Lachesis they are indicative of the persecution mania and obsession with evil. The fear of solitude represents the fear of separation from his environment, and the fear of thunderstorms is symbolic of the introversion of his feelings of anger and aggression.

He has great emotional reserves to fall back on in times of stress and does not suffer from disappointed love (25). His sensitivity accounts for feelings of nostalgia ('Homesickness', 27) and hatred (26). When suffering from exhaustion, he may become indifferent to his loved ones and averse to company (29); he finds a secluded place from where he can commune with the spirits ('Clairvoyance', 31 and 'Magnetized, desires to be', 32) and enjoy his own company, giving free rein to his creativity and thoughts ('Meditation', 37).

The lack of paranoid delusions of persecution (28) and sensitivity to horrible stories (33) is further confirmation of his feelings of unity with the world.

He does not have the characteristic mood swings of Lachesis (35) or the desire to moan and grumble all the time (36). Lachesis is torn between two wills: the desire to follow the dictates of her conscience and the desire to obey a superior evil power, and this conflict eventually wears her down and makes her tired of life (38) and suicidal (39). Phosphorus, on the other hand, may reach the same point for a different reason: his emotions seize up and he finds he can no longer feel anything; he has fearful premonitions of death and wishes to leave this life. However, the psoric dominates the syphilitic, and Phosphorus is the only remedy whose suicidal feelings are ameliorated by a good cry ('Suicidal disposition, weeping, amel.': *1*).

Staphysagria

For a more detailed discussion of this remedy the reader should refer to the chapter on Natrum Muriaticum.

Staphysagria does not have the anxiety on waking (4), fear on going to sleep (5), feelings of abandonment (6) and the dictatorial nature (9) that express Lachesis's fear of divine retribution for allowing her domineering and aggressive nature its full expression. Staphysagria has an exaggerated idea of her own importance ('Haughty', 2) and an exalted sense of injustice, and cannot express her anger because it clashes with her sense of honesty and uprightness; the male Staphysagria keeps a stiff upper lip and represses all feelings of moral indignation, although he trembles with rage and feels as if he is about to explode. Staphysagria believes ('Suspicious', 3) that she is undervalued, and this fills her with feelings of bitterness ('Malicious', 1) and blame ('Reproaches others', 8); but this is nothing compared with the resentment unleashed by unjust acts and words, and she becomes so paralysed with rage that her life becomes impossible.

She is too certain that she is right to fall prey to religious despair (11). Her mind becomes sluggish not on waking (12) but when she feels indignant. She has a good memory for what has happened (13), but the headache, like a block of wood in the forehead or occiput, which comes from grief or stress interferes with her memory for what she has read (14). She has no confusion as to her identity (15) but the weight of her problems makes her speak and think in a confused and incoherent way, with periodic spells of confusion.

She feels that the world is basically a hostile place and is always on the defensive; hence the tendency to find fault (18), contradict (19) and argue; in Lachesis these symptoms are examples of her talent for scathing criticism and hard competitiveness.

Her mind is dull, slow and confused and, not surprisingly, she has a marked aversion to mental work, although the remedy does not feature in any of the Work rubrics of Lachesis.

The fears of evil (23) and heights and the fear while walking are all various aspects of Staphysagria's worst fear, the fear of losing control.

She has ailments from disappointed love (25) and longs to recapture the better times she once knew (27) but, unlike Lachesis, is neither hateful (26) nor selfishly possessive; she becomes stuck in the past, grieving over unhappy memories and broken love affairs and nursing her wounded pride.

She does not have the Lachesis delusions of persecution (28), but has the delusion that she is great while others are low. She also believes that she is pursued, although not by enemies.

Staphysagria does not appear in the Excitability symptoms 30 to 33 and the symptoms 'Loathing, life', 38 and 'Suicidal disposition', 39 are not strong ones, as she is far too repressed to do anything about them.

Stramonium

Stramonium does not have the anxiety on waking (4), fear of going to sleep (5) and the disposition to blame (8) and dominate others (9) which describe the way that Lachesis tries to impose her will with her slanderous and accusing tongue. Her days are full of intrigue and jealousy; she wakes tense and anxious, as if preparing herself for combat, and is afraid of going to sleep for fear of divine retribution.

Nash says in his *Leaders in Homoeopathic Therapeutics* that Stramonium, Hyoscyamus and Belladonna are the three main remedies of delirium. Stramonium is characterised by the violence and intensity of its symptoms; the delirium is raging and the patient whistles, sings, laughs, prays piously or curses terribly with great loquacity. There is great restlessness in bed, with tossing and turning, changing position, lying crosswise then along it, curling himself up into a ball and sticking his head out beyond the pillow. Eventually, the tongue becomes dry and cracked and the mucous membrane of the mouth becomes inflamed; discharges are black and smell of decay, with the suppression of stools and urine. There is a loss of sight, hearing and speech, with fixed, staring eyes and profuse sweat which does not relieve.

As one would expect, the symptomatology of Stramonium is rich in delusions, sensations and deliriums. It is useful in cases of advanced mental conditions or mania states. However, a deeper analysis of its pathogenesis reveals how useful and frequently indicated it is in clinical practice.

The remedy is characterised by violence and sexual expression with great debility; the violence is extreme and uncontrollable, leading at times to acts of murder; however, Stramonium is more the victim than the perpetrator of violence, while Lachesis manipulates and controls with her domineering and critical nature. Stramonium is afraid of pushing people away and tries to suppress his aggressive impulses; but suppression leads to frustration and a terrible guilt complex, with the feeling that he has committed a dreadful mistake. Stramonium and Nux Vomica are the two most resentful ('Malicious', 1) remedies of our materia medica. If Stramonium's jealous (7) suspicions (3) are confirmed, he explodes with violent, unforgiving rage and wounded pride ('Haughty', 2). He accuses everybody of forsaking him (6) and pays a guilty price for his violence.

His religious despair (11) has a transcendental quality about it. He believes that he is a wretched soul who is incapable of doing his duty and is not worthy of salvation.

He is torn between good and evil and does not know who he is (15); he imagines he is divided in two and that one part of him is in communication with God while the other part is a devil. He is excitable and talkative (10), speedy (16) and disjointed (17) in speech. He has a weak memory, not for things that have happened or what he has read, but for names, people, what he has said and what he is about to say.

He is more introvertedly self-destructive than Lachesis and does not tend to criticise (18), blame (8) or contradict others (19).

To atone for the feelings of guilt, he works hard (20), fast (21) and efficiently, feeling much better when he has something constructive to do. Lachesis, by contrast, does not have Stramonium's perseverance (22).

Lachesis is afraid of evil because of her connections with the world of the supernatural and the delusions of persecution (28); in Barthel we find Stramonium under fear of evil (23), with other specific fears that distinguish him from Lachesis, such as the fear of dogs, being devoured by animals and being injured or murdered. Other characteristic fears of Stramonium are fear of the dark, solitude, water, suffocation and fear on waking.

Stramonium does not suffer from disappointed love (25), hatred (26) or nostalgia (27), as his feelings of resentment are not triggered by circumstances in his life but stem from his basically violent nature.

Unlike Lachesis, Stramonium is afraid of solitude and feels worse when alone; he has no wish to hide his motives and feelings and does not withdraw from people (29). Because of his strong persecution mania, he features in much of the delusions section. The struggles between good and evil create delusions that dogs are attacking him, that he is divided in two, as if cut through, that he is in direct communication with God and a devil at the same time; he feels utterly alone and unworthy of eternal glory, incapable of doing his duty. He believes that he is in danger and has every disease under the sun; his mind is filled with lascivious thoughts; he exposes himself and cannot stop talking and indulging in morbidly jealous thoughts; he prays desperately for the welfare of his soul.

Apart from clairvoyance (31), there is nothing trance-like about Stramonium, no desire to lose himself in meditation (37) or be magnetised (32). His violent and malicious behaviour is a consequence of neurological disturbances and uncontrollable impulsiveness rather than any evidence of deep-seated emotional problems, as he is neither sensitive to horrible stories (33), nor prone to jump on falling asleep (30).

Stramonium does not have the circulatory problems of Lachesis and is neither sad on waking (34) nor cheerful in the evening (35). Another difference is that he does not complain (36). He is his own worst enemy and eventually comes to reject life altogether (38); in one of his fevered crises, he tries to stab himself to death or throw himself from a window (39).

The following four remedies have five symptoms from the Minimum Characteristic Syndrome of Lachesis: Anacardium, Arnica, Ignatia and Pulsatilla.

Anacardium

For a more detailed discussion of this remedy, the reader should refer to the chapter on Lycopodium.

There are many similarities between Lachesis and Anacardium: they are both malicious (1), arrogant (2), wary of others (3) and talkative (10), with wandering speech (17), dullness on waking (12), difficulty in remembering what they have read (14), a contradictory disposition (19) and the capacity for hatred (26). They both feel pursued by enemies (28) and try to hide away (29); in addition, they are both clairvoyant (31), cheerful in the evening (35) and potentially suicidal (39), with thoughts of jumping off a high place.

However, Anacardium does not have jealousy (7), reproach of others (8), feelings of abandonment (6) or a domineering nature (9). This remedy is characterised by a perpetual conflict between the head and the heart, duty and desire, which is symbolised by the delusion that people are beside him. He is too unsure of himself to criticise others (18), although he will attack, both verbally and physically, anyone who dares criticise or contradict him.

He shares with Lachesis the feelings of hatred (26), the fear of evil and the delusions of persecution (28), and his behaviour can be cruel and immoral; other delusions are the feelings of being double, of the soul being separated from the body and that it is all a dream.

Arnica

Arnica is frequently used as a post-trauma remedy, although it is also very useful in chronic prescriptions. Kent says of this remedy: 'The Arnica patient is morose, wants to be let alone, does not want to be talked to, does not want to be approached. He does not want to be approached, both because he does not wish to enter into conversation, a mental state, and also because he does not wish to be touched on account of the great bodily soreness. These are the two most striking things in this medicine. Irritable, morose, sad, fearful, easily frightened, imagines all sorts of things, especially that he has heart disease ... that some deep-seated trouble is upon him. Full of nightmare, dreadful dreams ... He frequently rouses up in the night, grasps at the heart, has the appearance of great horror, fears some dreadful thing will happen ... thinks he is going to die suddenly ... It is also seen in persons who have gone through a railroad accident, or through some shock ... They rouse up in the night with a fear of sudden death ... the horrors they really went through are repeated ...' (*Lectures on Homoeopathic Materia Medica*, p. 142).

This remedy is amply described in the literature of materia medica, to which the reader should refer for a more complete picture. The following brief comparison is presented in the hope that it will encourage further study.

Arnica has symptoms 1, 2, 3, 9 and 10 from the Minimum Characteristic Syndrome of Lachesis; the significance of these symptoms in Lachesis has already been discussed. Arnica is a very sensitive remedy, with sensitivity to touch and all external impressions, like Phosphorus, Nux Vomica and Staphysagria. He does not want to be talked to or approached and prefers to be left alone; he resents ('Malicious', 1) the intrusion of the doctor, a friend of the family, and sends him packing; he is wary of all medical attention ('Suspicious', 3) and arrogantly ('Haughty', 2) maintains that he is not ill and does not need a doctor. He is argumentative, irritable, critical (18) and contradictory (19).

Arnica would make a good politician, with his extreme affability, insensitivity to suffering and domineering nature (9).

He has a terrifying fear that something dreadful is about to happen to him but does not fall prey to religious despair (11); he staunchly refuses all offers of help and insists that there is nothing at all wrong with him; he appears to be quite self-sufficient and independent, with a marked indifference to everything during a fever or chill; at times, however, he prays quietly for the salvation of his soul ('Prays quietly for her soul', C. Hering, *Materia Medica*, p. 4).

He has a dull and sluggish mind on waking, although it is more usual in this remedy to find dullness after receiving a blow to the head and ailments after emotional trauma. He not only forgets what he has read (14), but also cannot remember words, what he is about to say and what he has said; this may be either because he is not too bothered about communicating with others, or because he feels confused as if in a dream.

His moods fluctuate between depression and vacant apathy, and a state of crazed excitement and euphoria where he talks (10) nineteen to the dozen (16), in rambling speeches that go nowhere (17). He tries to overcome his 'unfitness for exertion and indifference to business' (J. F. Clarke, *Materia Medica*, p. 172) with sheer hard graft ('Industrious', 20).

The fear of evil (23) is a general expression of his fears of misfortune, being approached, touched, sudden death and high walls or buildings falling on him.

He does not have any particular problems in the area of relating to others and is not found in symptoms 25 to 27.

He does not have the delusion of being pursued by enemies (28), but has the delusion that he is about to be arrested; there are also delusions of seeing dead people with mutilated bodies and black spectres in the night. He is averse to company (29) both because he does not wish to be bothered and because he is fearful of being approached or touched.

In Arnica, the symptom clairvoyance (31) means a certain clarity of mind; in Hering's *Materia Medica* we find that he has a 'Mind clear like that of a clairvoyant' (p. 4).

He does not suffer in silence and is quite forthright in making his problems known ('Complaining', 36). The remedy is characterised by a great sensitivity to physical and emotional trauma, with hypochondriacal anxiety and anguished distress with the fever; he avoids other people, simultaneously complaining about his pains and denying that there is anything wrong. He is resentful, suspicious and arrogant, and retreats into non-committal amiability when he feels threatened or vulnerable.

Ignatia

For a more detailed discussion of this remedy the reader should refer to the chapter on Thuja.

Ignatia has five symptoms from the Minimum Characteristic Syndrome of Lachesis: resentment (1), pride (2), anxiety on waking (4), jealousy (7) and reproach of others (8), which describe Lachesis's state of emotional turmoil as she passes from grief to hatred to jealousy; with her manipulating ways and her inability to trust, she feels anxious when she wakes up to another day of struggle and loneliness.

As previously discussed in other chapters, Ignatia is a hysterical remedy with changeable and contradictory symptoms. Although she shares five of the core symptoms with Lachesis, there are clear differences between them, such as Ignatia's extreme sensitivity and the paradoxical, fluctuating desires and emotions.

She is obsessed by doubt and feelings of guilt, hence the despair of recovery and religious salvation (11).

Unlike Lachesis, Ignatia has no dullness on waking (12) and owes her failing memory and inability to think and comprehend to the instability of her emotions. Although Ignatia has no confusion of identity (15), she feels confused as if intoxicated or as if in a dream, rubrics that suggest a rather weak hold on reality. She may speak in a hurried (16) and rambling (17) way, due to her extreme sensitivity and changeability.

She can be critical (18) and contradictory (19) because of the emotional imbalance, rather than from any authoritarian desire to impose her will; the ailments from suppressed anger and silent grief describe her inability to articulate her feelings.

Ignatia is a sycotic remedy who is obsessively conscientious about her work (20) and ameliorated by occupation; she cannot bear being contradicted and is always in a hurry (21).

Ignatia's fear of robbers at midnight on waking (24) is similar to Natrum Mur.'s fear of emotional robbery; although she does not have the fear of going to sleep (5), she has the fear that she will never sleep again. Ignatia is an emotionally charged remedy with no fear of evil (23) or feelings of hatred (26), and she suffers with silent grief from disappointed love (25) and nostalgia (27).

She feels guilty that she has neglected her duty, has done wrong and is ruined and, for these reasons, chooses to avoid company (29).

Her sensitivity and feelings of guilt also account for the starting on failing asleep (30) and the effect that horrible stories have on her (33).

Lachesis's mood swings, frustration and despair bring about the cheerfulness in the evening (35) and loathing of life (38) that are not found in the tender and delicate Ignatia, whose emotions can change in a flash from the deepest grief to the most surprising and sudden violent rage if somebody tries to contradict or comfort her. She can do nothing to control her volatile emotions and guiltily sits, absorbed in memories of those who have hurt her, suffering her grief in silence, with much sighing and hysterical sobbing; in this state, she will withdraw completely from people (29) as any offer of comfort or support only serves to deepen her sorrow; she complains (36), thinks about nothing ('Meditation', 37) but misfortune and death and the idea of drowning her way out of her problems (39).

Pulsatilla

Pulsatilla is neither proud (2), afraid of going to sleep (5), domineering (9), loquacious (10) nor disposed to blame others (8). This remedy always needs a crutch, someone to lean on, to give her love and protection. The fear of being separated from her means of support makes her feel abandoned (6); she has a great fear of rejection and disapproval and is wary (3) and jealous (7) of others. She suffers her grief in silence, swallowing her feelings for fear of losing her loved one, but her troubles just keep on growing. Pulsatilla, who was once so mild and tender, can become full of resentment and bitterness ('Malicious', 1). Her whole approach to life is expressed in the anxiety and irritability she feels on waking (4). She tries to cover up her feelings of insecurity and uselessness by attending to her housewifely duties; she becomes capricious, vain, selfish, envious and suspicious and manipulates others with her tears and protests.

Her feelings of guilt lead to religious despair (11) and self-condemnation for her childish and selfish behaviour.

The rambling speech (17) is an expression of her changeability on a mental level, but she is not found in any of the other symptoms concerning the intellectual faculties. Her confusion is aggravated by mental effort and after eating and is relieved by walking in the open air.

Pulsatilla does not dare be critical (18) or contradictory (19) for fear of pushing away those on whom she depends, but it may enter her fickle head to raise her voice in tentative, fearful protest ('Complaining', 36) if something annoys her.

Unlike Lachesis, who spends a lot of energy in futile attempts to get things done (20, 22), Pulsatilla is careful, meticulous and slow, hurrying ('Hurry', 21) only at times when she feels that she has done wrong.

She has a fear of evil (23) because of her suspiciousness and guilty conscience, but no fear of robbers (24); in addition, she is afraid of darkness, ghosts and solitude.

It may seem surprising that Pulsatilla does not suffer from love disappointment (25), but this is so because any feelings of abandonment and grief are soon dispelled by a soothing word of comfort; and when none is forthcoming, she finds solace in happy memories of her childhood days (27). Although Pulsatilla is not found in the rubric 'Hatred' (26), like the Lycopodium woman who hates all men, the Pulsatilla man is afraid of women and avoids marriage until, eventually, he develops a real hatred of the female sex.

Like Lachesis, Pulsatilla has delusions of persecution (28); while Lachesis desires solitude to indulge her need to meditate (37) and practise clairvoyance (31), Pulsatilla needs to be alone to look for peace inside herself. She also needs people, is ameliorated by consolation and weeps when telling of her sickness.

Unlike Lachesis, she feels neither sad on waking (34) nor cheerful in the evening (35); but she complains in no uncertain terms (36) and demands attention and consideration; this is someone who takes and never gives, although she is aware of her self-centred, childish behaviour and begins to despair of her salvation (11) with doubts about the welfare of her soul. Eventually, she loses all interest in life (38) and turns to thoughts of suicide by drowning (39), a symbol of her desire to return to the womb.

The following three remedies have four symptoms of the Minimum Characteristic Syndrome of Lachesis: Calcarea Carbonica, Platinum and Sulphur. The reader should refer to previous chapters for a full comparative study of Calcarea Carbonica (see pages 87, 163–4 and 230).

Platinum

Platinum has symptoms 1, 2, 4 and 6 from the Minimum Characteristic Syndrome, but there is no mistrust (3), jealousy (7) or reproach of others (8).

Paschero says of this remedy: 'Platinum has alternating physical and mental symptoms and is prone to outbursts of hysterical tears and sardonic laughter. Despite the high sexual energy and lascivious dreams, she is emotionally cold and arrogant, and insults and despises her husband. The mental picture of Platinum is a combination of cruelty, pride and sexual excess.'

Platinum's delusions of grandeur clearly set her apart from Lachesis; she believes that she is so superior to other people that all feelings of mistrust, jealousy and reproach are simply beneath her; she does not concern herself with others, believing that nobody is capable of understanding her or appreciating the greatness of her spirit.

She feels dull and sluggish on waking (12) and has neither of the specific symptoms of memory (13, 14), although she is so indifferent to other people's opinions that she often forgets what she has heard. Her speech is erratic and rambling (17) and she makes no effort to explain the pearls of great wisdom that fall from her lips.

She feels nothing but contempt (18) for those who dare disagree with her opinions, will not deign to enter into an argument with her inferiors and cannot be bothered to contradict them (19) as it is not worth her time.

She is too proud and contemptuous to have any of the symptoms related to work.

Although Platinum has none of the specific fears of Lachesis (evil, robbers and thunderstorms), it is an extremely fearful remedy, of whom Clarke says: '*Anxietas praecordium* to an excessive degree, with great fear of death, which is believed to be very near, accompanied by trembling, palpitation of heart, and obstructed respiration. Sensation of dread and horror. Fear, with trembling of hands and feet and confusion of ideas, as if all persons approaching were demons.' (*Materia Medica*, p. 845). She is afraid of ghosts, people, men, that something will happen and that her husband will not return, and her fears are intensified before the menses.

She does not stoop to feelings of hatred (26), nostalgia (27) or the after-effects of a love disappointment (25). However, symptoms can be triggered off by scorn, grief, anger with anxiety, fear and indignation.

The aversion to company (29) stems from her feelings of isolation and separation from the family; almost all the sensations and delusions of Platinum are aspects of her basic delusions of grandeur; she believes that she is a great person of noble origins and that others are humble and low.

She believes that she is surrounded by devils and, in a fit of tearful rage, has a sudden impulse to kill her husband and children whom she loves. In fact, both remedies are capable of murdering their husbands: Lachesis out of jealousy and hatred, and Platinum out of arrogant contempt for someone who does not understand her. Both remedies can feel forsaken: Lachesis from jealousy, mistrust, a desire to possess and dominate and an obsession with evil and persecution, and Platinum from feelings of isolation, superiority, mocking contempt and disdain for the company of others.

The combination of egotism and indifference explains why Platinum does not appear in any of the excitability rubrics, unlike Lachesis who always has her head in the clouds.

Platinum has tremendous mood swings that come upon her for no apparent reason and without warning. One minute she can be as high as a kite, and then she can plunge to the depths of depression the next. One moment she is laughing, singing and dancing, then the next moment she explodes in a flood of angry tears; she feels completely alone, full of fear and nostalgia, and wants to be left alone. Plagued by remorse for the way she has treated others, she feels that even God has turned his back on her and despairs for her salvation (11). Eventually, she loses all interest in living (38) and complains loudly about her unhappy lot (36); she contemplates the idea of committing suicide (39), although her lack of courage and morbid fear of death get in the way. She falls into a crisis of despair, with alternating moods of arrogant promiscuity and religious piety.

Sulphur

This remedy has been discussed fully in previous chapters, and its characteristic symptoms distinguish it clearly from Lachesis. Sulphur's self-centred and conceited attitude to life accounts for the Lachesis core symptoms of arrogance (2), mistrust (3) and resentment (1). His attitude of indifference is not coloured by feelings of jealousy (7), abandonment (6), reproach (8) or the desire to dominate (9). He is motivated by lethargy and a weak will to manipulate circumstances to suit his convenience, and obstinately maintains an optimistic, if abstract, view on life.

In Sulphur, religious despair (11) stems from a guilty conscience, rather than from the metaphysical wanderings of Lachesis.

He cannot remember events because he is simply not interested ('Memory, weakness of, happened, for what has', 13), and his vagueness and confusion manifest as an identity problem (15); the outstanding characteristics of Sulphur are the morning aggravation and the confusion of ideas and objects.

He does not see eye to eye with society and his criticisms (18) serve to justify his rather complacent attitude; there is nothing of Lachesis's competitive spirit or wish to dominate in Sulphur, and neither contradictory (19) nor domineering (9) tendencies.

He is neither industrious (20) nor tempted to take on many different things (22), but can hurry himself up (21) to pacify his impatience and impulsiveness.

Unlike Lachesis, he is neither obsessed by evil nor persecution, and the fears of evil (23) and robbers (24) are indicative of his guilty conscience and fears of poverty and the future.

Sulphur will commit himself to nothing and no-one, and is too indifferent and apathetic to be affected by love disappointments (25) or nostalgia (27). He is entirely unconcerned with the world outside his head, although he cannot stand injustice and can be roused to hatred (26) of the person who has so offended: he can get carried away by egotism and impulsiveness, but anger soon gives way to remorse, with anxiety and fear.

He avoids company (29) because people bore and drain him; he is totally wrapped up in himself, with not a single persecutory thought in his head.

Apart from the starting on falling asleep (30), he has none of the Excitability symptoms that are evidence of Lachesis's state of nervous tension and clairvoyant sensitivity.

Sulphur has no sadness on waking (34). When he is forced to face up to the fact that he has achieved nothing with his life, he is overcome by guilty despair and tries to escape the harsh light of reality by dreaming ('Meditation', 37) about the castles in the air that might have been, until boredom finally descends upon him ('Loathing, life', 38) and he gives up the struggle ('Suicidal disposition', 39).

MISCELLANEOUS STUDIES

9

Calcarea Sulphurica

As a student of homoeopathy, I was always encouraged to use the repertory to find the logic behind each symptom in the materia medica.

The character of a remedy is perceived in the way it deals with life, how it reacts to stress and challenge and copes with circumstances and the environment. The essential nature and definition of a remedy is contained in a small, closely-knit group of symptoms that Paschero has termed the Minimum Syndrome of Maximum Value.

Once the minimum syndrome of the remedy has been defined, we then have a basis with which to compare it with others. Symptoms take on a new lease of life, and general guidelines can be established to facilitate our comprehension of the essential nature of each remedy, without which it is impossible to understand a case.

These ideas have enhanced my understanding of Kent's materia medica. For example, in the chapter on Calcarea Arsenicosa in his *Lectures on Homoeopathic Materia Medica*, he says: 'If this wonderful remedy is studied with the mind on Arsenicum and Calcarea, a broader knowledge will be gained' (p. 297); and in the chapter on Alumina, he says: 'When you have a good substantial proving of an oxide or a carbonate, and the mental symptoms are well brought out, you can use these, in a measure in a presumptive way, in prescribing another salt . . .'

It would seem that the only person who recognised the importance of Calcarea Sulphurica was the French homoeopath, H. Bernard, who gave a detailed description of its general and particular symptoms, but unfortunately gave little advice about its clinical application. Its mental symptoms have been practically ignored by the classical writers such as Hering, Clarke, Tyler, Duprat and Nash. Kent is the only one who has given us a clear description of the remedy, albeit a brief one. He says: '. . . similar to Pyrogen. An abscess that has ruptured and is slow to heal with a continuous discharge of yellow pus, is a strong indication for this remedy. The patient desires the open air; is sensitive to drafts; takes cold easily ... While the patient is cold in general, he often requires to be uncovered because of particular conditions. For instance, in croup and in headaches he feels the heat too much, but the pains of the body are often relieved by heat ... The patient is aggravated from exertion. His muscles are flabby ... When well-selected remedies act only a short time, and the symptoms agree, this remedy is one that should be thought of along with Sulphur, Psorinum and Tuberculinum ... Many of the symptoms are aggravated on waking. Many symptoms are aggravated by walking ... and becoming heated ... Great bodily weakness ...' Kent then goes on to give us a brief sketch of the mental picture: 'He becomes weak after anger and vexation ... He is easily made anxious ... Anxiety with fear during fever. Anxiety about the future. Anxious about his heart and his health in general ... Great sluggishness of mind. Continuously in a state of apprehension. Fear of death. Fear that some evil will befall him. Fear of insanity and fear of misfortune, and this comes on at night ... Always in a hurry ... hysterical. Impatient ... Easily offended or insulted. Prostration of mind. Quarrelsome, Restlessness ...' (pp. 303–305). But neither Kent's description nor the 87 symptoms in the Mind section of the *Repertory* give us a sense of the essential nature, the life and soul of the remedy.

The following material has been taken from four case histories of patients who received homoeopathic treatment over a long period of time.

CASE 1

A 4-year-old boy, Andres H., with dry, irritating eczema on the head and body which had not responded to allopathic treatment. The boy was methodical, jealous, warm-blooded, craved highly seasoned food and was intolerant of woollen clothing, as it made his skin itch. He was anxious about his family, feared that something bad would happen to them and was frightened of the dark. He had had severe nappy rash as a baby and episodes of croup. I prescribed Sulphur 200c. He was seen again four months later. The eczema had cleared within 15 days but his anxiety had increased, accompanied by a loss of appetite. He had also had another attack of croup which had been treated allopathically.

His mother had brought him back to see me because his head was again covered with eczema and scabs and the anal itching and intolerance to woollen clothing had returned. He had no appetite and was easily exhausted. It was clear that the Sulphur had merely suppressed the symptoms as, when the eczema had cleared, he had become worse in other ways, with a return of the croup and general weakness. Sulphur was nevertheless still indicated in that the patient was conscientious about trifles, aggravated by heat, the itching was aggravated by heat and he craved highly seasoned foods. However, the mental symptoms of jealousy, fear that something will happen and fear of the dark are not found in Sulphur. The fears are found in Calcarea, Causticum, Lycopodium and Phosphorus, and only Lycopodium has jealousy.

But Andres did not seem to be timid, dictatorial or lacking in confidence. He had the cautiousness of Causticum but not the great anxiety and sense of vulnerability; furthermore, Causticum does not have jealousy and is extremely rebellious, argumentative, weak and cowardly. He had the fears of Phosphorus and the anxiety for his family but was not restless, passionate, affectionate or hypersensitive and did not have the Phosphorus feelings of unity with the whole of creation. He had the fears of Calcarea and was a placid and sensible child. However, he was too meticulous for Calcarea, who is calculating and rational and believes that everything is as it should be.

It is interesting to note that when Andres had been at his healthiest he had had more characteristic symptoms of Calcarea, such as obesity, inflammation of the perineum and an umbilical hernia, which had been operated on, and the occasional attack of a croupy cough. However, Calcarea is chilly and sweaty on the head and feet, whereas he was warm-blooded and did not sweat.

From the repertorisation (opposite) it was clear that no single remedy covered the whole picture, although all the symptoms, except jealousy, are found in a combination of Sulphur and Calc. Carb. However, in his lectures on materia medica, Kent maintains that Calcarea Sulphurica is an important remedy for jealousy. Andres had the typical psoric anxiety and fear of Calc. Carb., the sycotic meticulousness of Sulphur and the jealousy of Calc. Sulph.

Sulphur had suppressed the eczema and caused the eruption of a croupy cough that does not, incidentally, appear in the Sulphur picture. Perhaps if I had seen him during the acute suffocating cough, with the desire for fresh air, I would have realised earlier which remedy was indicated. The administration of one dose of Calc. Sulph. brought about an immediate amelioration and he did not need another remedy for a year. His eczema, cough and mental symptoms were cured by the administration of the true simillimum.

Repertorisation

1) Fear, happen, something will
2) Fear, dark
3) Jealousy
4) Conscientious about trifles
5) Warm agg.
6) Desires, highly seasoned food
7) Skin, eruptions, itching,
   warmth agg.

Rubric Number	1 2 3 4 5 6 7
Calc. Sulph.	0 1 2 0 0 0 0
Calc. Carb.	2 2 0 0 0 0 0
Sulphur	0 0 0 2 2 3 2
Causticum	3 1 0 0 1 0 2
Lycopodium	1 2 0 2 2 0 2
Medorrhinum	0 2 0 0 0 0 0
Phosphorus	3 2 0 0 2 3 0

CASE 2

Señor Carlos B. He had always been healthy until four months previously a herpetic eruption had developed on his face and had been treated allopathically. One month later, after a prostate operation, he began with fever, vomiting, diarrhoea and disturbances of the nervous system which he believed to be the aftermath of the anaesthetic. He became very anxious and suffered severe migraine headaches with visual disturbances, mental dullness, restlessness and loss of consciousness after a bath or shower. He was worried that he had something seriously wrong with him, was afraid of the fainting spells and thought that he had never really recovered from surgery. He was placid, reserved, chilly, covered himself up well in bed but had warm hands and feet and desired highly seasoned food. He had always been a jealous man and, during the fits of nervous excitability, would become delirious with jealousy.

On repertorising the case, Lachesis was strongly indicated because of the jealousy and the aggravation from a warm bath, so I prescribed Lachesis 1M and 10M, but it did nothing. I then realised that the personality of Lachesis was very unlike the personality of my patient, who was neither malicious, arrogant, sarcastic, suspicious nor critical. Lachesis also has a great fear of death, especially at night, when she wakes choking and suffocating with a menopausal hot flush.

All this was quite unlike the placid, bland and apprehensive nature of the patient. Nux Vomica also covered all the symptoms but, unlike the patient, is impulsive, angry, sensitive and chilly and suffers from antiperistaltic contractions of the digestive system. The case was covered by Calcarea's fears and Sulphur's general symptoms, so Calcarea Sulphurica was indicated. The patient had two doses of the 1M three months apart, and was cured.

Repertorisation

1) Fear, disease, of impending
2) Jealousy
3) Horrible things, sad stories affect her profoundly
4) Faintness
5) Bathing, agg.
6) Desires, highly seasoned food

Rubric Number	1	2	3	4	5	6
Calc. Sulph.	0	2	0	0	3	0
Calc. Carb.	2	0	3	1	3	0
Sulphur	1	0	0	3	3	3
Ignatia	1	1	1	3	0	0
Lachesis	1	3	2	3	0	0
Nux Vomica	2	2	2	3	1	2
Phos. Ac.	2	1	0	2	0	0

('Faintness, warm bath': Lach: 2 – only remedy)

CASE 3

A 50-year-old lorry driver, Alberto M., suffering from painful attacks of arthritis every two or three months that affected his knees and ankles. He also had headaches on waking, and frequent backache. He was frightened of operations, wounds, cruelty, violence and accidents. Despite being a lorry driver, he did not like being away from home and felt lonely. He was very attached to his family and had little hope of finding a cure for his arthritis and great fear of the future. He was very warm-blooded, worse in the summer, in the sun and tolerated the cold well, except that with every attack of arthritis his head became hot and his feet cold. He was pleasant, placid and overweight, with mild eczema on the back for years which was very itchy; he always uncovered at night from the heat and was thirsty for large quantities of water. As a child, he was healthy and of average weight and until ten years ago had suffered from the occasional abscess or boil.

From repertorising the case it was evident that no single remedy covered the whole picture, although the patient's symptoms were fairly clear and well defined. Calcarea Carbonica has the fears and despair, while Sulphur has the physical generals and particulars. Both remedies were prescribed in the 1M and 10M at intervals of several months, but improvement was only partial and temporary. Calcarea Sulphurica has the fears of Calcarea and the general symptoms of Sulphur and brought about a permanent cure in the patient.

Repertorisation

1) Despair, recovery
2) Anxiety, future, about
3) Horrible things, sad stories,
   affect her profoundly
4) Company, desire for, alone,
   while agg.
5) Warm agg.
6) Head, heat, coldness, feet, with
7) Thirst, large quantities, for
8) Desires, highly seasoned food

Rubric Number	1	2	3	4	5	6	7	8
Calc. Sulph.	1	1	0	0	0	0	0	0
Calc. Carb.	3	3	3	1	0	2	0	0
Sulphur	0	1	0	0	2	2	3	3
Bryonia	2	3	0	0	2	0	3	0
Nux Vomica	1	2	2	0	0	0	0	2

CASE 4

Estela, aged 9. A case of chronic bronchitis, catarrh, recurrent tonsillitis and inflammation of the lymph glands, with bad breath and profuse, yellow nasal catarrh. She was very warm-blooded and sweated on the head during sleep. Her appetite was good and she craved highly seasoned food and salt. She was very jealous and impetuous. Over the course of 5 months she took Sulphur 200, 1M and 10M with no result. Her parents said that her temper had become worse and she had started to shout at them and at her sister. She had also become more impulsive, jealous and easily offended and had taken to shutting herself up in her room when angry.

I prescribed Natrum Muriaticum 10M. Two months later there had been no change in the bronchitis; she was still highly strung, bad-tempered, impulsive and jealous. Realising that the previous prescriptions had been mistaken, I enquired further into the nature of the new symptoms, as Estela was now 10 years old and entering adolescence. Her parents said that she got annoyed with her family for no apparent reason, but was happy and affectionate with friends and strangers. I combined this new information with the old symptoms that were still present.

Repertorisation

1) Jealousy
2) Impetuous
3) Aversion, members of
   family, to
4) Warm agg.
5) Head, perspiration, sleep,
   during
6) Desires, salt things

Rubric Number	1	2	3	4	5	6
Calc. Sulph.	2	0	0	1	0	1
Calc. Carb.	0	0	2	0	3	2
Sulphur	0	2	0	2	0	1
Lycopodium	0	0	0	2	2	0
Natrum Mur.	0	2	0	2	0	3
Nux Vomica	2	3	0	0	0	0
Sepia	0	3	3	0	2	0

I must admit that the symptoms I had selected for repertorisation were somewhat haphazard and disjointed, but let me assure the reader that I had followed Estela's development over the course of a year and these were the only symptoms that I could elicit. On a mental level, there was nothing else to go on initially, apart from the impulsiveness and jealousy. In cases like this, the general symptoms, such as warm-blooded sweating on the head during sleep and desire for salt – a symptom that is more remarkable and peculiar than the desire for highly seasoned food as the girl actually ate salt neat – are the most useful and should be considered as constitutional symptoms.

Now let us make our differential diagnosis. Sulphur was indicated at first; it is impulsive, warm-blooded and craves salt. But Sulphur is too egotistical to be jealous and refuses to get involved with life, preferring to take a back seat and play the indolent spectator. Furthermore, Sulphur did not act. Natrum Muriaticum was also apparently indicated for its impulsiveness, sibling jealousy, aggravation from the heat and craving for salt. But Natrum Mur. is a loner who is totally bound up with the past and feels full of resentment, wounded pride and regrets for what might have been – all mental characteristics that have nothing to do with Estela. Apart from its impulsiveness and jealousy, Nux Vomica has nothing else in common with Estela's case, being a very sensitive remedy, with great impatience, chilliness and antiperistaltic contractions of the digestive system. Sepia is impulsive, rejects her family and has head sweats during sleep. However, Estela has none of Sepia's fundamental indifference. Lycopodium is jealous, warm-blooded and has head sweats during sleep; but the jealousy in this remedy stems from a profound lack of confidence, which he tries to hide by being super-intelligent, meticulous, arrogant, bossy and intolerant of contradiction. None of this resonates with Estela's case.

Calcarea Carbonica does not have the first two symptoms, but does have the aversion to her family. Although Calcarea is chilly, it has a strong desire for salt and a marked tendency to sweat on the head during sleep, so is a close remedy for our patient, especially as it has the same pathological affinities of chronic bronchitis, frequent colds and recurrent tonsillitis. However, Estela is warm-blooded and impulsive, like Sulphur. Estela's extreme jealousy develops into an aversion to her family. Two doses of Calcarea Sulphurica 1M and 10M brought about a permanent cure of the physical symptoms and helped to resolve the family problems and the jealousy.

Calcarea Sulphurica is a great polychrest whose usefulness has been largely ignored. From my experience with over thirty Calc. Sulph. patients, I have reached the following conclusions.

These patients are constitutionally half-way between Calcarea Carbonica and Sulphur in that they are overweight, somewhat round-shouldered, with chubby hands and long fingers, warm-blooded and restless. Their general and mental symptoms, such as anxiety, impatience, impulsiveness, irritability and meticulousness, seem to indicate Sulphur. They also have the fears and sensitivity of Calc. Carb. with the characteristic nocturnal sweats, desire for salt, tendency to obesity and flab, chilliness, apathy and weakness. In the fourth case, although the fears were not present, we saw another Calc. symptom – aversion to the members of her family – a symptom that opens up a whole new dimension to this deep-acting remedy which, when used accurately, can bring about a long-lasting and rapid cure.

10

Sepia

REPERTORISATION EXERCISE

The minimum syndrome of maximum value of a remedy is the group of symptoms that provides a clear and characteristic definition of the remedy. The essence of Sepia is indifference to everything ('Indifference, everything, to': 2) and aversion to her family ('Aversion, members of family, to': 3); she is envious of her husband's masculinity and rejects him ('Aversion, husband': 3). Her indifference and feelings of dislike towards those who are close to her are represented by the desire for solitude ('Company, aversion to, amel. when alone': 3) and her wish to avoid people ('Company, aversion to, avoids the sight of people': 2) and lie with her eyes closed ('Company, aversion to, and lies with closed eyes': 1). Kind, reassuring words from well-meaning people either irritate her or make her cry ('Consolation agg.': 3); She feels trapped by the constraints of her femininity and is constantly engaged in battles with the opposite sex as she struggles to assert her independence. The symptoms 'Occupation, amel.': 3, 'Conscientious about trifles': 1, 'Contradiction, is intolerant of': 3 and 'Irritability, menses, before': 2 are all expressions of emotional aridity and the desire to win one over on men.

Repertorisation

The following nine symptoms have been repertorised:

Pseudo-psora
1) Indifference, everything, to
2) Aversion, members of family, to
3) Aversion, husband
4) Company, aversion to
5) Consolation agg.

Sycosis
6) Occupation, amel.
7) Conscientious about trifles
8) Contradiction, is intolerant of
9) Irritability, menses, before

303

Rubric Number	0 2 3 4 5	6 7 8 9
	Pseudo-psora	Sycosis
Aurum	0 0 0 2 0	1 1 3 0
Baryta Carbonica	0 0 0 3 0	1 2 0 0
Calcarea Carbonica	0 2 0 1 1	1 0 0 1
Ferrum Metallicum	0 0 0 2 0	2 1 2 0
Fluoricum Acidum	0 2 0 1 0	0 0 0 0
Ignatia	1 0 0 3 3	3 3 3 0
Lycopodium	0 0 0 2 1	1 2 3 2
Natrum Carbonicum	0 2 2 2 0	2 2 1 0
Natrum Muriaticum	0 0 1 3 3	0 0 0 2
Nux Vomica	0 0 0 3 1	2 2 2 2
Phosphorus	2 0 0 1 0	0 0 0 0
Sepia	2 3 3 2 3	3 1 3 2
Silicea	0 0 0 0 3	1 3 2 0
Thuja	0 0 0 2 1	1 2 1 0

Using the above table, it is not difficult to see which remedies are closest to Sepia.

Ignatia

Ignatia has six out of nine symptoms; the missing ones are the aversion to the family, husband and children, and the irritability before menses. Ignatia's general state of indifference to everything, aversion to company and aggravation from consolation all stem from emotional instability and sensitivity. Characteristics of Ignatia are the paradoxical reactions, emotional changeability and sensitivity. She is meticulous, energetic and intolerant of contradiction, but does not have the irritability before menses that is so symbolic of Sepia's wish to be seen as equal with men. Unlike Sepia, Ignatia can be sympathetic and affectionate and is often indicated in cases of hysteria, neurosis and compulsive behaviour.

Natrum Muriaticum

The essence of Natrum Mur. is a combination of disappointed love, repressed anger and resentment. While it has certain pseudo-psoric aspects in common with Sepia and shares the aversion to company, it lacks the basic indifference to everything. It has none of the sycotic compensatory symptoms except the irritability before menses that expresses a frustration with the constraints of her femininity.

Nux Vomica

Nux Vomica is often used as an acute remedy in a Sepia constitution. It does not have the first three pseudo-psoric symptoms that are concerned with emotional indifference. Nux is overexcitable, easily exhausted and intolerant of other people's attempts to make him feel better. In a sycotic case, however, it could be confused with Sepia as it has all the sycotic symptoms. There is an intense irritability about the remedy and he tends to pick quarrels with everyone. He is chilly, constipated with ineffectual urging and loves his food.

Natrum Carbonicum

This remedy is very close to Sepia but does not have the emotional indifference, aggravation from consolation and irritability before menses. Natrum Carb. is a weak, apathetic and lonely remedy ('Forsaken feeling': *1*) and suffers from depression, flatulence and indigestion; he is aggravated by the sun and desires solitude, peace and quiet; he is occasionally roused from his state of lethargy by a sudden noise ('Starting, noise, from': *3*) or gentle nostalgic music that makes him cry ('Weeping, music, from': *2*), especially when playing the piano ('Weeping, music, from, piano, of': *3*).

Lycopodium

Like Thuja, this remedy could easily be confused with Sepia in a sycotic case. However, unlike Sepia it lacks confidence and tries to cover this up by avoiding people and putting on a front of arrogance, egotism and extreme affability. He is intelligent, lively and energetic and does not tolerate the slightest contradiction because it increases his feelings of insecurity; he feels unworthy and unloved and tries to earn merit and recognition by being meticulous and industrious. The female Lycopodium feels irritable before menses because her drive to prove herself to be superior to men is thwarted at this time of the month. The Lycopodium wife is not emotionally frigid and loves her husband but rejects her children ('Children, dislikes her own': *2*).

Thuja

Egotism, anger, guilt and perversion are the fundamental elements of this sycotic remedy. Thuja avoids company and hates consolation because he tries to do all he can to hide his true nature from others.

11

Sulphur

FIRST YEAR MATERIA MEDICA
(Transcript of a lecture)

In the previous class, we were discussing a simple way of classifying different types of people. On either side of the figure of the so-called average person, represented by a two by four rectangle, we placed a small fat figure, represented by a circle, and a tall thin figure, represented by a long thin rectangle.

Using this model, we said that Sulphur was an example of the normal rectangle, someone who is well adapted to his environment, while the small fat one is the least well adapted and the tall thin one is over-adapted. However, it can also be said that Sulphur is the one who has the most problems in communicating with his surroundings. The French writers have always said that Sulphur is incapable of self-detoxification (this is not medical terminology). They talk about toxins, the ability or inability to produce and eliminate toxins, in a rather arbitrary fashion.

I am going to describe what happens and hopefully you will realise the usefulness of seeing and understanding the remedy in this way. I will start by discussing the pathological, rather than homoeopathic, aspects to give us a broad understanding of what is going on, and I will then go on to discuss the homoeopathic aspects. Sulphur's main area of disturbance centres around the circulatory system. It causes irregular distribution of circulation with congestion and flushes of heat. The French say that disturbances of circulation produce problems with the blood vessels which interfere with normal cell metabolism and its effects are felt in all orifices of the body. You already know that sulphur is an important element in liver and intestinal functions and that it was taken with honey in the olden days as a cure for liver malfunction and certain skin eruptions. It is still used today in ointments and as a cure for scabies. Some people still believe in the old wives' tale that says if you burn a wick of sulphur your pains will vanish; where there is a muscular contraction, the electrical discharge provoked by the friction will cause the wick to break.

When seen through a microscope, the structure of the mineral sulphur is chaotic and disordered, in contrast to the structure of arsenic which is wonderfully ordered. When shaken, sulphur heats up and explodes; hence the marked aggravation from heat, bursting pains and high temperature of the Sulphur patient. The Sulphur infant has nothing unusual about his appearance; he is warm-blooded with average-looking fingers, neither too long, like Phosphorus, nor too short, like Calcarea, and an average-sized head. The skin is unhealthy and the child tends to get overheated in certain parts of the body. For example, the top of his head and his feet are so hot to touch that you would think he is running a temperature. As soon as he is able to move, he will try to kick his feet free of his socks. Or he will put his feet on a cool patch of the bed and kick the covers off. It is the sluggish circulation that causes the aggravation from heat and rest, the over-heating of certain parts of the body and the relief from cold. The Sulphur adult will stick his feet out of the bed and complain that the soles of his feet are burning. This is a characteristic general symptom found in Sulphur and other remedies.

There are also great fluctuations of heat and cold. The headache is accompanied by cold feet and a burning head, as if all the blood rushes upwards into the head. There may also be the opposite, cold head and hot feet. There are spots of heat in different parts of the body. The discharges and skin eruptions that occur when the child falls ill are the body's attempts to cope with the internal imbalances. Small eruptions appear on the skin, minute vesicles that herald the onset of prickly heat, or miliaria rubra, where the sebaceous glands are blocked and there is intolerable itching. When the weather is hot, young children feel very hot, sweaty and itchy around the neck. The mother will say that her child cannot tolerate anything made of wool. Colds descend to the chest and are aggravated by anything that in-creases the congestion: heat, enclosed spaces and sleep position. The baby feels worse when lying down in his cot with the door closed, the nose becomes more inflamed with a burning coryza that irritates the nostrils. In cases of conjunctivitis, the first signs will be a dryish eczematous eruption followed by a burning, itching discharge that is worse from heat, in a closed room and from contact with clothes. There is great itching with the inflammations of skin and mucous membranes.

Another important and notable characteristic is the alternation between one condition and another, the interrelationship between what we call activated pathology.

In orthodox medicine it is important to find the cause, the aetiological factor. For example, to their way of thinking, a case of eczema may be due to an allergy, and it is necessary to find what the patient is allergic to. Once the offending article has been found, whether it be tomato, lettuce or woollen clothing, a course of antihistamines is then prescribed and the patient is put on a desensitisation programme to immunise the organism against the allergic process. But once that problem has been cured, it will not be long before the Sulphur patient produces another, with similar characteristics and in a different part of the body or affecting more internal organs. So, instead of the skin eruption, we get a case of diarrhoea. First thing in the morning, he is forced out of bed by an explosive, burning diarrhoea that smells of sulphur or rotten eggs.

Allopathic doctors would now do tests to discover the cause and may conclude that it is a neurological, intestinal or bacteriological problem; but they would make no connection between this and the previous skin condition. In allopathic thinking, every disease is caused by different factors, whereas in homoeopathy the human being is studied in its totality and the whole process of alternating conditions is taken into account. So the patient will say that if he has eczema, his diarrhoea is better and when the diarrhoea comes back, the eczema disappears; in other words, he only has one condition at a time. The alternating nature of symptoms is characteristic of Sulphur – diarrhoea alternating with skin eruptions, asthma alternating with skin eruptions, headaches alternating with skin eruptions, headaches alternating with asthma, headaches alternating with diarrhoea.

The Sulphur infant is susceptible to skin eruptions, colds and catarrh. The Calcarea infant has thick, foul milk crusts on the head, whereas Sulphur has dry, itching eruptions that alternate with other symptoms.

As the child grows, his personality becomes more developed; he is uncontrollable, restless, hyperactive, cheerful, optimistic, untidy, dirty, independent and a know-all. Sulphur is basically an incorrigible optimist at heart who believes that the world revolves around him – he is besotted with himself and indifferent to his surroundings, contented, cheerful, restless, a great thinker, philosopher and idler.

It is interesting to see the connections between the mental and physical states and how mental symptoms can represent physical conditions. The big problems that afflict this cheerful and self-satisfied individual is a sluggish circulatory system and a lethargic nervous system; these two problems tire him out and make his spine curve over in a manner that is typical of the tall thin Sulphur. Although traditionally it was thought that there were two constitutional pictures of Sulphur, there is in reality only one as the Sulphur character can adapt itself to many different people. In clinical practice we see both the tall, thin Sulphur, the Don Quixote type, a great painter and philosopher who spends his time lounging around bars thinking and making speeches, and the short, fat one, also a great one for pontificating, but who is much less romantic than the first type and more of a Calcarea. The former is psoric and the latter sycotic. Both types have a lot in common and suit a whole range of people.

The mental aspects of a remedy are a much more reliable guide to a remedy than the physical appearance, which is open to so much interpretation that it is impossible to differentiate one remedy from another by this means. Phosphorus can be short and fat just as Calcarea can be tall and thin. The physique may be an aid to diagnosis, but must never be used as a confirmatory symptom.

The materia medica will provide useful information about remedies, but it would be a mistake to try and diagnose a patient simply from his appearance, no matter if he is tall, fat, thin or short. In homoeopathy it is the totality that counts, and the most important aspects are the mental symptoms.

As I have already said, the Sulphur patient has a sluggish circulatory system and suffers from tremendous exhaustion. He is fatigued by everything that aggravates the congested circulation. This is true of everyone who suffers from circulatory problems but they will all have different characteristics that lead us to different remedies. For example, he feels worse on standing, as if all the blood rushes to the feet, in a stuffy room and in the heat of the summer; and feels better lying down, which ameliorates his circulatory problems, in the open air where he can be cool, but not while walking because he is too lazy and apathetic. Pulsatilla and Lycopodium also have sluggish circulations but they are ameliorated by walking and moving about because they need to keep busy. Sulphur is apathetic on both a mental and physical level; he is lazy and, in order to survive in a hostile world, he wraps himself in a great blanket and tells himself that he does not care about anything.

Psychologists would say that a person becomes indifferent when things mean too much to him, but we as homoeopaths must observe what is in front of our eyes. Sulphur is decidedly indifferent to everything, to all external things; these are very strong symptoms in Sulphur. He cares nothing for material possessions because he is a philosopher who is only concerned with the profound meaning of life.

It is the only remedy in black type that is indifferent to his appearance and does not care what clothes he is wearing. He looks dirty and unkempt, his shirt badly needs a wash, his nails need cutting and he smells dirty because his body is filled with toxins that his metabolism is unable to deal with; he has offensive sweat under the armpits, on the feet and genitalia. His skin smells dirty. The mother of a Sulphur baby says that she does not know what is wrong with her child, she washes and washes him but he still smells dirty. The skin looks dirty. The eczema itches and irritates and is aggravated by heat, enclosed spaces and woollen clothing; it alternates with other conditions and looks dirty and unwashed like an old man's scabies. These are the Sulphur eruptions.

The famous image of Sulphur is the ragged philosopher, the tramp who is blithely unaware of his dirty appearance, oblivious to the fact that he is infested by fleas and lice. He is indifferent to his surroundings and erects a barrier that protects him from the world, a barrier of dirt, rags and tatters, fleas, disgusting skin eruptions and offensive body odours.

Psychologists have always considered juvenile acne to be a screen behind which the young man can hide from the world and avoid growing up. While some people manage to grow out of this stage, others keep their acne for life.

Sulphur positively revels in the dirt – the dirtier he is the more comfortable he feels, but he cannot tolerate his own bodily smells. Disgust for his body odours is a typical symptom of Sulphur. When Sulphur, the poet and philosopher, becomes an old man, he looks back on his life and is overcome with remorse for the way he has behaved and throws himself into religion in an attempt to expiate his guilt. The repertory calls it anxiety of conscience, as if guilty of a crime, and it is one of the most important symptoms in Sulphur. The interesting thing is that he cannot tolerate his own bodily smells because he cannot tolerate himself and is full of self-condemnation and guilt. The opposite side of the coin is the belief that his rags and tatters are fine silk.

When you look at the repertory you will see that the delusions, sensations and illusions are characteristic in that they only appear in a few remedies. Some delusions are found in many remedies, but others are found in only two or three. Those which are found in only a few remedies give you the whole vital expression of the remedy. In Sulphur, for example, we see that although he is unconcerned by his physical appearance and is indifferent to his surroundings, he has the delusion that his rags are beautiful. In order to protect himself from his own shadow – his rigidity, egotism, indifference, apathy and lack of connection with the world – he says that his possessions are beautiful and weaves castles in the air which shield him from reality.

We all know the story of the fox and the grapes; they were just out of reach and he could not get at them, so he told everyone that he didn't want them anyway because they were sour. That fox must have been a Sulphur because he was too lazy to reach the grapes. When Sulphur realises that his worst fears have been confirmed and he has actually become a failure – his relentless optimism and air castles have all come to nothing – he makes great speeches about the fact that he knew all along that he was destined to fail. But before this happens, the fox says that the grapes were sour, meaning that he was not interested in them anyway. The fact is that he wanted to eat them but cannot accept that he has failed, so he lies. He consoles himself by telling himself that the grapes were sour, although they were ripe all along. He is incapable of admitting defeat and manipulates reality to suit himself.

A Sulphur patient of mine, a great Argentinian writer, told me that he hardly ever went to the beach because he did not want everyone to look at his unsightly physique. Apparently, if he did go he went fully dressed and spent the whole time sitting in a tent watching other people. It was as if he were watching the world through a pane of glass – he could not match up to other people, so he chose to isolate himself. 'I get my kicks from laughing at those fat women in their gross swimming costumes – they really ought to be shot,' he would say. 'Young women in bikinis are a delight to watch, but those disgusting old women just clutter up the beach and look awful.' He knew that he was no match for other men so decided to bow out of the competition altogether and make fun of other people in his typically derisory fashion. Sulphur is a particularly critical remedy.

Sulphur's mental symptoms are difficult to find in the materia medica, but come through clearly in the repertory.

The repertory is the bible of homoeopathy and there are many different versions. It contains all the symptoms of every remedy, although in practice we use only between two and six hundred of the two thousand remedies at our disposal, and can truthfully say that we are familiar with only about fifty of these.

Sulphur must have about four hundred mental symptoms and it is impossible to remember them all. So in the repertory, whether aided or not by a computer, we can find every characteristic trait of every remedy. For example, you could look in the repertory for all the remedies that are arrogant, and they would be classified in three grades according to whether the remedy has cured the symptom several times in clinical practice or whether the symptom occurs frequently or infrequently in the remedy.

When you have five or six strong mental symptoms that seem to define the psychological make-up of the patient, you can then do a repertorisation to find all the remedies that have the characteristic traits you have selected. You can then combine this with the characteristic physicals, generals, modalities and a few well-chosen particulars and you will find the remedy that covers all these symptoms. Then, if the essential nature of the remedy matches the essential nature of the patient, this is the remedy that the patient needs. That is homoeopathy in a nutshell: the search for a remedy that is capable of bringing about dynamic change in the depths of the organism on both a mental and physical level. In homoeopathy, all pathology is caused by the disturbance and faulty adaptation of the vital force. No matter if the problem is cancer, pneumonia, dysentery or meningitis, in every case it is caused by a disturbance on the dynamic level which brings about an alteration on the physical level, often with fatal consequences for the patient. From birth to death, the vital force does all it can to ensure our survival.

We were talking about Sulphur, who hides behind the covering of eczematous eruptions and protects himself from all involvement and commitment. Like the poet-writer whom I described earlier said, he entertains himself by criticising those he is unable to mix with.

This is the essential nature of Sulphur, although you will find that there are many mental symptoms in the repertory that may not fit into your understanding of the true picture. When you read materia medica you will inevitably find some characteristics that seem to have no connection with the others, and you will just have to memorise these. Eventually, you will build up a picture in your mind of the essence of a remedy by discussing with colleagues and tutors, memorising the facts and seeing real life versions of remedy pictures in the consulting room. All I am trying to do is make your work a little easier. You will see in the repertory, for example, that Sulphur's connection with the outside world is so tenuous that he does not appear in any rubric that would imply a relationship with other people. Take the rubric 'Anger, contradiction, from'; this implies a relationship with those who oppose his ideas. Every remedy will either have such a symptom or not, according to the nature of its inner dynamic.

For example, Lycopodium is a frequently used remedy that is arrogant, insecure and intolerant of contradiction. Why? Because it forces him to entertain the possibility that he may not be right after all; and, as he is always worried about whether he is right or not, he gets annoyed and tries to impose his ideas by shouting louder than anyone else because he is afraid of being contradicted. Silicea also has anger from contradiction. Why? Because he is shy, intimidated by people and insecure. He feels completely crushed by contradiction because it reinforces his belief that he is the one in the wrong.

Sulphur, on the other hand, does not care at all whether he is contradicted or not – he is just not interested. He has constructed a model of the world in his head, and as far as he is concerned, that is how the world is. He is quite unconcerned with what other people think.

Take another rubric, 'Ailments from grief'. This is for people who become ill after a grief of some sort. To find the indicated remedy, you have to look at how the person has become ill, as everyone is different. The Pulsatilla way, for example, is to feel forsaken, unhappy, tearful, in great need of affection, reassurance and tender, loving care.

Sulphur, in contrast, is not affected by grief. Let us look at what this means for a moment. When we say that he is not affected by grief, we mean that to be unaffected by grief is peculiar or extraordinary in the circumstances. In other words, grief is not a symptom when it is appropriate to the situation. If someone told you that his wife and children had died, his house had been burnt down and his dog had been kidnapped, you would expect him to be depressed; grief would be a normal reaction to the situation and where it was not present, Sulphur might be a possible prescription.

If Pulsatilla is prescribed for a grief, it is because the grief is exaggerated, out of proportion; the healthy person would have no need for these ailments from grief. For example, if I put everything I own into a box and then discover that I have lost it and will never get it back, you would expect me to rant and rave, because I have lost everything I own; this is a normal reaction to the situation and not 'Anger from contradiction'. Feelings become symptoms only when there is no logical explanation for them.

You will notice that Sulphur does not appear in the rubrics 'Ailments from grief', 'Complaints from fright' and 'Ailments after anger', because he thinks and behaves in accordance with his inner reality; he has an unshakable belief that the world is the way he thinks it is. Sulphur appears mainly in rubrics that affect his ego. Take the rubric 'Ailments after mortification', for example. This describes someone who overreacts all the time to the trivial injustices and petty irritations of everyday life by feeling absolutely mortified, eaten up and destroyed.

Sulphur has 'Ailments after mortification' because it has to do with his ego. He also has some fears; the fear of robbers, because they threaten to take something away from him and the fear of ghosts, because of the guilt. He has no fear of solitude. If you were left all alone in the middle of the Sahara desert, you would expect to feel frightened. But the symptom 'Fear, alone, of being' refers to someone who cannot bear to be alone in the house for a whole day, or even for a single moment when he is ill, for no justifiable reason. On the other hand, the patient who is afraid of being left on his own because he is a heart patient who will die if he moves a muscle is justifiably afraid. This is not so much a fear of solitude as a need to have someone near. We can only use this symptom in a patient who is frightened of being alone for no apparent reason. Fear of solitude is not the same as fear of being alone; it describes the patient who is afraid of living completely on his own, although he may not be afraid of being on his own for a while in a room.

Take, for example, the case of a woman who cannot separate from her husband although she does not love him and has no financial problems. She puts up with him, not because he is worth it, not because she loves him and not because she needs help with the children; she simply cannot conceive of living alone. That is what is meant by a fear of solitude. To give meaning to any given symptom, we must have a complete understanding of the patient's whole attitude to life, and the best symptoms are those that are clearly expressed and have no logical explanation. When the patient says that he does not know why he is the way he is, that is an important symptom in the case and should be taken into consideration.

The Sulphur patient erects a barrier to protect him from his fear. The most important thing in his life is himself, in the most narcissistic, egotistical way possible. He has a confirmed belief in himself as a wise and wonderful being. But you may wonder how he can be so sure of himself if the repertory says that he lacks self-confidence. Obviously, this is the other side of the coin. He covers up his profound feelings of insecurity with a great show of supreme self-confidence. He knows that he cannot rely on his weak and lethargic body with its sluggish circulation, and this makes him feel insecure. So he consoles himself by picking holes in other people and allowing himself to be admired for his leadership qualities, although he is quite indifferent to others and unconcerned about his own faults. But he knows, deep down, that he does not have a leg to stand on and the older he gets, the less control he has, until his whole edifice begins to crumble and we see the emergence of insecurity, guilt, failure, religious fanaticism and fervent prayers for the salvation of his soul. He becomes overcome with guilt and remorse for the way he has treated others, frightened that he has lost his way and convinced that he is doomed to eternal condemnation.

In the Sulphur child, however, we see the smart alec, master of invention, creation and discussion, who knows all there is to know about everything. When contradicted or opposed, he may get angry at first, but soon shrugs it off and goes on to something else. He lives in a fantasy world where hard work has no place. The mother will tell you that her son is an idle good-for-nothing who refuses to apply himself to his studies. If you ask the son why he does not study, he will tell you that he does and that he knows it all anyway. As he is intelligent, all he has to do is give a cursory glance to the work to pass his exams. His mother nags him about the state of his books and he will tell her to stop going on at him, that he is bored with her constant nagging. He is happy enough with things as they are, but on a physical level he feels tired, weak and lethargic all the time.

The general symptoms of the remedy must be studied in depth. The information you will find in the materia medica is useful but limited as it is too materialistic to be of any real value. This is not what homoeopathy is all about. It is useful in what it says about the appearance of the patient and the general modalities, and tells you what you need to know about the remedy in general terms.

For example, as far as the general modalities are concerned, Sulphur is warm-blooded, although he may be chilly, and the symptoms are aggravated by all forms of heat: hot weather, warm stuffy rooms, warm clothing and the heat of the bed.

However, not all Sulphurs are the same. Some will be aggravated more by a warm room or the heat of the bed. They become congested, overheated and tired and may faint while standing in an enclosed place like a church. Sulphur, Pulsatilla, Lycopodium and Phosphorus all have fainting, with amelioration from fresh air and aggravation from humid, cloudy weather. As far as the time modalities are concerned, Sulphur is worse on waking in the morning and does not want to get out of bed. He can fall asleep anywhere and everywhere, like a cat. He feels as if intoxicated and tries to sleep it off, but with his sluggish circulation and the accumulation of lactic acid and anhydrous carbon in the muscles, he either wakes feeling tired or cannot wake up at all in the morning. This is what is meant by 'Waking, difficult'.

Mornings are the worst time of day for a Sulphur. In the early hours of the morning, he is forced out of bed by an attack of diarrhoea. When he gets up and slowly starts to move around, he begins to feel better as the lactic acid and anhydrous carbon start to circulate once more and he takes in some oxygen. He eats some breakfast but does not like the milk; he drinks more than he eats because he is not hungry; his stomach feels heavy, the tongue is coated and his belches smell of rotten eggs. He has two or three glasses of water for breakfast. In the tall thin Sulphur, everything feels as if it is drooping, and the stomach feels as if it is falling to the floor, especially between 10 and 11 a.m. The stomach feels empty at this time and he has to have a nibble of something. At lunch time, the Sulphur child consumes vast quantities of water, maybe four or five glasses. He has a swollen belly from all the liquid he has drunk, and is always getting diarrhoea.

One of my grandchildren is not a Sulphur but a Calc. Sulph. and he is like this only a bit tougher. When he comes home from school, he is the only child with his shirt and tie all dishevelled, the shirt half out of his trousers, looking an absolute mess. He has been in school for three years and is friends with everyone. He is as dirty as only he knows how to be. When he runs, he gets very red in the face and gulps his drinks down one after the other, and then does not want to eat because his stomach is too full from all the drink.

Sulphur often has a small appetite and a large thirst. The adult tries to tempt his appetite with strong flavours. His system is overloaded with toxins, his intestines and liver are not functioning properly and in order to stimulate the digestive system into action, he needs to eat highly flavoured food; so he develops a craving for rich, spicy food with lots of flavour. You must remember this about Sulphur: desire for highly seasoned food with lots of sauce and hot spices. After a meal, his stomach swells up, he becomes very drowsy and has to have a nap. This is also a remedy of great periodicity. Frequently, he will get an aggravation of his illness every 8 or 15 days, and there is alternating between one illness and another.

The most characteristic food desires and aversions of Sulphur are the desire for highly seasoned food, sweets, large quantities of drink, and aversion to, or desire for, milk. You will find many opposite symptoms in the repertory such as a strong desire for sweets, aggravation from sweet things and aversion to sweets; excessive heat in bed and also shivering. The strongest symptoms are the desire for sweet things, salty food, butter, fatty food and highly seasoned food.

Other general modalities are that he cannot stand upright because everything is falling down and a marked aggravation from standing. Which particular symptoms can you remember? Starting with the head, the heat of the head is very marked. Most of the time, although there are exceptions, the top of the head is hot when he has a headache and the feet are cold. When he has a cold, there is a lot of greenish mucus that tastes sweetish and irritates and burns the nostrils. He feels better in the open air, is aggravated by enclosed spaces and the appearance of a cold alternates with deeper pathology. The lips are dry, cracked and very red, and the tongue and outside edge of the mouth burn and sting. All orifices of the body, the anus, the nostrils, are reddened. In other words, the borderline between the body and the outside world is in a permanent state of irritation, burning and itching. Whether these symptoms are relevant or not depends on their context in the patient's whole picture.

For example, here is a Sulphur in the consulting room. He says:

'I have been suffering from asthma for 20 years. I always have to use some inhaler or other, and it keeps it at bay.'
'And how does it affect you ?'
'I'm fed up with it because it tires me out and I never feel well.'
'What else?'
'I'm very warm-blooded. Especially when I get an attack, I have to get out into the fresh air, I feel better outside and I get the asthma worse at certain times of the year, mainly when it's hot. And when I eat hot, spicy food.'
'Is it stress-related?'
'Not really. Maybe when something upsets me. But I notice it when I eat something and when the weather is heavy or humid and hot. That's when I feel bad.'
'What else?'
'Headaches. My head feels heavy and hot. The strange thing is, when I have the asthma I don't get the headaches. And when the asthma is better, I get the headaches. When I don't get headaches, if I eat something that disagrees with me I get tired.'
'What else in your medical history?'
'Well, I had the normal childhood diseases. My mother says I had

eczema for a long time on the elbows. My feet were always very sweaty and smelly.'

'Did you get treatment for this?'

'Yes, with alum. And ointment for the eczema that made it go away.'

'How long did you have it for?'

'Until I was fifteen.'

'Do you still get it?'

'Sometimes I still get it on my neck. But I feel better when I get it, not so tired.'

'Are you affected by the weather?'

'I don't feel the cold. In winter I just wear a shirt, that's all. Sometimes I feel cold but more often than not I feel hot and I can't bear to be in a stuffy environment.'

'How do you sleep?'

'OK. Sometimes I wake at 3 or 4 in the morning and can't get back to sleep again. I don't like that when it happens. I keep my body covered up but leave the feet outside the blanket. Sometimes my feet get so hot in summer that I have to put them in a bucket of water! It helps if I leave them outside the blanket, but then they get cold and I have to bring them in under the covers until they heat up again. My skin is very dry, and I've got warts that itch and sting. When I was a child, I used to get very smelly and sweaty.'

'How would you describe yourself?'

'Easy-going, contented. My wife would say that I am very hot-tempered. I rant and rave for a bit and then I forget about it.'

'Tell me more about your wife.'

'She's very selfish! Always thinking of herself. I come home tired after a long day's work and and all I want is to put my slippers on and read the paper in peace and quiet. I don't want to have to tidy up after me, I'm too tired.'

'Do you like being on your own?'

'I love it, doctor. I love my own company. I can get on with my things, do a bit of woodwork, that sort of thing.'

'What do you do if you're not doing your woodwork?'

'Have a rest. Go to sleep.'

'Can you rest without doing anything?'

'Yes, I love my rest. I really look forward to my little siestas. On Sundays I like the wife to cook, to do me some nice ravioli with a nice sauce.'

Sulphur

This is Sulphur. Easy-going, happy with his lot, selfish, engrossed in himself. This is what needs to be treated in the patient. Later on in life, he will see that things have not worked out as he had hoped and he begins to realise the things he has done wrong. He says:

'My wife became ill. The doctor advised her to go to Cordoba but I insisted on going to Mar del Plata. She never went out when I didn't want her to. I know that was wrong of me and I feel bad about it. I know that I have not been as helpful to my friends as I could have been. I feel bad about that and wish I could do something to make it better.'

'Do you do something about it?'

'Well, I can't now because I'm not well enough.' He is always thinking of the wrong things he has done, but he never actually does anything about it. 'The world is a bad place, doctor. Look at the British, look at the President, look at the evangelists, look at the philosophers ... I think something ought to be done.'

'What do you do about them?'

'I can't do anything at all. But the world has to change. Things are getting very bad, nobody respects anybody.'

'Do you respect people?'

'I do what I can.' He spends his whole time criticising, speculating about the world and feeling guilty. This is Sulphur.

The female Sulphur would talk something like this:

'How do you feel about your life?'

'I have lost my children and my husband. I am all alone.'

'How would you describe yourself?'

'Well, doctor, that's life, you just have to come to terms with things. I see my friends for a chat and we go to see a film and I'm happy with my lot.' Sulphur has a fundamental, unshakable optimism and keeps himself apart from the reality of everyday living, unaffected by changing events and surroundings. This attitude is typical of Sulphur: great optimism for no apparent reason. 'Do you get upset at all?'

'Yes, I cry a lot when I see a sad film.'

But it is quite obvious that despite all this emotion, she is actually incapable of lifting a finger to help anyone else. She will weep at the beauty of the countryside or about a sick child, but it is too much effort to do anything to help. Sulphur can be sentimental but never giving, he is too selfish for that. The most characteristic trait is egotism and indifference to others. A healthy Sulphur can be generous to others. A sick Sulphur does not have to have all the symptoms of the remedy, but he must have the characteristic ones. The female patient is warm-blooded, optimistic, industrious, easily irritated and hurried; she shouts a lot and bustles about restlessly, but there is an unmistakeable apathy about her and her presenting complaint is usually something like tiredness, eczema or a sluggish circulation.

This picture is enough to begin with. Gradually, things that seem difficult at first will get easier as you get to know other remedies and compare them with one another.

Bibliography

Allen, H. C., *Keynotes and Characteristics of the Materia Medica with Nosodes.*

Allen, H. C., *Materia Medica of the Nosodes with Provings of the X-Ray.*

Allen, T. F., *Encyclopedia of Pure Materia Medica.*

Barthel, H. and Klunker, W., *Synthetic Repertory.*

Bernard, H., *Traité d'homéopathie.*

Clarke, J. H., *Dictionary of Practical Materia Medica.*

Duprat, H., *Traité de matière médicale homéopathique.*

Farrington, E. A., *Clinical Materia Medica.*

Farrington, H., *Homoeopathy and Homoeopathic Prescribing.*

Gallavardin, J.-P., *Psychisme et homoéopathie.*

Gathak, N., *Chronic Disease – its Cause and Cure.*

Gypser, K.-H. (ed.), *The Minor Writings of J. T. Kent.*

Hahnemann, S. C. F., *Chronic Diseases.*

Hahnemann, S. C. F., *Materia Medica Pura.*

Hahnemann, S. C. F., *Organon of Medicine.*

Hering, C., *Guiding Symptoms of the Materia Medica.*

Kent, J. T., *Lectures on Homoeopathic Materia Medica.*

Kent, J. T., *Lectures on Homoeopathic Philosophy.*

Kent, J. T., *New Remedies, Clinical Cases, Lesser Writings, Aphorisms and Precepts.*

Kent, J. T., *Repertory of Homoeopathic Materia Medica.*

Nash, E. B., *Leaders in Homoeopathic Therapeutics.*

Paschero, T. P., *Homeopatía.*

Tyler, M. L., *Homoeopathic Drug Pictures.*

Voisin, H., *Matière médicale homéopathique clinique.*

Appendix I: Rubrics Referred to in the Repertorisation Tables

	Kali-c.	Lach.	Lyc.	Med.	Nat-m.	Sil.	Thuj.
The great majority of the rubrics below are from Kent's *Repertory*. Two rubrics are marked as from the *Synthetic Repertory*. Also, the author has created new rubrics and added some remedies to existing Kent rubrics – both groups are marked with [EFC].					Solid bullet points indicate that a rubric is part of the MCS of the given remedy. The rubrics with hollow bullets are not in the MCS but they are also discussed in detail.		
Affectionate						●	
Ailments from: anticipation [*Synthetic Repertory*]						●	
Anger, ailments after, with silent grief					●		
Anticipation, complaints from			●	●			
Anxiety, conscience, of				●	○	○	●
Anxiety, fear, with	●						
Anxiety, future, about							●
Anxiety, morning, waking, on		●					
Anxiety, salvation, about			○				
Anxiety, time is set, if a				○			
Bad news, ailments				○			
Capriciousness	○						
Censorious, critical		○					
Chaotic							○
Clairvoyance		○					
Company, aversion to		○	○		●		●
Company, desire for	●		○				
Company, desire for, alone, while agg.						○	
Complaining		○					
Concentration, difficult						○	
Concentration, difficult, on attempting to, has a vacant feeling					○		
Confidence, want of self	●		●			●	
Confidence, want of self [EFC]				○			
Confusion of mind						○	
Confusion, dream, as if in							○
Confusion, identity, as to his		○					
Confusion, walking, while, open air amel.			○				
Conscientious about trifles				●		●	●
Conscientious about trifles [EFC]				○			
Consolation agg.	●				●	○	○
Contradict, disposition to		○	●				
Contradiction, is intolerant of			●			○	●
Contrary	●		●				○

Appendix I

Appendix I: (continued)

The great majority of the rubrics below are from Kent's *Repertory*. Two rubrics are marked as from the *Synthetic Repertory*. Also, the author has created new rubrics and added some remedies to existing Kent rubrics – both groups are marked with [EFC].				Solid bullet points indicate that a rubric is part of the MCS of the given remedy. The rubrics with hollow bullets are not in the MCS but they are also discussed in detail.			

	Kali-c.	Lach.	Lyc.	Med.	Nat-m.	Sil.	Thuj.
Delusions, people, behind him, some one is				o			
Delusions, persons, come in, look at her, whisper and say 'come' [EFC]				o			
Delusions, pursued, thought he was, enemies, by		o					
Despair, recovery	o						
Despair, recovery [EFC]				o			
Despair, religious (of salvation etc.)		•		•			•
Dictatorial		•	•				
Discontented, himself, with	o						
Dream, as if in a				o	o		
Dullness	o			•			
Dullness, head, from weight on vertex [EFC]				o			
Dullness, mental exertion, from						o	
Dullness, sluggishness, difficulty of thinking and comprehending							o
Dullness, waking, on		o					
Dwells on past disagreeable occurrences			o		•		
Estranged, family, from her					o		
Excitement, bad news, after	o						
Excitement, horrible things, after hearing		o					
Excitement, night							o
Fear, alone, of being	•		o				
Fear, approaching him, of others							o
Fear, dark				o			
Fear, disease, of impending	o						o
Fear, disease, of impending [EFC]				•			
Fear, evil, of		o					
Fear, happen, something will						o	
Fear, happen, something will [EFC]				o			
Fear, insanity, of [EFC]				o			
Fear, robbers, of		o				o	
Fear, sleep, to go to		•					
Fear, stomach, arising from	o		o				
Fear, strangers, of							o
Forsaken feeling	o	•					

Appendix I

Appendix I: (continued)

<table>
<tr><td>The great majority of the rubrics below are from Kent's Repertory. Two rubrics are marked as from the Synthetic Repertory. Also, the author has created new rubrics and added some remedies to existing Kent rubrics – both groups are marked with [EFC].</td><td>Solid bullet points indicate that a rubric is part of the MCS of the given remedy. The rubrics with hollow bullets are not in the MCS but they are also discussed in detail.</td></tr>
</table>

	Kali-c.	Lach.	Lyc.	Med.	Nat-m.	Sil.	Thuj.
Fright, complaints from						O	
Frightened easily					O	O	
Grief, ailments from					O		
Hatred		O			O		
Haughty		●	●				
Homesickness		O			O	O	
Hurry	O	O		●	O		O
Hysteria					O	O	
Impatience	O						
Impetuous	●						
Indifference, pleasure, to					O		
Indifference, society, when in	O						
Industrious		O					
Irritability, children, in						O	
Irritability, menses, before	O		O				
Irritability, waking, on			O				
Jealousy		●					
Loathing, general	O						
Loathing, life		O	O		O		O
Loquacity		●					
Love, ailments, from disappointed		O			●		
Magnetized, desires to be		O				O	
Malicious		●			●		
Meditation		O					
Memory, weakness of, expressing one's self, for	O					O	O
Memory, weakness of, stating her symptoms, great difficulty [EFC]					O		
Memory, weakness of, happened, for what has		O					
Memory, weakness of, names, for proper			O	O			
Memory, weakness of, read, for what has		O					
Memory, weakness of, words, for							O
Mildness						O	
Mirth, evening		O					
Mistakes, speaking, intend, what he does not						O	

Appendix I: (continued)

The great majority of the rubrics below are from Kent's *Repertory*. Two rubrics are marked as from the *Synthetic Repertory*. Also, the author has created new rubrics and added some remedies to existing Kent rubrics – both groups are marked with [EFC].	Solid bullet points indicate that a rubric is part of the MCS of the given remedy. The rubrics with hollow bullets are not in the MCS but they are also discussed in detail.

	Kali-c.	Lach.	Lyc.	Med.	Nat-m.	Sil.	Thuj.
Mistakes, writing, in							o
Mistakes, wrong words, using			o				
Moaning	o						
Mood, alternating	o		o				
Mortification, ailments after			o		o		
Obstinate	o					●	
Occupation, amel.				●			●
Offended, easily					o		
Procrastinate, desire to [EFC]					o		
Prostration of mind			o			o	
Quarrelsome	o						o
Reproaches himself							o
Reproaches others		●			o		
Restlessness, anxious	o						
Restlessness, night					●		
Sadness, morning, waking, on			o				
Sensitive, noise, slightest, to [*Synthetic Repertory*]						o	
Speech, hasty			o				
Speech, wandering			o				
Starting, noise, from	o		o	o	o	o	
Starting, sleep, on falling			o				
Stomach, apprehension in							o
Suicidal disposition		o		o			o
Suspicious		●					●
Sympathetic					o		
Talk, indisposed to							o
Thinking, complaints, of, agg.					o		o
Thoughts, persistent							o
Thoughts, unpleasant subjects, haunted by	o						
Thoughts, vanishing of					o		
Time, passes too slowly					o		
Timidity						●	
Touched, aversion to being	o						

Appendix I: (continued)

The great majority of the rubrics below are from Kent's *Repertory*. Two rubrics are marked as from the *Synthetic Repertory*. Also, the author has created new rubrics and added some remedies to existing Kent rubrics – both groups are marked with [EFC].					Solid bullet points indicate that a rubric is part of the MCS of the given remedy. The rubrics with hollow bullets are not in the MCS but they are also discussed in detail.	

	Kali-c.	Lach.	Lyc.	Med.	Nat-m.	Sil.	Thuj.
Undertakes, many things, perseveres in nothing		○					
Unobserving	○						
Violent						○	
Weeping, alternating with laughter						○	
Weeping, ameliorates symptoms				○			
Weeping, involuntary						○	
Weeping, music, from							○
Weeping, remonstrated with, when	○						
Weeping, spoken to, when					○		
Weeping, telling of her sickness, when	○				○		
Weeping, thanked, when			○				
Work, impossible					○		

Appendix II

Appendix II: The Minimum Characteristic Syndrome for each of the Seven Remedies

Kali Carbonicum
Anxiety, fear, with
Company, desire for
Confidence, want of self
Consolation agg.
Contrary
Fear, alone, of being
Impetuous

Lachesis
Anxiety, morning, waking, on
Dictatorial
Fear, sleep, to go to
Forsaken feeling
Haughty
Jealousy
Loquacity
Malicious
Reproaches others
Suspicious

Lycopodium
Anticipation, complaints from
Confidence, want of self
Conscientious about trifles
Contradict, disposition to
Contradiction, is intolerant of
Dictatorial
Haughty
Occupation, amel.

Medorrhinum
Anticipation, complaints from
Anxiety, conscience, of
Dullness
Fear, disease, of impending
Hurry
Restlessness, night

Natrum Muriaticum
Affectionate
Anger, ailments after, with silent grief
Company, aversion to
Consolation agg.
Dwells on past disagreeable occurrences
Love, ailments, from disappointed
Malicious

Silicea
Ailments from: anticipation [*Synthetic Repertory*]
Confidence, want of self
Conscientious about trifles
Obstinate
Timidity

Thuja
Anxiety, conscience, of
Anxiety, future, about
Company, aversion to
Conscientious about trifles
Contradiction, is intolerant of
Occupation, amel.
Suspicious

INDEX OF REMEDIES

– NOTES –

Other Books in the Beaconsfield Homoeopathic Library

Classical Homoeopathy, Dr Margery Blackie, 1986, reprinted 1990 with Repertory. The complete teaching legacy of one of the most important homoeopaths of our time. 0906584140

Everyday Homoeopathy (2nd Edition), Dr David Gemmell, 1997. A practical handbook for using homoeopathy in the context of one's own personal and family health care, using readily available remedies.
0906584442

Homoeopathic Prescribing, Dr Noel Pratt, revised 1985. A compact reference book covering 161 common complaints and disorders, with guidance on the choice of the appropriate remedy. 0906584035

Homoeopathy, Dr T. P. Paschero (in translation) 1997. A major work by one of the great Argentinian masters. 0906584418

Homoeopathy as Art and Science, Dr Elizabeth Wright Hubbard, 1990. The selected writings of one of the foremost modern homoeopaths. 0906584264

Homoeopathy in Practice, Dr Douglas Borland, 1982, reprinted 1988 with Symptom Index. Detailed guidance on the observation of symptoms and the choice of remedies. 090658406X

Homoeopathic Treatment of Beef and Dairy Cattle, The, C. E. I. Day, MRCVS, 1995. Describes how homoeopathy may be used in the care of cattle, both as individuals and in a group. 090658437X

Homoeopathic Treatment of Eczema, The, Robin Logan, FSHom, 1997. A textbook on the homoeopathic treatment of this condition.
0906584477

In Search of the Later Hahnemann, Rima Handley, FSHom, DPhil, 1997. A study of Hahnemann's hitherto unknown Parisian casebooks.
0906584353

Insights into Homoeopathy, Dr Frank Bodman, 1990. Homoeopathic approaches to common problems in general medicine and psychiatry. 0906584280

Introduction to Homoeopathic Medicine (2nd Edition), Dr Hamish Boyd, 1989. A formal introductory text, written in categories that are familiar to the medical practitioner. 0906584213

Other Books in the Beaconsfield Homoeopathic Library

Materia Medica of New Homoeopathic Remedies, Dr O. A. Julian, paperback edition 1984. Full clinical coverage of 106 new homoeopathic remedies, for use in conjunction with the classical materia medicas. 0906584116

Mental Symptoms in Homoeopathy, Dr Luis Detinis, 1994. A comparative study of the Mind rubrics in Kent's *Repertory*. 0906584345

Studies of Homoeopathic Remedies, Dr Douglas Gibson, 1987. Detailed clinical studies of 100 major remedies. Well-known for the uniquely wide range of insights brought to bear on each remedy. 0906584175

Tutorials on Homoeopathy, Dr Donald Foubister, 1989. Detailed studies on a wide range of conditions and remedies. 0906584256

Typology in Homoeopathy, Dr Léon Vannier, 1992. A study of human types, based on the gods of Antiquity, and the remedies which are relevant to them. 0906584302